Advances in Kinesiology and Sports Science

Advances in Kinesiology and Sports Science

Editor: Tilly Martin

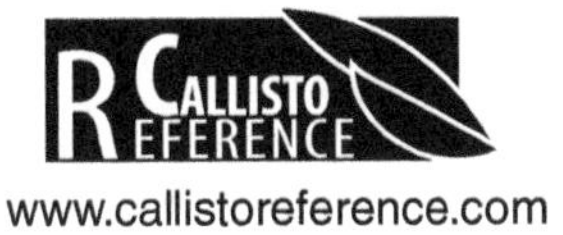

www.callistoreference.com

Callisto Reference,
118-35 Queens Blvd., Suite 400,
Forest Hills, NY 11375, USA

Visit us on the World Wide Web at:
www.callistoreference.com

ISBN: 978-1-64116-337-8 (Hardback)

Cataloging-in-Publication Data

Advances in kinesiology and sports science / edited by Tilly Martin.
p. cm.
Includes bibliographical references and index.
ISBN 978-1-64116-337-8
1. Kinesiology. 2. Sports sciences. 3. Sports medicine. 4. Sports. I. Martin, Tilly.
QP303 .A28 2020
613.7--dc23

Table of Contents

Preface

This book has been an outcome of determined endeavour from a group of educationists in the field. The primary objective was to involve a broad spectrum of professionals from diverse cultural background involved in the field for developing new researches. The book not only targets students but also scholars pursuing higher research for further enhancement of the theoretical and practical applications of the subject.

The scientific study of human and non-human movement is known as kinesiology. It encompasses the physiological, psychological and biochemical dynamic principles and mechanisms of movement. The branch of kinesiology which deals with the human health is known as human kinesiology. It studies biomechanics and orthopedics, sports psychology, and strength and conditioning. Human kinesiology also includes methods of rehabilitation such as physical and occupational therapy, and sports and exercise. Sports science is a field that observes the functioning of a healthy body during exercise. It studies how physical activities such as sports promote the health and performance of the whole body. It encompasses various areas such as biokinetics, biomechanics and anatomy. This book discusses the fundamentals as well as modern approaches to kinesiology and sports science. It presents researches and studies performed by experts across the globe. Those in search of information to further their knowledge will be greatly assisted by this book.

It was an honour to edit such a profound book and also a challenging task to compile and examine all the relevant data for accuracy and originality. I wish to acknowledge the efforts of the contributors for submitting such brilliant and diverse chapters in the field and for endlessly working for the completion of the book. Last, but not the least; I thank my family for being a constant source of support in all my research endeavours.

Editor

1

Prediction of Kick Direction from Kinematics during the Soccer Penalty Kick

Yumeng Li (Corresponding author)
Department of Kinesiology, University of Georgia, Athens, Georgia, USA
330 River Rd, Athens, GA30605, USA
E-mail: yumengli@uga.edu

Marion J.L. Alexander
Faculty of Kinesiology and Recreation Management, University of Manitoba, Winnipeg, Canada
306 Max Bell Center, Winnipeg, R3T 2N2, Canada
E-mail: marion.alexander@umanitoba.ca

Cheryl M. Glazebrook
Faculty of Kinesiology and Recreation Management, University of Manitoba, Winnipeg, Canada
319 Max Bell Center, Winnipeg, R3T 2N2, Canada
E-mail: cheryl.glazebrook@umanitoba.ca

Jeff Leiter
Pan Am Clinic, Winnipeg, Canada
75 Poseidon Bay, Winnipeg, R3M 3E4, Canada
E-mail: jleiter@panamclinic.com

Abstract

Background: Speed and direction of the ball are key factors in successful soccer penalty kicks. The kinematics that contribute to the kick direction are unclear. **Purpose:** The purpose of the study was (1) to compare the differences in instep kick kinematics between left and right kick directions; (2) to determine the significant factors that predict kick direction. **Method:** Four digital video cameras (80 Hz) collected data from eleven experienced female soccer players during instep penalty kicks to the left and right. Video analysis software (Dartfish Team Pro 6.0) was used to process and analyze the video files. **Results**: Paired t-tests indicated that several variables before ball contact were different. The linear regression included three variables (support foot orientation, support foot position behind the ball and approach angle) to best predict kick directions (R^2 = 75.6%, $p < .01$). **Conclusion:** The results may be useful for goalkeepers to anticipate kick direction before ball contact to gain a better chance to save the penalty kick.

Keywords: Instep kick, Anticipation, Goalkeeping

1. Introduction

For a penalty kick in soccer the player kicks a stationary ball located 11 m away from the goal line. Two types of kicks are commonly used during penalty kicks: side-foot kick and instep kick (Nunome, Asai, Ikegami, & Sakurai, 2002). The side-foot kick is frequently used to gain accuracy, whereas instep kick is used to increase ball speed (Nunome et al., 2002). The ball speed can be up to 30 m/s (Andersen & Dörge, 2011), resulting in only 0.3 – 0.4 seconds from ball contact to when the ball passes the goal line. The level of difficulty in penalty defense was highlighted by Bar-eli, Azar, & Ritov, (2007) who analyzed 286 penalty kicks in top leagues and worldwide championships. They reported that 80% of the penalty kicks resulted in a goal being scored (Bar-eli, Azar, & Ritov, 2007).

In order to increase the chance to save penalty kicks for goalkeepers, several strategies were proposed by previous authors. Kuhn (1987) described late strategy and early strategy. The late strategy indicated that goalkeepers move to one side or another at the moment of ball contact or immediately afterwards, whereas the early strategy involved moving before ball contact (Kuhn, 1987). The late strategy was suggested as a better strategy with a higher rate of successful saves (Kuhn, 1987; Morya, Bigatao, Lees, & Ranvaud, 2005). Another specific strategy was proposed by Bar-Eli et al. (2007). They suggested the optimal strategy for goalkeepers may be to stay in the center of the goal. The probability of saving the penalty kick is higher when the goalkeeper remains in the center (33.3%) compared to jumping to the left (14.2%) or right (12.6%) (Bar-eli et al., 2007).

Goalkeepers should also strive to anticipate ball direction using visual cues before ball contact (Lees & Owens, 2011). Savelsbergh and colleagues (2002) investigated differences in anticipation and visual search behavior between expert and novice goalkeepers during the penalty kick. They found that experts were more accurate in predicting the direction of the penalty kick and waited longer before initiating a response (Savelsbergh, Williams, Van Der Kamp, & Ward, 2002). Savelsbergh et al. (2002) suggested the ball areas (including support leg, kicking leg and ball) were more informative compared to arms, trunk and pelvis area, particularly as the moment of ball contact approached. This finding was also supported by Dicks and colleagues (2011) in which they suggested goalkeepers would benefit from learning to ignore early information (e.g. approach) and use later information that is just before the initiation of the kicking action.

On the other hand, high ball-speed and accurate cunning direction (e.g. corner of the goal) would give little chance for goalkeepers to save penalty kicks. There are various studies focused on factors that can contribute to ball speed (Dörge, Andersen, Sørensen, & Simonsen, 2002; Katis & Kellis, 2010; Nunome et al., 2002). However, there are few studies investigating kick directions in penalty kicks (Scurr & Hall, 2009; van der Kamp, 2006). Most of these studies focused on the kick accuracy. To our knowledge, there is only one study that quantitatively described the postural cues in kicking that may be used by goalkeepers to save penalty kicks (Lees & Owens, 2011). These authors compared the movement of three different kicks: low side-foot kick to the left corner (relative to the kicker), low side-foot kick straight ahead and a low instep kick straight ahead. They suggested that the support foot orientation on the ground is the best cue to predict kick direction (Lees & Owens, 2011). However, due to the limits of using a laboratory space, the researchers did not study kicks to the right. Players tend to kick the ball to the side of the goal and almost 40% penalty kicks are to the right (Bar-eli et al., 2007). To our knowledge, there has been no study comparing the differences in the instep kick movements involved in altering kick directions, so the key factors that contribute to kick direction are still unclear. Therefore, the purpose of the present study was (1) to compare the differences in instep kick kinematics between two kick directions: left and right; (2) to determine the significant kinematic factors that predict kick direction. Understanding of the relationship of these factors may be useful in preparing goalkeepers to anticipate kick direction before ball contact, giving them increased time in which to react and stop the ball. We hypothesize that kicking leg, support foot and pelvis kinematics would display differences between different kick directions and those kinematic variables could be used to predict the kick direction.

2. Methods

2.1 Participants

Eleven female participants (height 166 ± 8 cm, weight 61 ± 7 kg, age 21 ± 1 yr) were recruited from the university soccer team. All participants were right foot dominant players without any injuries in the six months prior to the study. All participants were skilled with an average of 13.4 ± 1.9 years of experience in soccer training. Consent forms were signed by the participants, following the university ethics protocol. The participants wore their own outdoor soccer cleats to perform the instep kicks.

2.2 Instrumentation

Four digital video cameras (80 Hz, 640 × 480 pixels, shutter speed = 1/500 s, Fijifilm EXR) were used to film the kick movements (Figure 1). One camera was set up five meters on the right side the ball and perpendicular to the sagittal plane of the kick movement. Because the participants were all right-foot dominant, the camera was on the right side to capture the movement that occurred in the sagittal plane. Another camera was set up behind the net of the goal, which captured the participants' movement that occurred in the frontal plane. The third camera was suspended 3.5 meters above the ground and directly above the ball. This camera was mounted on a lightweight tripod that was securely fixed on the end of a steel pipe. The other end of the pipe was anchored on the ground. This overhead view camera captured the movement that occurred in the transverse plane. The fourth camera was behind the ball. This camera captured the pathway of the ball to the goal in order to determine successful trials to analyze. This camera setup and arrangement ensured the relatively good quality of each frame in the video, so that all movements of interest could be viewed and analyzed. A 'T' shape tape marker was placed on the ground close to the penalty spot to define right (+)/left (-) x-axis and posterior (+)/anterior (-) y-axis. The x-axis was parallel to the goal line. The tape was videotaped by all cameras as a calibration object.

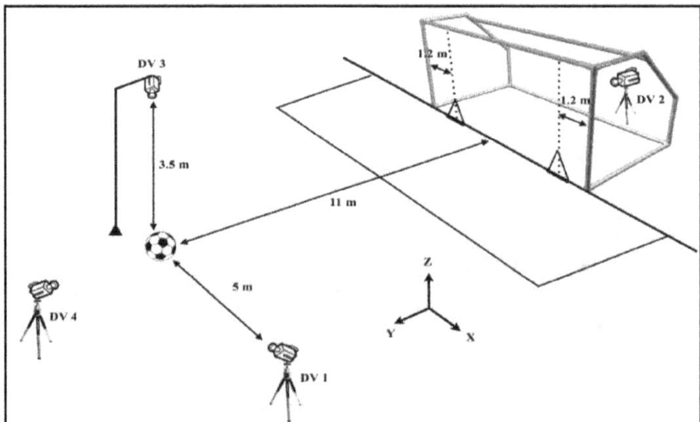

Figure 1. Schematic representation of the data collection set-up.

2.3 Testing Procedure

Prior to the data collection, 15-mm diameter, reflective tapes were placed on participants' anterior superior iliac spine (ASIS) to track the pelvic orientation and improve the digitizing consistency and accuracy. The participants performed about ten minutes of warm-up instructed by their coach including jogging on the field, dribbling the ball and short distance passing. The data were collected on an outdoor soccer field with artificial turf. The goal size was Federation Internationale de Football Association (FIFA) standard: 7.3 m wide by 2.4 m high. A FIFA standard sized ball was located at the penalty spot. The participants were instructed to shoot at a target area within the goal using an instep kick as fast and accurately as possible with the right foot. Two target areas (right and left) were defined by the goal post and the vertical axis of a pylon (Figure 1). The pylon was positioned 1.2m inside of the left and right goal posts and was 25 cm high. Participants chose their own preferred approach pattern. Kick direction was alternated every trial and initial direction was counterbalanced across participants. To minimize fatigue, participants took a 20 second break after each trial. The first three trials that place the ball successfully in the target area on each side were selected for further analysis.

2.4 Data Processing and Analysis

The Dartfish Team Pro 6.0 (Dartfish, Fribourg, Switzerland) was used to process and analyze the video files. Digitized video clips were from 5 frames before the last step of approach to 5 frames after ball contact. Fourteen points were manually digitized for both sides of the body: the estimated joint center of shoulder, hip, knee and ankle; and toe (tip of the shoe), heel and ASIS. One additional digitized point was the ball center. Test-retest intra-class correlation indicated a high reliability of digitizing process ($\alpha = .95 - .98$). A 12 Hz fourth-order Butterworth low pass filter was used to filter the raw coordinates data. The cut-off frequency was determined using the residual analysis (Winter, 2009). The kicking phase was defined from kicking foot toe-off to ball contact during the last step of approach. For the sagittal plane, kicking side hip and knee flexion/extension angle and angular velocity were calculated. Hip and knee angles were calculated using relative angles, in which 0° is the neutral position; flexion is positive and extension is negative. Joint angular velocities were calculated as the first time-derivatives of joint angles. In order to create the ensemble average curve across all participants, the sagittal plane kinematics during the kicking phase were normalized to 21 points period (0 – 20). Each time interval represented 5% of the phase, and then all the trials were averaged. For the transverse plane, pelvic orientation (PLO), support foot orientation (SFO), approach angle (APA), distance from support foot heel to ball center in x and y direction (DSBx and DSBy) and ball speed were measured/calculated at the instant of the support foot touchdown from the overhead view camera. PLO was measured from the vector between the two ASISs relative to the x-axis (Figure 2). SFO was measured from the vector between toe and heel relative to the y-axis. APA was measured from the orientation of the vector that represented the trajectory of the toe in the transverse plane before touchdown relative to the y-axis. The trajectory of the toe was tracked from three frames before touchdown to the touchdown from the overhead camera. The horizontal ball velocity was calculated as the average speed during the first three frames after ball contact using the finite-difference method (Winter 2009, p.77). The kick direction angle was measured from ball center trajectory to y-axis in the transverse plane after ball contact. For the frontal plane, trunk lateral lean (TKL) and support leg lean (SLL) were measured at the instant of support foot touchdown from the front view camera. TKL was measured from the trunk vector to global vertical axis. The trunk vector was defined as the vector joining the midpoint of the two shoulders and the midpoint of the two ASIS. SLL was measured from the vector between hip and ankle joint to global vertical axis.

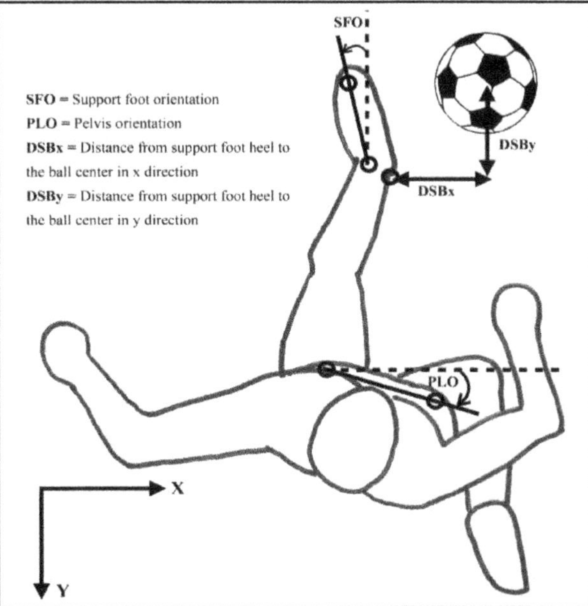

Figure 2. Measurements of kinematic variables at support foot touchdown from the overhead camera. Counterclockwise angle is positive

2.5 Statistical Analysis

Peak values of hip and knee angles and angular velocities, and frontal and transverse plane kinematics at support foot touchdown were tested using paired t-tests between the two kick directions. Stepwise multiple linear regression was used to test whether the kinematic variables predict kick direction angle. Only the variables that were significantly different between the two kick directions were included in the regression analysis. The criterion for statistical significance was $p < 0.05$ for all analyses.

3. Results

3.1 Sagittal Plane Kinematics

The joint angles and angular velocities for right (kicking side) hip and knee are presented in Figure 3. Support foot touchdown occurred at 43% (SD = 3%) during kicks to the right and at 45% (SD = 3%) during kicks to the left. The peak joint angles and angular velocities in the sagittal plane are presented in Table 1. Paired t-tests indicated that peak knee extension angular velocity was significantly higher in the kicks to the left. No other significant differences were observed.

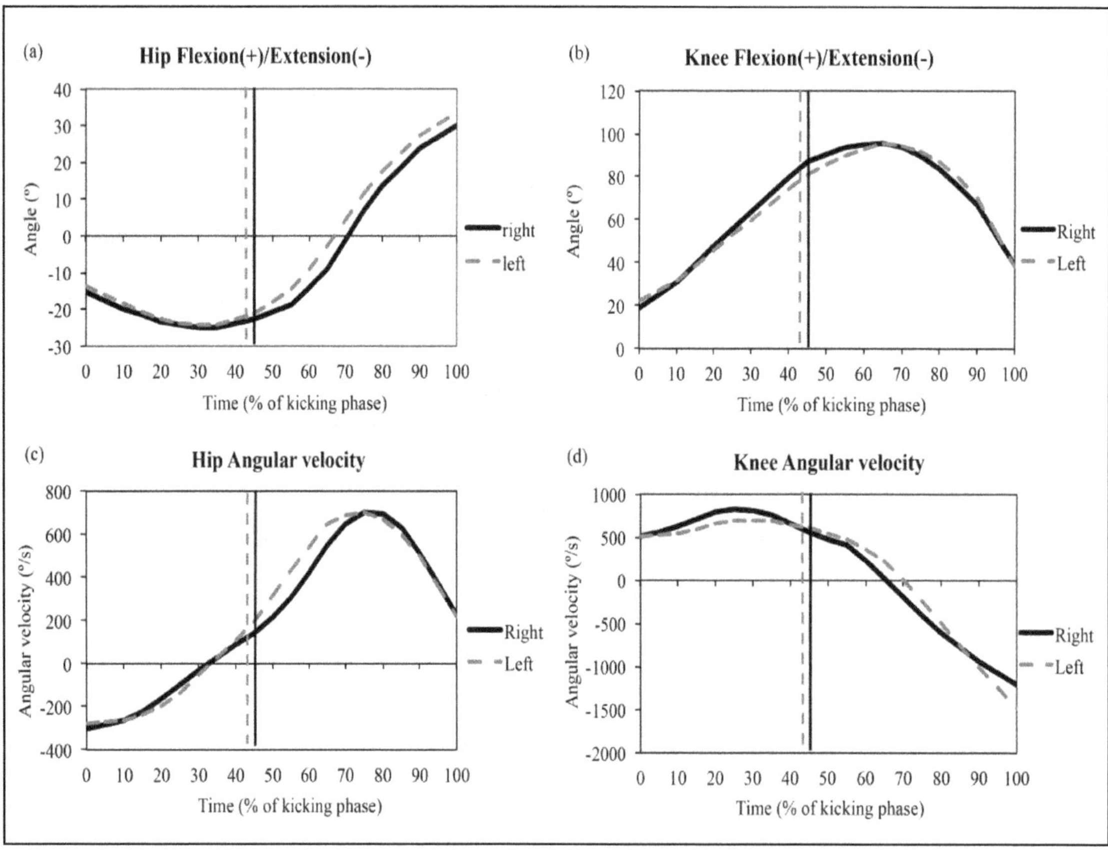

Figure 3. Ensemble average for hip and knee joint angles (a, b) and angular velocities (c, d). 0% of kicking phase corresponds to toe-off of the right foot (kicking side); 100% corresponds to ball contact. The support foot touchdown occurred at 43% and 45% of kicking phase during the left and right kicks, respectively (shown in vertical lines).

3.2 Transverse and Frontal Plane

Kinematic variables in the transverse and frontal plane, and the ball speed and direction measured from the transverse plane are presented in Table 1. The support foot and pelvis pointed more to the left when kicking to the left. In addition, the support heel was significantly closer to (less DSBx) and farther behind (greater DSBy) the ball when kicking to the left. The APA was significantly less for the left kicks. The support leg exhibited significantly less lean for the left kicks. No other statistically significant differences were found.

Table 1. Lower extremity, pelvis, and ball kinematics (mean ± SD) displayed in the two kick directions.

	Variables	Right	Left	t-value	p-value
Sagittal plane	Hip extension (°)	-26 ± 6	-25 ± 7	0.354	0.731
	Knee flexion (°)	97 ± 17	97 ± 16	0.149	0.885
	Hip flexion ω (°/s)	819 ± 162	822 ± 146	0.074	0.942
	Knee extension ω (°/s)	-1208 ± 204	-1490 ± 321	3.390	*0.007
Transverse plane	SFO (°)	-3 ± 11	17 ± 8	12.816	*<0.001
	PLO (°)	-24 ± 9	-11 ± 6	6.746	*<0.001
	DSBx (cm)	36 ± 8	30 ± 8	6.708	*<0.001
	DSBy (cm)	5 ± 10	17 ± 8	6.591	*<0.001
	APA (°)	26 ± 7	8 ± 6	11.178	*<0.001
Frontal plane	TKL (°)	8 ± 3	7 ± 2	1.691	0.122
	SLL (°)	28 ± 8	22 ± 7	4.279	*0.002
Ball kinematics	Ball speed (m/s)	17.7 ± 1.9	17.5 ± 2.0	1.061	0.314
	Kick direction (°)	-15 ± 3	14 ± 3	28.584	*<0.001

For hip and knee joint, flexion is +; extension is -. ω = angular velocity. SFO = support foot orientation, PLO = pelvis orientation, DSB = distance from support foot heel to ball center, APA = approach angle, TKL = trunk lateral lean, SLL = support leg lean. The positive sign for SFO indicated the support foot pointed to the left relative to the y axis. The positive sign for the DSBy indicated the heel is behind the ball center. The positive sign for TKL and SLL indicated leaning away from the ball. Right kick direction is negative angle; left is positive. * $p < 0.05$.

3.3 Regression Model

The kinematic variables that were significantly different between two kick directions included SLL, SFO, PLO, peak knee extension angular velocity, DSBx, DSBy and APA and these were entered to the linear regression model. Through the stepwise procedure, there were three variables that were included in the final regression model: SFO, DSBy and APA. These three variables explained 75.6% of the variance of kick direction angles (R^2 = 75.6%, p < .001). The part correlation squared were 13.7%, 6.3% and 9.0% for SFP, DSBy and APA, respectively, which indicated how much R^2 would decrease if that variable was removed from the regression model (Abdi, 2007). The regression equation produced was as follow:

Kick direction angle = $0.42 \times (SFO) + 0.37 \times (DSB_y) - 0.62 \times (APA) + 2.47$

4 Discussion

4.1 Support Foot Orientation

The results of the present study are consistent with reports by previous authors who found that the support foot tends to point toward the desired kick direction (Lees & Owens, 2011). That is, the SFO positively correlated with the kick direction angle, which indicates that the ball direction would be altered in the same direction as the support foot. The orientation of the support foot may influence the pelvic axial rotation and further affect the kick direction. The proper orientation of the support foot may allow for proper pelvic orientation, which then facilitates a greater range of pelvic rotation needed to achieve maximal velocity of the kicking leg (Lees, Asai, Andersen, Nunome, & Sterzing, 2010). The pelvis had more retraction angle (greater PLO) and less SFO (more to the right side) in kicks to the right compared to the left. Therefore, SFO could be a useful cue for goalkeepers to predict the kick direction during a penalty kick. SFO appears to be a consistent cue because it barely changed from the support foot touchdown to ball contact (Lees & Owens, 2011), and may be relatively easy to detect by goalkeepers from the frontal view. The support foot touchdown occurred at about 45% of the kicking phase, which left about 125 ms until ball contact. The averaged ball speed in the present study was approximately 17.5 m/s, which left about 630 ms from contacting the ball to passing the goal line. With an averaged response time of 200 ms (from receiving visual cues, e.g. SFO, to initiating the diving movement; Dicks, Button & Davids, 2010) and an averaged horizontal (medial-lateral) diving speed of 3 – 4 m/s (Suzuki, Togari, Isokawa, Ohashi, & Ohgushi, 1987), a goalkeeper could cover ±1.7 to ± 2.2 m (47% – 60% of the goal width) in the medial-lateral direction of the goal. SFO may be beneficial to the goalkeepers who were using the late strategy and give them extra time to anticipate kick direction, but not too early as to be used as deception for penalty takers (Dicks et al.,

2011). However, SFO in the instep kick should be differentiated from those in the curved kick. In a curved kick, the support foot pointed to the right of the desired ball direction (Alcock, Gilleard, Hunter, Baker, & Brown, 2012).

4.2 Support Foot Touchdown Position

The distance from support heel to the ball center at touchdown was found to be different between directions. The support foot touchdown position has been known as a factor that affects the height of the ball trajectory and swing leg orientation (Lees et al., 2010). To our knowledge, there has been no study investigating the role of the support foot touchdown position on kick direction. The linear regression model suggested that the DSBy could significantly predict kick direction. DSBy positively correlated with kick direction angle, which indicates that the more backward the support heel touchdown the more toward the left side the ball would go. Even though the effect of touchdown position on the ball direction may be subtle, along with the SFO, it may provide information to predict the kick direction. It is likely that if the support foot touchdown is behind the ball and points towards the left side, the ball will probably go to the left. If the support foot touchdown is in front of the ball and points towards the right, the ball will probably go to the right. Therefore, we suggested that future penalty defense training for goalkeepers may focus on searching visual information from penalty taker's support foot touchdown. Our suggestion was supported by Savelsbergh et al. (2002) who used an eye-tracking system and observed that the expert goalkeepers spent longer fixating on the kicking leg, support leg and ball areas.

4.3 Approach Angle

A 30 – 45° approach relative to the desired ball direction produces maximal ball speed (Isokawa & Lees, 1988). An angled approach can position the body to gain greater hip and knee flexion and enables the kicking leg to be tilted in the frontal plane so that the foot can be placed further under the ball, thus enabling better ball contact (Lees & Nolan, 1998). The players altered APA depending on kick direction. In the present study, the APA was significantly greater in the kicks to the right side, meaning that APA is a potentially valuable source of information for goalkeepers. The regression model indicated that the APA negatively correlated with kick direction, which means that the greater APA the more to the right side the ball would go. Though APA is a significant predictor, however, there may be difficulties to use APA as information to predict the kick direction. Firstly, the desired APA varies from player to player. A previous study reported self-selected APA was 30.3 ± 15.2° with range of 39° during instep kick (Scurr & Hall, 2009). Secondly, the approach angle may be difficult to detect from the front view or judge as large or small by goalkeepers due to lack of consistent reference. Thirdly, Dicks et al. (2011) argued that the APA was an early piece of information that can be used as deception for penalty kickers to fool the goalkeepers. Therefore, APA may be a less consistent or reliable predictor compared to SFO and DSBy for anticipating kick direction. When APA was removed from the regression model, the explained variance would drop to about 67% (dropped by 9% from 75.6%).

Other variables (e.g. PLO, TKL, SLL and peak knee extension angular velocity) could likely account for the unexplained variance of kick direction (about 24%). However, these variables are difficult to detect or judge by goalkeepers during such a fast kick movement; thus, less valuable for anticipating kick direction.

4.4 Limitations

One limitation of the present study is the conventional two-dimensional (2D) analysis that was used in the study. Nunome & Ikegami (2006) observed a distortion in knee angular velocity 50 ms before ball contact by the 2D analysis compared with 3D. They suggested this distortion was likely caused by computing angular velocities from quasi-planar projection (Nunome & Ikegami, 2006). However, it is unclear that such distortion displayed in the present study. Another potential limitation is the relatively low number of participants and trials for each participant, which may increase the type II error. Even with the low sample size, however, several significant differences were observed. A final limitation is that the present study did not examine the kinematics of kicks to the center of the goal. It has been reported that 28.7% of kick directions in skilled players were to the center (Bar-eli et al., 2007). For future studies, analyzing more directions would provide more insight to role of kinematics in predicting kick direction.

5. Conclusion and Practical Applications

In this study, differences in kinematics were observed between penalty kick directions. Support foot orientation along with support foot placement behind the ball may be the most useful cues to anticipate kick direction for goalkeepers in penalty defense. The support foot tended to point towards the desired kick direction and planted further behind the ball in the left kicks. Other factors may be less informative to be used as visual cues.

References

Abdi, H. (2007). Part (semi partial) and partial regression coefficients. In Neil Salkind (Ed.), *Encyclopedia of Measurement and Statistics* (735-737). Thousand Oaks (CA): Sage.

Alcock, A. M., Gilleard, W., Hunter, A. B., Baker, J., & Brown, N. (2012). Curve and instep kick kinematics in elite female footballers. *Journal of Sports Sciences*, *30*(4), 387–394. http://dx.doi.org/10.1080/02640414.2011.643238

Andersen, T. B., & Dörge, H. C. (2011). The influence of speed of approach and accuracy constraint on the maximal speed of the ball in soccer kicking. *Scandinavian Journal of Medicine & Science in Sports*, *21*(1), 79–84. http://dx.doi.org/10.1111/j.1600-0838.2009.01024.x

Bar-eli, M., Azar, O. H., & Ritov, I. (2007). Action bias among elite soccer goalkeepers : The case of penalty kicks. *Journal of Economic Psychology*, *28*, 606–621. http://dx.doi.org/10.1016/j.joep.2006.12.001

Dicks, M., Button, C., & Davids, K. (2010). Effects of availability of advance visual information on association football goalkeeping performance during penalty kicks. *Perception*, *39*(8), 1111–1124.

Dicks, M., Uehara, L., & Lima, C. (2011). Deception, Individual Differences and Penalty Kicks: Implications for Goalkeeping in Association Football. *International Journal of Sports Science and Coaching*, *6*(4), 515–522. http://dx.doi.org/10.1260/1747-9541.6.4.515

Dörge, H. C., Andersen, T. B., Sørensen, H., & Simonsen, E. B. (2002). Biomechanical differences in soccer kicking with the preferred and the non-preferred leg. *Journal of Sports Sciences*, *20*(4), 293–299.

Isokawa, M., & Lees, A. (1988). A biomechanical analysis of the instep kick motion in soccer. *Science and Football: Proceedings of the First World Congress of Science and Football*, 449–455.

Katis, A., & Kellis, E. (2010). Three-dimensional kinematics and ground reaction forces during the instep and outstep soccer kicks in pubertal players. *Journal of Sports Sciences*, *28*(11), 1233–1241. http://dx.doi.org/10.1080/02640414.2010.504781

Kuhn, W. (1987). Penalty-kick strategies for shooters and goalkeepers. In *Science and football: proceedings of the First World Congress of Science and Football, Liverpool, UK* (pp. 489–492).

Lees, A., & Nolan, L. (1998). The biomechanics of soccer: a review. *Journal of Sports Sciences*, *16*(3), 211–234. http://dx.doi.org/10.1080/026404198366740

Lees, A., Asai, T., Andersen, T. B., Nunome, H., & Sterzing, T. (2010). The biomechanics of kicking in soccer: a review. *Journal of Sports Sciences*, *28*(8), 805–817. http://dx.doi.org/10.1080/02640414.2010.481305

Lees, A., & Owens, L. (2011). Early visual cues associated with a directional place kick in soccer in soccer. *Sports Biomechanics*, *10*(02), 125–134. http://dx.doi.org/10.1080/14763141.2011.569565

Morya, E., Bigatao, H., Lees, A., & Ranvaud, R. (2005). Evolving penalty kick strategies: World Cup and club matches, 2000–2002. In *Science and football V. Proceedings of the fifth world congress of science and football* (p. 510).

Nunome, H., Asai, T., Ikegami, Y., & Sakurai, S. (2002). Three-dimensional kinetic analysis of side-foot and instep soccer kicks. *Medicine and Science in Sports and Exercise*, *34*(12), 2028–2036. http://dx.doi.org/10.1249/01.MSS.0000039076.43492.EF

Nunome, H., & Ikegami, Y. (2006). Kinematics of soccer instep kicking: A comparison of two-dimensional and three-dimensional analysis. *Proceedings Of International Symposium On Biomechanics In Sports*, 2611–2614.

Savelsbergh, G., Williams, A., Van Der Kamp, J., & Ward, P. (2002). Visual search , anticipation and expertise in soccer goalkeepers Visual search, anticipation and expertise in soccer goalkeepers. *Journal of Sports Sciences*, (20), 279–287.

Scurr, J., & Hall, B. (2009). The effects of approach angle on penalty kicking accuracy and kick kinematics with recreational soccer players. *Journal of Sports Science & Medicine*, *8*(2), 230–234.

Suzuki, S., Togari, H., Isokawa, M., Ohashi, J., & Ohgushi, T. (1987). Analysis of the goalkeeper's diving motion. In T. Reilly, A. Lees, K. Davids, & W. J. Murphy (Eds.) *Science and Football.* Proceedings of the 1st World Congress of Science and Football, Liverpool, UK, 13-17 April (pp. 468-475). Routledge Revivals.

Van der Kamp, J. (2006). A field simulation study of the effectiveness of penalty kick strategies in soccer: late alterations of kick direction increase errors and reduce accuracy. *Journal of Sports Sciences*, *24*(5), 467–477. http://dx.doi.org/10.1080/02640410500190841

Winter, D. A. (2009). *Biomechanics and motor control of human movement*. Hoboken, N.J. : Wiley, c2009.

2

The Use of Simulation Training to Accelerate the Rate of Forward Ice Skating Skill Acquisition

Nathan J Washington
School of Science and Health, Western Sydney University, PO box 2751, Sydney New South Wales, Australia
E-mail: n.washington@westernsydney.edu.au

Sera Dogramaci
New South Wales Institute of Sport, Figtree Drive, Olympic Park, Sydney, NSW, Australia
E-mail: sera.dogramaci@nswis,gov.au

Kylie A Steel (Corresponding author)
School of Science and Health, Western Sydney University, PO box 2751, Sydney New South Wales, Australia
E-mail: k.steel@westernsydney.edu.au

Eathan Ellem
School of Science and Health, Western Sydney University PO box 2751, Sydney New South Wales, Australia
E-mail: e.ellem@westernsydney.edu.au

Abstract

Background: Australia's interest and participation in ice hockey is increasing, however a lack of access to facilities means familiarity with this sport is limited, and so too is the facilitation of skill development within an ecologically valid context. **Objective:** While numerous methods may be employed to address this, one resource which remains relatively unexplored is the StrideDeck Treadmill, therefore the purpose of this study was to investigate the effectiveness of this equipment with specific reference to the biomechanical changes for skating ability. **Methods:** N = 16 male athletes (Mage = 15.0 ± 0.76 yrs) from a junior league competition participated in this intervention based study. n = 9 were assigned to the training intervention (StrideDeck) once a week, while the control group (n = 7) continued their normal training routines. Further, monthly sprint tests both on the StrideDeck and an on-ice protocol were conducted to track progress via kinematic analysis. **Results:** Data analysis revealed no significant overall effects for on-ice sprint skating performance after StrideDeck training; however there were significant kinematic differences between StrideDeck and ice conditions. **Conclusions:** Therefore while the StrideDeck may have merit in regard to physiological paramters, the results of this study do not support its use as a skill acquisition tool in regard to increasing skating ability.

Keywords: Simulation training, skill acquisition, treadmill, ice skating, ice hockey skating, ice skating stride

1. Introduction

Research has demonstrated the development of expertise in movement execution is influenced by factors such as feedback, instruction, and practice type (e.g., deliberate practice) (Ericsson & Lehmann, 1996; Baker & Young, 2014). Other factors that should also be considered are access to coaches, equipment, and facilities (Baker & Young, 2014). However, in Australian contexts there are limitations to these resources; as such athletes must employ a variety of strategies and resources to accelerate their learning. For example, simulation training is a practice method designed to replicate the movements or environment associated with the context it is attempting to emulate (Cha et al., 2012). It is also a training method that is essential in cases where accessing specific environments is limited or there is a high risk of injury, thus impeding the mastery of a skill (Cha et al.2012).

Simulation training in sporting contexts helps athletes develop necessary skills that can be transferred into competition, thus improving the proficiency of skill execution and reducing error (de Groot et al., 2011). For example, ball projection machines replicate ball trajectories in sports such as cricket, volleyball, and tennis which can increase skill acquisition and execution (Pinder et al., 2011). Further, motor sport employs virtual simulators to enhance the driver's decision making skills, thus decreasing the risk of accidents and track hiring costs (de Groot et al., 2011). Such environmental constraints are evident within ice hockey, specifically the availability of ice rinks for skating practice. Australian ice hockey players lack access to a sufficient number of ice rinks which is disadvantageous for players. For example, Australia (ranked 36th) is limited to 10 indoor rinks for 4,264 players (426.4 players per rink) (International Ice Hockey Federation (IIHF), 2015), whereas Canada (ranked 1st) have 2,631 indoor and 5,000 outdoor rinks for 721,504 players (94.5 players per rink) (IIHF, 2015). Given restrictions in rink accessibility, Australian ice hockey players face different challenges compared to northern hemisphere (Soberlak & Côté, 2003). For instance, skating in ice hockey is the most important movement skill when gauging success in competitive leagues (Bracko, 2004). Furthermore, talent scouts pay significant attention to skating when determining potential players for team selection (Hansen & Reed, 1979). Ice hockey players need to be confident and powerful skaters in order to focus on strategy and tactics during high velocities in a game situation (Upjohn et al.2008); and maintain efficiency given the average skating distance is between 3km-5km per game (Montgomery et al., 2004). Therefore, the importance of skating combined with the lack of access to facilities to promote skating development reduces world ranking progression with top competitors such as Canada and United States of America.

Several simulation training methods currently exist that emulate ice surfaces, such as synthetic ice panels, slide boards, and skating treadmills, which provide glide-like properties to help enhance skating mechanics (Stidwill et al.,2010; Pies et al.,1998; Dreger, 1997; Nobes et al.2003). This allows skaters to replicate the movement patterns performed on ice in a different environment, thus continuing their skating development. Despite the prevalence of simulation tools and equipment focusing on the skating component, there is a lack of evidence observing the effectiveness of simulation training in ice hockey skating.

The current study utilises the StrideDeck Treadmill (SDT) (Figure 1.), which is a portable piece of equipment that focuses on the forward stride component of skating, which accounts for 85% of total skating time in ice hockey (Stamm, 2010). Therefore, the purpose of this study was twofold, firstly, to assess whether incorporating the SDT within regular training sessions increases skill acquisition of skating, and secondly whether any increases in performance translate to improve on-ice hockey sprint times.

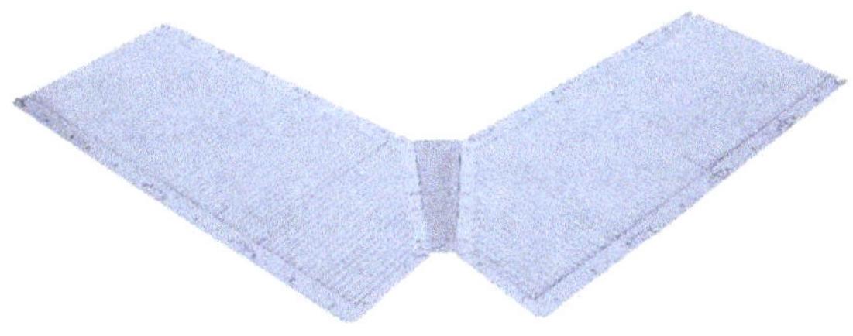

Figure 1. StrideDeck Treadmill

2. Methods

2.1 Participants

Sixteen male athletes (M_{age} = 15.0 ± 0.76 yrs, M_{height}164.3 ± 7.52 cm, M_{weight} 57.9 ± 7.38 kg) from an Australian junior ice hockey team volunteered to participate in this study. Athletes varied in their level of ice hockey expertise (state representative = 6, social = 10), with n = 9 and n = 7 players randomly allocated to training and control groups respectively. Each group contained a mix of attacking and defending players, however goaltenders were excluded from the study. Data collection for this study took place during the winter competition season (May to September) at the local ice rink participants used for training. Ethics approval was gained from Western Sydney University's Human Research Ethics committee, with athletes and their parent/guardians providing informed consent prior to participating in the study.

2.2 Protocol

The training group implemented the StrideDeck Treadmill (SDT) prior to each on ice practice session, while the control group continued their regular practice. To test if the SDT had any effect on skating performance athletes underwent on ice sprint tests every four weeks (four sprinting tests took place over the course of the study) to track progress and observe any improvements that may have occurred. Further, to determine if the SDT is a viable skating training apparatus, a biomechanical comparison was implemented to assess kinematic differences between strides in SDT and sprint test protocols.

Participants wore their full on-ice equipment during SDT training sessions, including skates, helmets, with hockey stick in hand (Figure 2). Rubber skate guards were worn on the SDT to protect the skate blades as the plastic rollers create friction resulting in an increase in wear. Prior to SDT sessions, athletes completed a familiarisation period with the treadmill which involved performing 10 consecutive strides. During SDT sessions, athletes engaged in forward stride motion for two minutes, this meant athletes maintained a consistent pace with full leg extensions.

Athletes then increased the extension rate to a higher intensity for an additional minute, resulting in a total intervention time of three minutes. Training and control groups completed four on-ice sprint tests throughout the season. Baseline forward straight line sprinting time was based on the International Ice Hockey Federation Skills Challenge Manual (IIHF, 2015). Participants were required to sprint as fast as possible from the starting line to the finishing line (100ft/30.48m distance).The forward sprint was filmed using a tripod mounted Sony High Definition video camera recording 50fps (Sony Corporation, Tokyo, Japan) allowing a biomechanical comparison between on-ice and SDT to take place. The forward stride consists of three phases, beginning when the blade has made initial contact with the ice, progressing through the glide, push-off, and recovery phases (De Boer et al., 1986). Timing commenced as soon as the participant initiated movement from the starting line until their torso crossed the finish line. The result of the two trials of the forward sprint were recorded, then averaged to produce a mean time for forward skating.

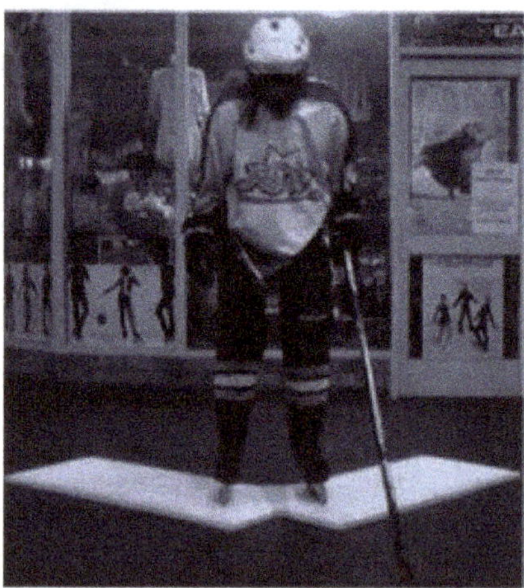

Figure 2. Subject on StrideDeck Treadmill with full equipment as well as skate guards

2.3 Analysis

A biomechanical comparison between on-ice and SDT was completed using Kinovea software (version 0.8.15, Kinovea, France). This additional analysis was employed to determine whether the stride leg angles performed on the SDT were similar to the sprint testing protocol. Further, analysis measured stride kinematics across four SDT sessions and sprint tests to measure if any changes occurred over time.

Using the Kinovea software, common landmarks were measured for both legs, specifically leg adduction (medial), leg abduction (lateral), and ankle flexion angles (Figure 3). Measurements were taken when the athletes were striding at a high intensity in the final minute on the SDT.

Statistical analysis was conducted SPSS (version 22.0) to assess whether significant changes occurred in skating sprint performance after SDT sessions when compared to the control group. A linear mixed model was applied for the dependant variable of forward sprint time (FWD). Fixed factors were group (Training and Control) and session (pre/post ice), with participant being a random factor. Further, the dependant variables for biomechanical analysis were medial, lateral, and ankle flexion angles. Fixed factors were leg (left and right) and session (pre/post ice and SDT). Moreover, a final analysis was conducted that determined whether significant changes occurred in SDT performance only. Four sessions were analysed in total, with analysis focusing on the above kinematic dependant variables in each session (SDT1, SDT2, SDT3, SDT4). An alpha level of p = <.05 was set as the criterion for significance for all statistical procedures.

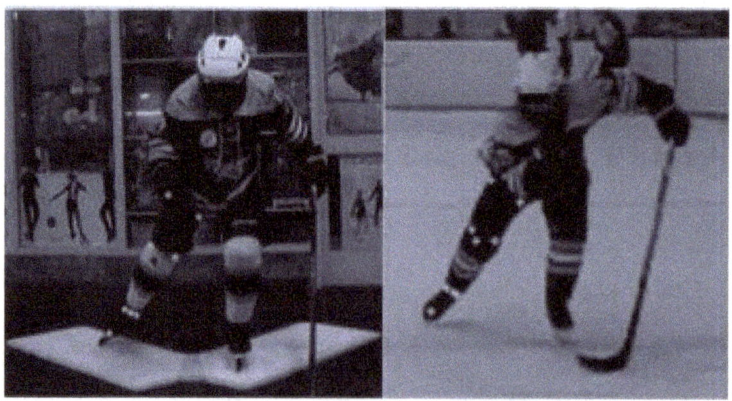

Figure 3. Kinematic markers identify the movements analysed. Medial/ leg adduction, lateral/leg abduction, and foot/ ankle

3. Results

3.1. Sprint Test

Analysis of sprint times returned no significant main effects for Group $F(1, 15) = 1.16$, $p = .299$ or session $F(3, 29) = 0.54$, $p = .659$, nor was there a significant Group x Session interaction $F(3, 29) = 1.12$, $p = .359$. While training and control groups returned differences between pre- and post-tests, these times were not significant (Table 1).

Table 1. Differences between the training and control groups based on session

	Group	
Session	Training	Control
Pre-Test	5.22 (0.41)	5.58 (0.39)
Post-Test	5.24 (0.39)	5.41 (0.58)

Note. Mean sprint time for training and control groups in pre- and post-tests when groups were combined, data presented as mean time (standard deviation).

3.2 Kinematic comparison between ice and SDT

Analysis of medial kinematic data returned a significant overall effect for Session $F(3, 462) = 36.06$, $p = < .001$ (Figure 4), as well as a significant Session x Leg interaction $F(3, 461) = 9.45$, $p = <.001$. When legs were combined, there were significant differences in average medial angles between ice and SDT sessions (Table 2). Further, the significant interaction is attributable to differences between left and right legs in pre-ice, as well as post-deck sessions (Table 3).

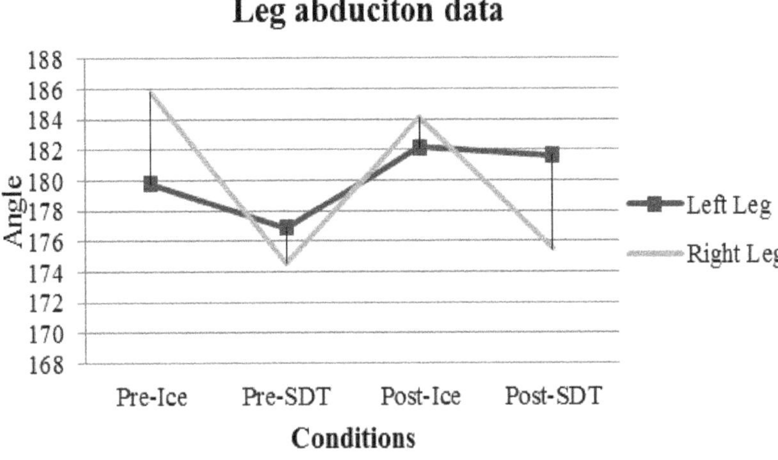

Figure 4. Medial kinematic angle differences between legs on different conditions

Table 2. Kinematic data based on session (Pre-Post) and condition (Ice vs SDT)

	Angle		
Session	Medial	Lateral	Ankle
Pre-Ice	174.79 (5.17)$_{1,2}$	182.78 (4.85)$_{1,2}$	150.98 (5.80)$_{1,2,3}$
Post-Ice	174.69 (4.92)$_{3,5}$	183.12 (4.48)$_{3,5}$	147.05 (5.37)$_{2,4,6}$
Pre-Deck	183.48 (5.013)$_{1,3,4}$	175.71 (4.62)$_{1,3,4}$	161.76 (5.53)$_{1,4,5}$
Post-Deck	179.01 (5.013)$_{2,4,5}$	178.54 (4.62)$_{2,4,5}$	156.89 (5.53)$_{3,5,6}$

Note. Summary of kinematic variables across ice and StrideDeck sessions with legs combined, subscript numbers indicate significance between sessions for a given variable only, not between variables, data presented as mean angle (standard deviation).

Table 3. Presents data demonstrating session and leg interaction.

		Angle		
Session	Leg	Medial	Lateral	Ankle
Pre-Ice	L	177.14 (5.69)	179.76 (5.60)	155.17 (6.66)
	R	172.43 (5.69)	185.80 (5.60)	146.78 (6.66)
Post-Ice	L	175.34 (5.07)	182.15 (4.71)	148.84 (5.64)
	R	174.03 (5.43)	184.10 (5.24)	145.25 (6.24)
Pre-Deck	L	182.30 (5.43)	176.89 (5.24)	163.05 (6.24)
	R	184.65 (5.43)	174.54 (5.24)	160.48 (6.24)
Post-Deck	L	176.21 (5.43)	181.62 (5.24)	155.35 (6.24)
	R	181.81 (5.43)	175.46 (5.24)	158.43 (6.24)

Note. Summary of Session x Leg kinematic variables, data presented as mean angle (standard deviation).

Analysis of lateral kinematic data returned a significant overall effect for Session $F(3,462) = 18.88$, $p = <.001$, as well as a significant Session x Leg interaction $F(3,461) = 9.39$, $p = <.001$ (Table 3). When legs were combined, there were again significant differences in average lateral angles between ice and SDT sessions (Table 2).

Analysis of ankle kinematic data returned a significant overall effect for Session $F(3,462) = 49.27$, $p = <.001$, Leg $F(1, 460) = 8.77$, $p = .003$ (Figure 5), as well as a significant Session x Leg interaction $F(3,461) = 5.39$, $p = <.001$ (Table 3). When legs were combined, again there were significant differences in ankle angles between ice and SDT sessions (Table 2). When sessions were combined, there was a greater angle in the right ($M = 155.60$, $SD = 5.14$) compared to the left ankle ($M = 152.74$, $SD = 5.18$).

3.3 StrideDeck session kinematic analysis

Analysis of medial kinematic SDT data returned significant overall effects for Session $F(3, 385) = 11.65$, $p = .005$ and Leg $F(1, 385) = 50.90$, $p = < .001$, as well as a significant Session x Leg interaction $F(3, 385) = 5.62$, $p = <.001$. Further, analysis of lateral kinematic SDT data returned significant overall effects for Session $F(3, 385) = 4.79$, $p = .003$ and Leg $F(1, 385) = 27.57$, $p = < .001$, as well as a significant Session x Leg interaction $F(3, 385) = 2.69$, $p = .046$. Moreover, analysis of ankle kinematic SDT data returned significant overall effects for Session $F(3, 385) = 8.05$, $p = < .001$, as well as a significant Session x Leg interaction $F(3,385) = 4.98$, $p = .002$ (Figure 6).

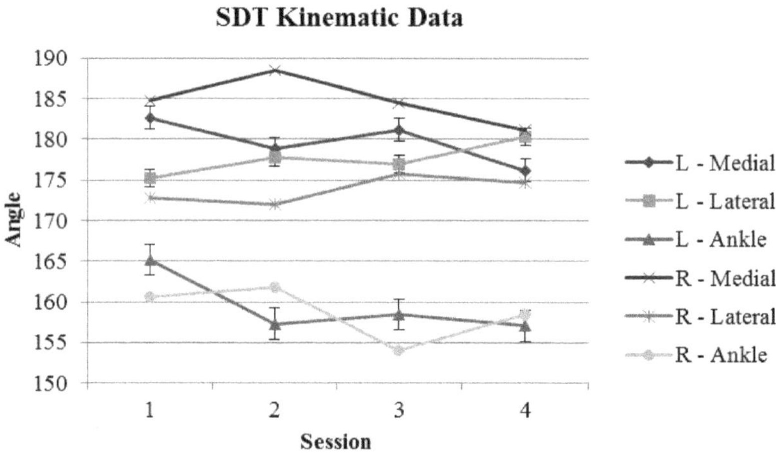

Figure 5. Ankle kinematic angle differences of legs on different conditions.

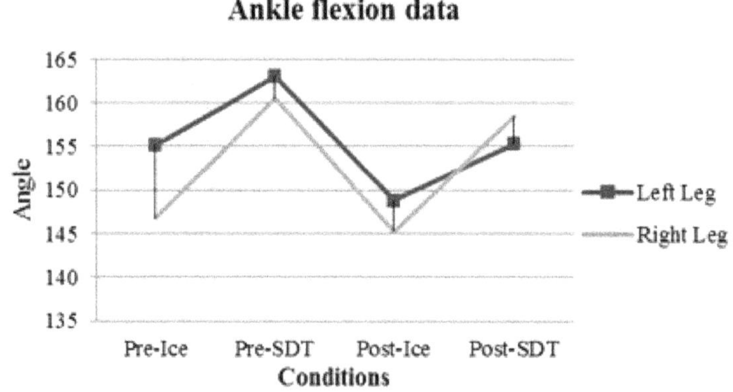

Figure 6. SDT kinematic data only for all angle variables across four sessions.

4. Discussion

The aim of this study was to assess whether the StrideDeck Treadmill (SDT) improved ice skating performance using a pre-post intervention design. The outcome was measured based on improvements in forward ice skating sprint times. While there were no significant improvements in skating performance between pre- and post- sprint tests, there were kinematic trends for post-SDT and post-ice conditions. However, this demonstrated the SDT did not sufficiently contribute to enhanced sprint skating ability.

While there were no significant findings for sprint time, there were significant kinematic differences between medial and lateral angles for all sessions when comparing skating surfaces. This demonstrated movement patterns on the SDT did not reflect that of skating on ice; this may be due to the changes in mechanics associated with high skating velocities. Marino (1977) found while athletes are skating in sprint intensity, they spend more time in single support leg phase than double support leg phase. This was evident in the sprinting kinematic of the current study when measuring the push-off leg angles on the ice. The athletes opposing leg would be in the recovery phase whereas on the SDT the opposite leg that was being measured was positioned on the ground to balance the skater. However, the length of time spent in double support phase was not measured here; therefore it is unclear whether this affected results.

In addition to the significant findings for medial and lateral angles, ankle flexion angles were significantly different between the SDT and ice skating. Participants wore rubber skate guards to protect the blades of the boot when performing on the SDT; resulting in an increase in friction between the guards and the rollers. The increased resistance may have disrupted the athlete's movement pattern, resulting in a greater level of self-organisation to overcome the resistance, which also affected and led to significant differences in medial and lateral angles (Magill, 2010). Similar movement pattern disruption was also found due to the disparity in the surface coefficient of friction in a study carried out by Stidwill et al., (2010). The subjects had a more upright trunk angle with increased stride frequency on synthetic ice surfaces compared to ice conditions. Although these were minor differences in the study (Stidwill et al. 2010) this demonstrated the effect resistance can have on the movement pattern when executed on frictionless surfaces (i.e., ice).

High velocity speeds play a significant role in increasing joint range of motion, with Lafontaine (2007) and Buckeridge et al., (2015) suggesting joint motion amplitude is proportional to increases in velocity. Further, Chang et al., (2009) as well as De Koning et al., (1995) found skaters had to accommodate high skating speed with increased hip abduction angles and rate. Without the extension rate demonstrating the intensity between the two surfaces, the range of motion is compromised on the SDT, therefore resulting in significant differences across all measurements in comparison to ice conditions (Table 2.).

The glide phase contributes to the velocity of ice skating, with the gliding motion utilising the stretch shortening cycle (Upjohn et al., 2008). This is executed with a forward trunk lean which applies more weight on the gliding skate. By increasing knee flexion (eccentric contraction) a player can use the elastic stored energy to apply more force in the push-off (concentric contraction) resulting with an increased stride length (Upjohn et al., 2008; Stamm, 2010). The design of the SDT did not allow a glade phase to occur, this further illustrates why there was a lack of kinematic differences between the SDT and on-ice.

Kinematic measurements could be more reliable in future studies by employing kinematic markers placed on the skaters to increase the accuracy of estimations in analysis. Moreover, measurements were only taken from the frontal plane; whereas additional data could be collected from the sagittal plane, thus providing insight to stride length and analysis of the recovery phase. Despite study measurement limitations, supported literature demonstrates that skating mechanics on both SDT and ice are significantly different, and these findings are supported by previous ice skating biomechanical studies (De Boer et al. 1986; Marino, 1977).

When considering motor control, Maslovat et al., (2004) suggest practice conditions should match test conditions as closely as possible, thus leading to an increase in performance in the latter. This is true in simulation training studies where transfer of skill acquisition from a training environment to real environments are evident due to the familiarity in neuromotor processes, decision-making, and correct skill execution volume (de Groot et al., 2011; Pinder et al.,2011; Del Sal et al.2009; Willaert et al., 2012; Bekker & Lotz, 2009). However, this did not occur in the current study as there were significant differences in movement patterns between SDT and ice. The design of the SDT may not have allowed participants to perform normal skating movement patterns. Athletes are able to perform the gliding phase and manoeuvres on ice, whereas this is impossible on the SDT. Practicing incorrect movement patterns can inhibit the motor skill which enforces why the SDT had produced no transfer of skills onto real environments (Kottke et al. 1978).

It should be noted that adequate time is needed for subjects to become familiarised with an apparatus otherwise testing performance may not be representative of their ability (Lockwood & Frost, 2007). Lockwood and Frost (2007) found that it had taken subjects up to six weeks to become familiar and skate efficiently on the skating treadmill. Considering skaters in this study were only exposed to the SDT once a week for a period of four weeks, this may not have afforded enough time for subjects to become familiar with the device.

5. Conclusion

Overall, the SDT resulted in significant biomechanical differences, e.g., differences in leg abduction, adduction, and ankle flexion when compared to ice conditions; however this did not translate to improved sprint ability on ice. It is likely the motor patterns for the SDT compare to on-ice sprinting are dissimilar, thus the associated mechanics for each surface do not correlate with each other. We therefore suggest that the SDT in its current form does not provide suitable platform for skill development, though may be useful for improved fitness. Future studies could possibly assess whether the SDT can be utilised as a fitness method to increased skating endurance.

Acknowledgment

We are thankful to the Canterbury ice hockey team for volunteering their time to participate. We are also grateful for the New South Wales Institute of Sport for providing the equipment and supporting our study.

References

Baker, J., & Young, B. (2014). 20 years later: Deliberate practice and the development of expertise in sport. *International Review of Sport and Exercise Psychology*, *7*(1), 135-157.

Bekker, J., & Lotz, W. (2009). Planning formula one race strategies using discrete event simulation. *The Journal of the Operational Research Society, 60*(7), 952-961.

Bracko, R. (2004). Biomechanics powers ice hockey performance. *Biomechanics,* 47-53.

Buckeridge, E., LeVangie, M., Stetter, B., Nigg, S., & Nigg, B. (2015). An on-ice measurement approach to analyse the biomechanics of ice hockey skating. *PLoS ONE, 10*(5).

Cha, M., Han, S., Lee, J., & Choi, B. (2012). A virtual reality based fire training simulator integrated with fire dynamics data. *Fire Safety Journal, 50*, 12-24.

Chang, R., Turcotte, R., & Pearsall, D. (2009). Hip adductor muscle function in forward skating. *Sports Biomechanics, 8*(3), 212-222.

De Boer, R., Schermerhorn, P., Gademan, J., de Groot, G., & van Ingen Schenau, G.J. (1986). Characteristic stroke mechanics of elite and trained male speed skaters. *International Journal Sport Biomechanics, 2*, 175-185.

Del Sal, M., Barbieri, E., Garbati, P., Sisti, D., Rocchi, M., & Stocchi, V. (2009). Physiologic responses of firefighter recruits during a supervised live-fire work performance test. *Journal of Strength and Conditioning Research, 23*(8), 2396-2404.

de Groot, S., Mulder, M., & Wieringa, P. (2011). Car racing in a simulator: Validation and assessment of brake pedal stiffness. *Teleoperators & Virtual Environment, 20*(1), 47-61.

De Koning, J., Thomas, R., Berger, M., de Groot, G., & van Ingen Schenau, G.J. (1995). The start in speed skating: From running to gliding. *Medicine and Science in Sports and Exercise, 27*, 1703–1708

Dreger, R. (1997). Using skate-treadmills to train hockey players for speed. *Strength & Conditioning Journal, 19*(6), 33-35.

Ericsson, K., & Lehmann, A. (1996). Expert and exceptional performance: Evidence of maximal adaptation to task constraints. *Annual Review of Psychology, 47*(1), 273-305.

Hansen, H., & Reed, A. (1979). Functions and on-ice competencies of a high caliber hockey player—a job analysis. In *Science in Skiing, Skating, and Hockey. Proceedings of the International Symposium of Biomechanics in Sports* (pp. 107-115). Del Mar, CA: Academic Publishers.

International Ice Hockey Federation (IIHF), (2015), Country profiles. Retrieved from: http://www.iihf.com/iihf-home/countries/australia/

International Ice Hockey Federation (IIHF), (2015). Skills manual challenge: Test 3. Retrieved from: http://www.ihi.is/gogn/skill_challange.pdf

Kottke, F., Halpern, D., Easton, J., Ozel, A., & Burrill, C. (1978). The training of coordination. *Archives of Physical Medicine Rehabilitation, 59*, 567-572.

Lafontaine, D. (2007). Three-dimensional kinematics of the knee and ankle joints for three consecutive push-offs during ice hockey skating starts. *Sports Biomechanics, 6*(3), 391-406.

Lockwood, K., & Frost, G. (2007). Habituation of 10-year-old hockey players to treadmill skating, *Sports Biomechanics, 6*(2), 145-154.

Magill, R. (2010). *Motor Learning and Control: Concepts and Applications* (9th ed.). New York: McGraw Hill-Int.

Marino, G. (1977). Kinematics of ice skating at different velocities. *American Alliance for Health, Physical Education and Recreation, 48*(1), 93-97.

Maslovat, D., Chus, R., Lee, T., & Franks, I. (2004). Contextual interference: Single task versus multi-task learning. *Motor Control-Champaign, 8*(2), 213-233.

Montgomery, D., Nobes, K., Pearsall, D.J., & Turcotte, R. (2004). Task analysis (hitting, shooting, passing and skating) of professional hockey players. In D.J Pearsall and A.B Ashare (Ed.), Safety *in Ice Hockey: Fourth Volume* (pp. 288-295). West Conshohocken, PA: ASTM International.

Nobes, K., Montgomery, D., Pearsall, D. J., Turcotte, R. A., Lefebvre, R., & Whittom, F. (2003). A comparison of skating economy and on-ice and on the skating treadmill. *Canadian Journal of Applied Physiology, 28*(1), 1-11.

Pies, N., Provost-Craig, M., Neeves, R., & Richards, J. (1998). Cardiopulmonary responses to slideboard exercise in competitive female ice skaters. *Journal of Strength and Conditioning Research, 12*(1), 7-11.

Pinder, R., Renshaw, I., Davids, K., & Kerhervé, H. (2011). Principles for the use of ball projection machines in elite and developmental sport programmes. *Sports Medicine, 41*(10), 793-800.

Stamm, L. (2010). *Laura Stamm's Power skating* (4th ed.). United States: Human Kinetics.

Stidwill, T., Pearsall, D. J., & Turcotte, R. A. (2010). Comparison of skating kinetics and kinematics on ice and on a synthetic surface. *Sports Biomechanics, 9*(1), 57-64.

Soberlak, P., & Côté, J. (2003). The developmental activities of elite ice-hockey players. *Journal of Applied Sport Psychology, 15*, 41-49.

UpJohn, T., Turcotte, R., Pearsall, D., & Loh, J. (2008). Three-dimensional kinematics of the lower limbs during forward ice hockey skating. *Sports Biomechanics, 7*(2), 206-221.

Willaert, W., Aggarwal, R., Herzeele, I., Cheshire, N., & Vermassen, F. (2012). Recent advancements in medical simulation: Patient-specific virtual reality simulation. *World Journal of Surgery, 36*(7), 1703-1712.

3

Emotional Labour in Teaching Secondary Physical Education

Ye Hoon Lee
Department of Health, Physical Education, and Recreation, University of North Alabama, PO box 5073, Florence, AL, USA
E-mail: ylee6@una.edu

Hyungil Harry Kwon (Corresponding author)
Department of Physical Education, Chung-Ang University, #202, bldg. 305, Chung-Ang Univ., 84, Heukseok-ro, Dongjak-gu, Seoul, South Korea
E-mail: hkwon@cau.ac.kr

Hwajung Oh
Physical Education Laboratory, Chung-Ang University, #1419, bldg. 303, Chung-Ang Univ., 84, Heukseok-ro, Dongjak-gu, Seoul, South Korea
E-mail: ohpapsy@gmail.com

Abstract

Background: Teaching physical education is an emotion-laden context which requires physical education teachers to engage in emotional labor in order to foster their well-being, as well as student's outcomes. **Objective:** The purpose of this study was to investigate the predictability of emotional labour strategies on job satisfaction and emotional exhaustion among secondary physical education teachers in South Korea. Specifically, the four forms of emotional labour (i.e., surface acting, deep acting, genuine positive expression, and genuine negative expression) were hypothesized to have different influences on job satisfaction and emotional exhaustion. **Method:** A total of 225 full-time physical education teachers were invited to participate in the paper-pencil survey. The questionnaires contained items measuring the four forms of emotional labour, emotional exhaustion, and job satisfaction which had been modified to fit the physical education setting. **Results:** The results indicated that surface acting, genuine positive expression, and genuine expression was significantly associated with emotional exhaustion whereas only genuine positive expression was significantly associated with job satisfaction and emotional exhaustion. Finally, emotional exhaustion mediates the relationship between surface acting and job satisfaction, genuine positive expression and job satisfaction, and genuine negative expression and job satisfaction. **Conclusion:** These results suggest that emotional labour plays a critical role on physical education teachers' well-being and job attitude.

Keywords: emotional regulation, physical education teacher, genuine expression, Asian culture, surface acting

1. Introduction

1.1 Introduce the problem

Teaching is a highly emotional practice (Sutton, 2005) in that teachers often face emotionally challenging incidents every day when dealing with difficult and hostile students, medical emergencies, or angry parents (Tuxford & Bradley, 2015). These emotional challenges have been found to influence teachers' well-being, mental health, and job attitude, as well as students' learning outcomes (Chan, 2006). Thus, it is critical for teachers to identify how to cope with emotional demands. Emotional labour, a term first coined by Hochschild (1983), is defined as the process of both regulating one's inner feelings and expressing appropriate emotions at work (Grandey, 2000). Teachers need to purposefully modify and display appropriate emotions in their interaction with students as it has the potential to strengthen their ability to deal with emotional challenges and teaching effectiveness (Sutton, 2005). Emotional labour can be a crucial construct in the physical education (PE) domain as it could identify an effective coping strategy to enhance occupational well-being (e.g., less job burnout and greater job satisfaction) and organisational outcomes (e.g., teaching effectiveness and teacher-student relationship). The significance of the construct can be even greater when we consider that the unique physical structure of the PE context (e.g., a large open space) could elicit a higher degree of emotional challenges (Koustelios & Tsigilis, 2005). In fact, displaying positive emotions in PE context were found to provide multiple benefits for PE teachers and students (see Stuhr, Sutherland, & Ward, 2012). For example, in their in-depth interview with two PE teachers, Stuhr and his colleagues (2012) found that displaying positive emotion affected student performance by creating more teacher-student relationship and increasing student's participation. However, few studies have examined what would cost to their well-being during their endeavor to modify inner feelings to display positive emotion (i.e., emotional labour).

Further, despite the growing concern about emotional labour in teaching, most emotional labour studies tended to focus on Western cultures (e.g., Barber, Grawitch, Carson, & Tsouloupas, 2011; Keller, Chang, Becker, Goetz, & Frenzel, 2014; Taxer & Frenzel, 2015; Tsouloupas, Carson, Matthews, Grawitch, & Barber, 2010), which implies that there has been relatively little attention to Asian cultures. It is possible that the findings may differ from Asian cultures because of differences in culture and school norms. For example, Korean students and teachers tended to perceive fewer unexpected events, probably because of the holistic reasoning common in East Asia, and thus experienced fewer fluctuations in their emotional status (Choi & Nisbett, 2000). Thus, it may be meaningful to examine the relationship between Asian PE teachers' emotional labour strategies and its consequences.

1.2 Changes in Teacher-Student Relationship in the Korean Educational Context.

Education in South Korea is viewed as a critical element for one's success; there is an old proverb saying, "Students should not step over the teacher's shadow". It means teaching is honored as one of the most glorious professions and students need to respect their teachers. The proverb is firmly rooted in the long Confucian tradition inherent in Korean society, which has shaped the strong hierarchical relationship between elders and young people. In fact, the Korean society considers that a hierarchical structure is the best way to achieve organisational goals effectively. Thus, older people or people in higher positions are typically expected to take responsibility for managing young people or people in lower positions, whereas lower-status people have to obey the higher status people (Lee, Fraser, & Fisher, 2003). It is not surprising that this is also reflected in the school system, which is 'hierarchical' and 'monotonous'. That is, teachers hold a higher position and even the same authority as parents, while students, who hold a relatively low position, should obey them (Lee, 2007).

However, this situation recently has faced dramatic change, as students increasingly consider themselves recipients of educational services and the majority of parents have become dissatisfied with the quality of education (Kim, 2003). As a result, the hierarchical relationship between teachers and students and teacher's authority has weakened. Consequently, students have begun to challenge teachers' authority, which has led teachers to experience negative emotions and job burnout (Park & Lee, 2012). In a recent national survey, approximately two-thirds of Korean teachers felt that they were treated by students and their parents in a disrespectful manner, which in turn led to lower job satisfaction and increased turnover intention in the future (Korean Federation of Teachers Association, 2012).

Further, Korean government has recently implemented a new sport policy which led PE teachers to exhibit a higher burnout level than those participants in the past (Ha, King, & Naegar, 2011). The rapid and dramatic changes in their authority and working environment caused them to experience increased unpleasant emotions in their daily work. Thus, a greater need exists for Korean teachers to engage in emotional labour to regulate negative emotions and behaviors in a disciplinary situation than there has been in past decades. Although the changes in teacher-student dynamics can be witnessed almost everywhere in the world, such changes are more dramatic in Korea compared to other cultures because Korean culture traditionally followed Confucian hierarchy in all aspects of life.

1.3 Review of Literature

1.3.1 Grandey and Gabriel's conceptual framework of emotional labour

Grandey and Gabriel (2015) have recently presented a conceptual framework of emotional labour consisting of antecedents, consequences, and moderators. According to the framework, emotional labour is the combination of emotion requirements of the situation, the one's internal regulation process, and outward emotion performance. That is, these three components are working together to constitute the overall emotional labour construct (Lee & Chelladurai, 2015). Specifically, surface acting and deep acting were identified as different types of internal regulation process. The framework also identified individual characteristics (e.g., personality, motivation, and emotional ability) and situational characteristics (e.g., aroused emotions, customer reaction) as antecedents. Employee well-being (job satisfaction and burnout/health) and organisational well-being (interpersonal relationship performance, job performance) were identified as consequences of emotional labour. Finally, several relational factors (e.g., emotional intelligence, identification, and relationship quality) and contextual factors (e.g., job autonomy, financial compensation, and perceived organizational and supervisor support) were included as the moderating factor in the relationship between emotional labour and the proposed consequences.

Emotional requirements of the situations are known as display rules (Hochschild, 1983) which serve as the standards that guide appropriate emotional display. For example, service employees typically follow positive display rules (e.g., kindness and enthusiasm) to please their customers, whereas it is recommended for bill collectors to display negative emotions (e.g., anger) to be effective on their jobs. In the teaching context, it is expected that teachers need to follow two distinctive display rules, which makes the process of emotional labour more difficult. That is, teachers need to determine judiciously which emotions to display at given situations, as sometime they need to display positive emotion (supportive display rules) to encourage students, whereas they should express negative emotion (disciplinary display rules) to discipline students (Barber et al., 2011).

Surface acting involves the process of modifying only outward expressions regardless of their true feelings, whereas deep acting involves the process of modifying "actual feelings" to display appropriate emotions. Thus, individuals who utilize surface acting essentially "fake" the appropriate emotional display, whereas those who utilize deep acting try to genuinely experienced the desired emotions and display them accordingly (Grandey, 2000). Ashforth and Humphrey (1993) introduced genuine expression as the third category of emotional labour, because they considered the previous two categories to be insufficient to represent the breadth of the emotional labour process at work. They argued that employees could feel the desired emotions and display them accordingly in automatic ways. For example, teachers may truly feel and express enthusiasm toward their subject matter, and the expression of such enthusiasm is different from deep acting because it requires no modification process. Regulating emotions, albeit automatically, requires labour in order to be consistent with situational requirements. That is, displaying appropriate emotions in response to organisational requirements in a given situation is considered labour, regardless of whether or not one regulates one's emotions spontaneously (Diefendorff, Croyle, & Gosserand, 2005). Later, Discrete Emotions Emotional Labour Scale (DEELS) was developed by Glomb and Tews (2004), in which genuine expression was divided into the two sub-categories – genuine positive expression and genuine negative expression – in order to understand emotional labour in more comprehensive way.

1.3.2 Emotional Labour and Emotional Exhaustion

Emotional exhaustion, defined as a chronic fatigue state of emotional depletion (Maslach & Jackson, 1986), is considered the "central quality of burnout and the most obvious manifestation of this complex syndrome" (Maslach, Schaufeli, & Leiter, 2001; p. 402). Teaching was found to be highly vulnerable to emotional exhaustion because it involves a high degree of interpersonal dimension (Sutton, 2005). Ample studies have shown that emotionally exhausted teachers experienced decreased job satisfaction and quality of teaching, which in turn negatively influenced students' academic achievement (Blandford, 2000; Ha et al., 2011).

Researchers have frequently found a positive relationship between surface acting and emotional exhaustion among teachers (Barber et al., 2011; Chang, 2009; Taxer & Frenzel, 2015; Tsouloupas et al., 2010). Individuals utilizing surface acting are required to devote significant psychological effort in the process of suppressing their true feelings. This effort, along with the psychological strain of emotional dissonance, depletes one's emotional resources, which in turn lead to emotional exhaustion (Hochschild, 1983). However, compared to surface acting, deep acting does not generate emotional dissonance but instead elicits a feeling of authenticity, because it entails a match between a felt emotion and a displayed emotion (Brotheridge & Grandey, 2002).

Unlike surface acting and deep acting, there is little evidence regarding the effect of genuine positive expression and genuine negative expression on emotional exhaustion. Taxer and Frenzel (2015) found negative association between genuine positive expression and emotional exhaustion. Based on such scarce empirical evidence, further exploration is warranted. We hypothesized that PE teachers' genuine positive expression would be negatively associated with emotional exhaustion because it does not generate emotional dissonance and psychological effort. Finally, regarding the relationship between genuine negative expression and emotional exhaustion, Taxer and Frenzel (2015) found a significant positive association between American teachers' genuine negative expression and emotional exhaustion. A number of scholars in health psychology and medical science have found that frequent expressions of negative emotions (e.g., anger and sadness) had a negative impact on individual health, and were associated with a range of chronic illnesses, from cardiovascular disease to diabetes and asthma (Haukkala, Konttinen, Laatikainen, Kawachi, & Uutela, 2010). Accordingly we posit that

H1: Surface acting will be positively associated with emotional exhaustion.
H2: Deep acting will be negatively associated with emotional exhaustion.
H3: Genuine positive expression will be negatively associated with emotional exhaustion.
H4: Genuine negative expression will be positively associated with emotional exhaustion.

1.3.3 Emotional Labour and Job Satisfaction

Job satisfaction, defined as "a pleasurable or positive mental state resulting from the appraisal of one's job or job experience" (Locke, 1976, p. 1300), is included in this study. Although research on job satisfaction among PE teachers has received limited attention, it has been considered a critical element in teaching due to its association with organizational outcomes including productivity and profit, turnover intention, and actual turnover behavior (see Koustelios & Tsigilis, 2005). Empirical evidence has shown inconsistent results in the relationship between different types of emotional labour and job satisfaction for teachers (Taxer & Frenzel, 2015; Yin, 2015; Zhang & Zhu, 2008). For example, Zhang and Zhu (2008) found that surface acting significantly predicted job satisfaction negatively, whereas other studies found no association between them (Taxer & Frenzel, 2015; Yin, 2015). Further, Zhang and Zhu (2008) and Yin (2015) found a positive association between deep acting and job satisfaction, whereas Taxer and Frenzel (2015) found no association. Based on such scarce empirical evidence, further exploration is warranted.

Further, it has been found that teachers' genuine positive expression, which theoretically requires no psychological effort and generates no emotional dissonance, was positively associated with job satisfaction, as it is an automatic process (e.g., Taxer & Frenzel, 2015; Yin, 2015). On the other hand, previous literature has also found that frequent expressions of anger have a negative impact on individuals' job attitudes, because those inner negative emotions entail unpleasant feelings (Baumeister & Exline, 2000), which in turn result in decreased job satisfaction (Taxer & Frenzel, 2015). Accordingly, we posit that among Korean PE teachers,

H5: Surface acting will be negatively associated with job satisfaction.
H6: Deep acting will be positively associated with job satisfaction.
H7: Genuine positive expression will be positively associated with job satisfaction.
H8: Genuine negative expression will be negatively associated with job satisfaction.

1.3.4 Emotional Exhaustion as a Mediator

Based on the previous evidence regarding the relationship between emotional labour and teacher well-being outcomes, we expected that the association between the four forms of emotional labour and job satisfaction would be mediated by emotional exhaustion. Previous studies have shown that emotional exhaustion is a negative circumstance, and teachers who experience emotional exhaustion are less likely to have job satisfaction (Ha, et al., 2011; Koustelios & Tsigilis, 2005). For example, Ha and his colleagues (2011) found that job burnout negatively affected job satisfaction and with emotional exhaustion contributing the most compared to other components of burnout among Korean PE teachers. Thus, this study attempted to test whether emotional exhaustion mediates the relations between the four forms of emotional labour and job satisfaction. Accordingly, we posit that among Korean PE teachers

H9: Emotional exhaustion will mediate the relationship between surface acting and job satisfaction.

H10: Emotional exhaustion will mediate the relationship between deep acting and job satisfaction.

H11: Emotional exhaustion will mediate the relationship between genuine positive expression and job satisfaction.

H12: Emotional exhaustion will mediate the relationship between genuine negative expression and job satisfaction.

1.4 Purpose of the Study

In summary, this study tested a part of Graney and Gabriel's (2015) conceptual framework by conducting an empirical examination of the relationship among the four forms of emotional labour, emotional exhaustion, and job satisfaction, and the mediating effect of emotional exhaustion among Korean physical education teachers. It is posited that different forms of emotional labor is associated with emotional exhaustion and job satisfaction. More specifically, the purpose of this study was three-fold: (a) to examine the relationship between the four forms of emotional labour and emotional exhaustion; (b) to examine the relationship between the four forms of emotional labour and job satisfaction; and (c) to examine the mediating role of emotional exhaustion in the relationship between the four forms of emotional labour and job satisfaction.

Further, Stuhr and his colleagues (2011) suggested that future PE research need to examine the role of positive emotions and "deep acting (p. 179)" to expand the physical education field. Emotional labour is the recent construct which can shed light on understanding how to intentionally generate and display positive emotions while eliminating the accompanying harmful effect derived by such process. Although the role of positive emotions have been studied in sport science, emotional labor has received relatively little attention in either kinesiology or Asian context. Thus, this study will contribute to kinesiology and emotional labour literature by introducing an unexplored construct of emotional labour and its predictability for Asian cultures.

2. Methods

2.1 Participants

225 full-time PE teachers from 12 different middle schools in Seoul and vicinity were invited to participate in the study. This study chose a convenience sampling method in order to obtain sufficient number of participants for statistical analysis. Among the total participants, 161 (71.9%) teachers were male and 63 (28.1%) teachers were female. According to Ministry of Culture, Sports, and Tourism (2014), the total number of middle school PE teachers in Korea are 8,304 in 2013. They reported that among them, 6,749 (81.2%) were males and 1,555 (18.8%) were. Their mean age was 32.40 (SD = 8.75), ranging from 20 to 62. Job tenure as a PE teacher ranged between 1 and 34 years with a mean value of 12.33 years.

2.2 Procedure

Before the main study, researchers conducted a pilot study with 10 PE teachers to establish the validity and the reliability of the questionnaires. Participants were asked to complete the questionnaires and based on their comments and feedbacks, the survey items were modified to improve the validity of the survey. For the main study, two trained research assistants visiting the schools explained the purpose of the study, conducted the face-to-face survey, and gathered the data. The research obtained the approval from the Human Subjects Institutional Review Board at the university in order to protect human subjects.

2.3 Instrument

2.3.1 Surface acing and deep acting.

The surface acting and deep acting were measured by Brotheridge and Lee's (2003) Emotional Labor Scale (ELS). The four items of surface acting and four items of deep acting were anchored with five-point Likert scale ranged from 1 (never) to 5 (always). The original items were modified so that the items could be applicable to PE teachers and PE teaching context. In employing the scale, participants were asked to respond to the stem "On an average day at schools and PE classes, how often do you do each of the following when both teaching and interacting with students?" Sample items for surface acting are "Pretend to have emotions that I don't really have". Sample items for deep acting are "Really try to feel the emotions I have to show as part of my job". The scale showed an acceptable internal reliability alpha of .76 for surface acting and .90 for deep acting (Brotheridge & Lee, 2002).

2.3.2 Discrete emotion emotional labour scale.

Regarding genuine positive expression and genuine negative expression, a shorter version of Discrete Emotion Emotional Labor Scale (DEELS, Glomb & Tews, 2004) was utilized. Four items of discrete positive emotions (i.e., contentment, enthusiasm, liking, and happiness) and four items of negative emotions (e.g., anger, anxiety, frustration, and sadness) were adapted from DEELS. Although the original subscale includes 5 items of discrete positive emotions (i.e., liking) and 10 items of negative emotions (i.e., disliking, aggravation, fear, irritation, distress, hate), panels of the study consisted of one sport pedagogy professor, one sport management professor, and two experienced PE teachers concluded that some of the items were not applicable to teaching context. Additionally, negative emotions were chosen based on typical unpleasant emotions in teaching listed by Chang (2009). A sample item asked "How often do you genuinely express enthusiasm when you feel that way?" Respondents can choose from 1 (I never genuinely express this) to 5 (I genuinely express this many times a day). The scale showed an acceptable internal reliability alpha of .84 for genuine positive expression and .87 for genuine negative expression (Mahoney et al., 2011).

2.3.3 Emotional exhaustion.

This study utilized the shorter version of emotional exhaustion subscale of the Maslach Burnout Inventory (Maslach & Jackson, 1986). A sample item is "I feel used up at the end of the day". The words "recipient" and "people" were replaced by "students", whereas "work" was replaced by "teaching". In previous study, the scale showed a good internal reliability alpha of .83 with the sample of teachers (Barber et al., 2011).

2.3.4 Job satisfaction.

PE teacher's job satisfaction was measured by the modified version of Job Satisfaction Subscale of Michigan Organisational Assessment Questionnaire (Cammann, Fichman, Jenkins, & Klesh, 1979). A higher mean score indicates higher satisfaction with the job. A sample item is "My job is enjoyable". The reliability of the items was Cronbach alpha of .85 in Ha, King, and Naegar's (2011) study with the sample of Korean secondary PE teachers.

2.4 Data Analyses

The descriptive statistics were calculated for the research variables along with their reliability estimation (i.e., Cronbach's alpha) using SPSS 21.0. To satisfy the basic assumption of structural equation modeling (SEM), normality of the data were checked using skewness and kurtosis. After the normality of the data was examined, both measurement models and structural models were tested using AMOS 21.0. A confirmatory factor analysis (CFA) was conducted on the latent variables in order to check convergent and discriminant validity of the variables. The researchers assessed structural coefficients of the relationship in order to test the proposed structural relationship. Regarding mediation analysis, Iacobucci, Saldanhan and Deng (2007) has argued that structural equation analyses has a great advantage to test mediation hypotheses compared to comparing a series of different models. Thus, the researchers utilized structural equation modeling to test mediation analysis in that both direct and indirect relations were tested simultaneously. Specifically, a bootstrapping procedure (using 1,000 re-samples) were performed to test the whether there were significant mediating effects in the proposed relationship. The researcher used the well-established maximum likelihood estimation such as χ^2/df ratio, CFI, TLI, and NFI to evaluate the fit of the model. Kline (2005) suggested that χ^2/df ratio less than 2.0 was considered good. For NFI, CFI and TLI, values higher than .90 are considered to have an acceptable and values greater than .95 indicate a good fit to the data. In addition, RMSEA and SRMR values less than .06 indicates a close fit and values less than .08 indicates a reasonable fit of a model (Hu & Bentler, 1999).

3. Results

3.1 Descriptive Statistics, Reliability, and Validity

Descriptive statistics including mean scores, standard deviation, skewness, and kurtosis were calculated to detect any outliers and invalid data. A total of 225 responses were utilized for further data analyses. Alpha coefficients, descriptive statistics (means, standard deviations, skewness, and kurtosis) and correlation coefficients for all variables are presented in Table 1.

Table 1. Descriptive Statistics and Correlations among Study Variables

	1	2	3	4	5	6
1. Surface Acting	(.72)					
2. Deep Acting	.14**	(.86)				
3. Genuine Positive Expression	-.11	.19**	(.90)			
4. Genuine Negative Expression	.30**	-.08	.12	(.69)		
5. Emotional Exhaustion	.19**	-.15**	-.09	.28**	(.79)	
6. Job Satisfaction	-.01	.24**	.33**	-.20**	-.44**	(.84)
Mean	3.38	3.73	3.47	1.74	2.29	4.01
Standard deviation	.67	.64	.89	.51	.67	.71
Skewness	-.45	-.90	-.17	1.19	.26	-.48
Kurtosis	.23	1.77	-.76	2.54	-.02	.13

Note. α coefficient on the diagonal. Bivariate correlations among the study variables are significant at * $p < .05$ ** $p < .01$

3.2 Confirmatory Factor Analysis

Then, the convergent and discriminant validity of all constructs were tested using CFA. Results of confirmatory factor analysis showed a good model fit, $\chi^2/df = 160.78/98 = 1.64$, $p < .05$; RMSEA (90% CI) = .053 (.038-.068); SRMR = .043; NFI = .95; TLI = .94; CFI = .95. Regarding individual contributions of items to their assigned factors, the items all defined the latent variables well ranged from .45 to .91, the cut-off point suggested by Stevens (1996). Further, discriminant validity of the constructs were satisfied as the average variance extracted for two constructs exceeded the square of the correlation between the constructs as suggested by Fornell and Larcker (1981).

3.3 Structural Equation Modeling

Finally, all hypotheses (as shown in Figure 1.) were tested using structural equation modeling. Overall, the goodness-of-fit statistics indicated that the structural model showed a good fit, $\chi^2/df = 442.76/243 = 1.82$; RMSEA (90% CI) = .061 (.052-.069); SRMR = .063; NFI = .94; TLI = .94, CFI = .95. Regarding the relationship with emotional exhaustion, the results shown in figure 1 indicate that surface acting ($\beta = .24$; $p<.001$), genuine positive expression, ($\beta = -.16$; $p=.004$) and genuine negative expression ($\beta = .37$; $p<.001$) were directly associated with emotional exhaustion, whereas deep acting ($\beta = -.05$; $p>.05$) were not associated with emotional exhaustion. Thus, H1, H3, and H4 were supported, whereas H2 was not supported. Further, it was found that only genuine positive expression ($\beta = .22$; $p<.001$) had a significant direct relationship with job satisfaction whereas neither surface acting ($\beta = .05$; $p>.05$), deep acting ($\beta = .10$; $p>.05$), nor genuine negative expression ($\beta = -.06$; $p>.05$) were directly associated with job satisfaction. Thus, H7 were supported, whereas H5, H6, and H8 were not supported.

3.4 Mediation Analysis

H9 to H12 suggests that the relationship between the four forms of emotional labour and job satisfaction is mediated by emotional exhaustion. Figure 1 shows that direct path between surface acting and job satisfaction was not significant. However, if both paths from the independent variable to the mediator and from the mediator to the dependent variable are significant, we can confirm the mediation relationship. In this study, both paths were significant, $\beta_{\text{surface acting}\rightarrow\text{emotional exhaustion}}=.24$, $p<.01$, $\beta_{\text{emotional exhaustion}\rightarrow\text{job satisfaction}}=-.60$, $p<.01$. The total standardized indirect effect was -.12, $p<.05$ (Table 2). Additionally, the mediation path from genuine negative expression to job satisfaction was also significant in that $\beta_{\text{genuine negative expression}\rightarrow\text{emotional exhaustion}}=.37$, $p<.01$, $\beta_{\text{emotional exhaustion}\rightarrow\text{job satisfaction}}=-.60$, $p<.01$. The total standardized indirect effect was -.22, $p<.01$ (see Table 2). Thus, we can conclude that the relationship between surface acting and job satisfaction, and genuine negative expression and job satisfaction was fully mediated by emotional exhaustion. Finally, the direct path from genuine positive expression to emotional exhaustion and job satisfaction were both significant in that $\beta_{\text{genuine positive expression}\rightarrow\text{emotional exhaustion}}=-.16$, $p<.01$, $\beta_{\text{genuine positive expression}\rightarrow\text{job satisfaction}}=.22$, $p<.01$, $\beta_{\text{emotional exhaustion}\rightarrow\text{job satisfaction}}=-.60$, $p<.01$. Thus, the relationship between genuine positive expression and job satisfaction was partially mediated by emotional exhaustion. Therefore, H9, H11, and H12 were supported.

Table 2. Mediation analysis

Variable	direct effect β	indirect effect β	BC 95% Confidence Interval
SA	Not significant	-.12**	-.25 to -.01
GPE	.22**	.18**	.05 to .31
GNE	Not significant	-.22**	-.39 to -.10
EE	-.60**	n/a	n/a

Note. β values are standardized coefficients. Dependent variable is job satisfaction. * $p < .05$ ** $p < .01$

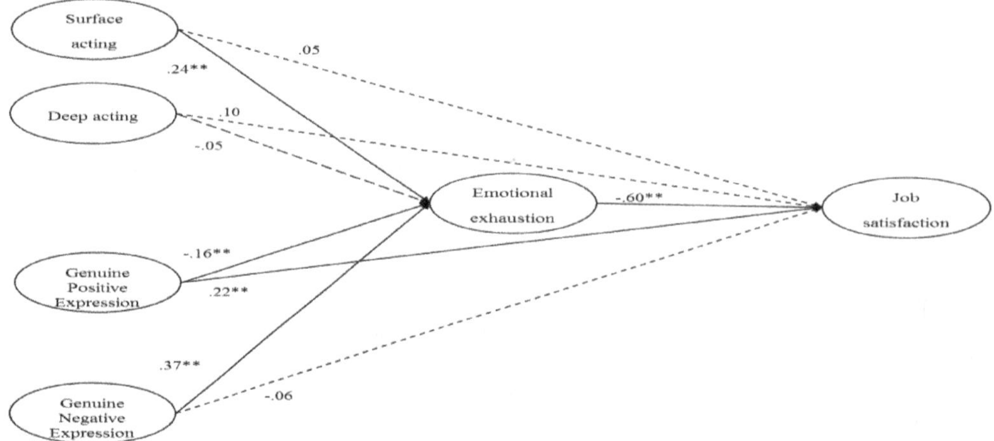

Figure 1. Structural equation model showing the mediating relationship among surface acting, deep acting, genuine positive expression, genuine negative expression, emotional exhaustion, and job satisfaction

Note. Solid lines represent significant relationships; dotted lines represent nonsignificant relationships. * $p < .05$. ** $p < .01$

4. Discussion

This study tested a part of Grandey and Gabriel's (2015) conceptual framework of emotional labour by examining the relationship between the four forms of emotional labour and individual outcomes of job satisfaction and emotional exhaustion, and to test the mediating role of emotional exhaustion in these relationships among Korean PE teachers. The results partially supported the hypotheses of the study, making important theoretical contributions to the literature on emotional labor literature.

Regarding the direct relationship between the four forms of emotional labour and emotional exhaustion, surface acting, genuine positive expression, and genuine negative expression were significantly associated with emotional exhaustion. That is, PE teachers who chose to fake their inner feelings and express either their true positive or negative feelings are either more or less likely to be emotionally exhausted. Unlike deliberate emotional labour strategies (i.e., surface acting and deep acting) which requires psychological efforts, genuine positive expression is an automatic process and does not require efforts and create dissonance (Muraven & Baumeister, 2000). Thus, those who utilize genuine positive expression will be less likely to experience emotional exhaustion whereas those who engage in surface acting will be more likely to experience emotional exhaustion. This is consistent with the findings of Barber et al. (2011), Chang (2009), Taxer & Frenzel (2015), Tsoulouspas et al. (2010), and Yin (2015).

In partial support of our hypothesis regarding the direct relationship between the four forms of emotional labour and job satisfaction, only genuine positive expression was significantly associated with job satisfaction. That is, PE teachers who naturally experience and express positive emotions are more likely to satisfy with their jobs. This is consistent with the findings of Taxer & Frenzel (2015), Yin (2015), and Zhang & Zhu (2008).

Although this study found no direct relationship between surface acting and job satisfaction, we found that the relationship was fully mediated by emotional exhaustion. As hypothesized, the relationship between emotional exhaustion and job satisfaction was significant (Koustelios & Tsigilis, 2005). Further, it was found that surface acting became influential, affecting emotional exhaustion even though it had no direct impact on job satisfaction. Thus, our result demonstrated that although surface acting may not affect job dissatisfaction directly, it would decrease PE teachers' satisfaction toward their jobs by making them emotionally exhausted. Similarly, although genuine negative expression had no direct impact on job satisfaction, PE teachers' job satisfaction would be decreased by making them emotionally exhausted.

The current study makes several practical contributions. Our results suggest that PE teachers who suppress their true emotions or display true negative emotions will be emotionally exhausted and be dissatisfied with their job to a significant degree. As a countermeasure, Korean school administrators may need to implement emotional labour training programs in order for PE teachers to avoid a surface acting strategy and genuine negative expression as emotional labour is a skill that can be taught and developed through practice and repetition (Grandey, Fisk, Matila, & Jansen, & Steiner, 2005). For example, a program can be designed to compel PE teachers to deliberately experience the situation that generates aversive mood in PE context (through video clip or articles). Then those teachers learn how to cope with the aversive emotions in more appropriate way. Through repetition, the regulating process may become more stable and require less effort from time to time.

Without the intervention program, PE teachers also need to develop their own coping strategies in order to manage negative emotions and express genuine positive emotions intentionally. For example, Stuhr and his colleagues (2012) found that PE teachers can elicit positive emotion climate by active listening, showing concern and encouraging students.

Sutton (2005) also provided relevant emotional regulation strategies for teachers. First, PE teachers can keep an emotion teaching diary to identify common patterns in timing and situations where positive and negative emotions are aroused and. Second, PE teachers can ask students about the consequences of emotional expression during the class and help them identify how different kinds of emotions influence students differently. Third, it is necessary for PE teachers to create an environment that helps them trigger positive emotions and calmness. For example, previous research has suggested that situational stimulus in everyday life has a potential to activate and influence emotional status and behaviors (see Aarts & Dijksterhuis, 2003). By extension, PE teachers should post certain cues around them to activate their willingness to express appropriate emotions. The cues may include a personalized "Keep Calm and Carry On poster", a picture of a landscape, or soft music that generates peace of mind.

Finally, Sutton (2005) addressed specific strategies to prevent negative emotions from becoming fully developed and to manage negative emotions during the class. Preventive strategies to defuse potential problem situations include stepping back and telling a joke. When negative emotions already have been elicited, PE teachers can use self-talk and reappraise the situation by reminding themselves that disruptive students are kids, or that they may be stressed out due to excessive parental demands. Several behavioral strategies can also help PE teachers deal with negative emotions, such as moving away from the situation or taking a deep breath and not taking students' comments or behavior personally.

4.1 Limitations and recommendations for future research

Methodologically, this study was cross-sectional study and used self-reported data from convenience sampling. Which might generate the common method bias. Thus, it should be cautious to infer the causality and directions among variables. That is, it is possible that the direction of the relationship is either the opposite or reciprocal. For example, emotional exhaustion may lead PE teachers to perform more surface acting as they depleted most of their psychological resources to engage in a cognitive reappraisal process (i.e., deep acting). Future research may implement an experimental study or a longitudinal study in order to confirm such reciprocal relationships. Additionally, this study used all questionnaires from other domains after the revision process; thus, future studies may need to develop new scales that can represent PE context in more clear way. Further, future studies may utilize a mixed method (Carson, 2009), combining quantitative and qualitative research techniques in order to collect multiple kinds of data, which allows for the "opportunity to compensate for inherent method weaknesses, capitalize on inherent method strengths, and offset inevitable method biases" (Greene, 2007, p. xiii).

Moreover, we focused on only two outcome variables of teacher well-being based on Grandey and Gabriel's (2015) conceptual framework, job satisfaction and emotional exhaustion. Future research should attempt to examine other key variables associated with teaching in terms of antecedents (i.e., affective event, emotional intelligence, affectivity, and personality), teacher well-being (i.e., physical health and organizational commitment), and teaching effectiveness (i.e., the quality of teacher-student relationships, students' perceived organizational climate, students' satisfaction, and students' trust toward teachers). Further, in terms of the effect of emotional labour on individual outcomes, these relationships might be moderated by several variables, including emotional intelligence, perceived social support, job autonomy, financial reward, and the teacher-student relationship quality.

Particularly, emotional intelligence, defined as the individual's ability to perceive, understand, utilize, and manage emotions in the self and others (Mayer & Salovey, 1997) can be a critical construct which has a particular implication to the study of emotional labour (Grandey & Gabriel, 2015; Lee, Chelladurai, & Kim, 2015). According to Opengart (2000), emotional intelligence involves cognitive ability to understand and mange emotions, whereas emotional labour is a behavioral process of expressing emotions outwardly. Thus, high emotional intelligence teachers possibly can perform more effective or highly advanced emotional labour strategies. Future research may need to examine the relationship between emotional intelligence and emotional labour strategies as an antecedent.

5. Conclusion

In summary, this study contributes to the both emotional labour and kinesiology literature by testing Grandey and Gabriels' (2015) conceptual framework and examining both direct and indirect relationship between the four forms of emotional labour and the individual outcomes (i.e., emotional exhaustion and job satisfaction). Thus, our research confirms the part of of Grandey and Gabriel's (2015) conceptual framework of emotional labour and identifies emotional exhaustion as an important mediator. Our study shows that PE teachers' emotional labour has significant implications for their individual outcomes. Thus, Korean school administrators need to consider developing an intervention program to decrease emotional exhaustion and enhance job satisfaction for PE teachers; which in turn influence student's learning experience. Further, Korean PE teachers need to understand the benefit of positive emotions during the class while the process might have double-edge effects on their personal well-being. We hope that this study can help PE teachers create a desirable working environment and identify health-beneficial coping strategies in their workplace.

References

Aarts, H., & Dijksterhuis, A. (2000). Habits as knowledge structures: Automaticity in goal-directed behavior. *Journal of Personality and Social Psychology, 78,* 53–63.

Ashforth, B. E., & Humphrey, R. H. (1993). Emotional labor in service roles: The influence of identity. *Academy of Management Review, 18*(1), 88-115.

Barber, L., Grawitch, M., Carson, R., Tsouloupas, C. (2011). Costs and benefits of supportive vs. disciplinary emotion regulation strategies in teachers. *Stress and Health, 27*(3), 173-187.

Baumeister, R. F., & Exline, J. J. (2000). Self-control, morality, and human strength. *Journal of Social and Clinical Psychology, 19*, 29-42.

Blandford, S. (2000). *Managing Professional Development in Schools. London: Routledge* .

Brotheridge, C., & Grandey, A. (2002). Emotional labor and burnout: Comparing two perspectives of "people work." *Journal of Vocational Behavior, 60,* 17–39.

Brotheridge, C. M., & Lee, R. T. (2002). Testing a conservation of resources model of the dynamics of emotional labor. *Journal of Occupational Health Psychology, 7*(1), 57-67.

Cammann, C., Fichman, M., Jenkins, D., & Klesh, J. (1979). *The Michigan Organizational Assessment Questionnaire.* Unpublished manuscript, University of Michigan, Ann Arbor.

Chang, M. (2009). An appraisal perspective of teacher burnout: Examining the emotional work of teachers. *Educational Psychology Review, 21*, 193-218.

Choi, I., & Richard, N. (2000). Cultural psychology of surprise: Holistic theories and recognition of contradiction. *Journal of Personality and Social Psychology, 79*(6), 890-905.

Diefendorff, J. M., Croyle, M. H., & Gosserand, R. H. (2005). The dimensionality and antecedents of emotional labor strategies. *Journal of Vocational Behavior, 66,* 339-357.

Fornell, C., & Larcker, D. F. (1981). Evaluating structural equation models with unobservable variables and measurement error. *Journal of Marketing Research, 18*, 39-50.

Glomb, T. M., & Tews, M. J. (2004). Emotional labor: A conceptualization and scale development. *Journal of Vocational Behavior, 64*, 1-23.

Grandey, A. A. (2000). Emotion regulation in the workplace: A new way to conceptualize emotional labor. *Journal of Occupational Health Psychology, 5,* 95–110.

Grandey, A., & Gabriel, A. (2015). Emotional labor at a crossroads: Where do we go from here? *Annual Review of Organizational Psychology and Organizational Beh*avior, 2, 323-349.

Grandey, A., Fisk, G., Matilla, A., Jansen, K., & Steiner, D. (2005). Is "service with a smile" enough? Authenticity of positive displays during service encounters. *Organizational Behavior and Human Decision Processes, 96*(1), 38-55.

Greene, J. (2007). *Mixed methods in social inquiry*. New York: Wiley.

Ha, J., King, K. M., & Naeger, D. J. (2011). The impact of burnout on work outcomes among South Korean physical education teachers. *Journal of Sport Behavior, 34*(4), 343-357.

Haukkala, A., Konttinen, H, Laatikainen, T., Kawachi, I., Uutela, A. (2010). Hostility, anger control, and anger expression as predictors of cardiovascular disease. *Psychosomatic Medicine, 72*(6), 556-562.

Hochschild, A. R. (1983). *The Managed Heart: Commercialization of Human Feeling*. Palo Alto, CA: University of California Press.

Hu, L., & Bentler, P. M (1999). Cutoff criteria for fit indexes in covariance structure analysis: Conventional criteria versus new alternatives. *Structural Equation Modeling, 6*, 1-55.

Iacobucci, D., Saldanhan, N., & Deng, X. (2007). A mediation on mediation: Evidence that structural equations models perform better than regression. *Journal of Consumer Psychology, 17*(2), 139-153.

Keller, M., Chang, M., Becker, E., Goetz, T., & Frenzel, A. (2014). Teachers' emotional experiences and exhaustion as predictors of emotional labor in the classroom: an experience sampling study. *Frontier Psychology, 5*, 1-10.

Kim, M. (2003). Teaching and learning in Korean classrooms: The crisis and the new approach. *Asia Pacific Education Review, 4*, 140–150.

Kline, R. (2005). *Principles of Structural Equation Modeling*. New York, NY: Guildford Press.

Korean Federation of Teacher's Association. (2012). *Teacher's day.* http://www.kfta.or.kr/news/view.asp?bName=news&sdiv=1& num=4874.

Koustelios, A., & Tsigilis, N. (2005). The relationship between burnout and job satisfaction among physical education teachers: a multivariate approach. *European Physical Education Review, 11*(2), 189-203.

Lee, S. (2007). The relations between the student-teacher trust relationship and school success in the case of Korean middle schools. *Educational Studies, 33*(2), 209-216.

Lee, Y., Chelladurai, P., & Kim, Y. (2015). Emotional labor in sports coaching: Development of a model. *International Journal of Sports Science and Coaching, 10*(2-3), 561-575.

Lee, S., Fraser, B., & Fisher, D. (2003). Teacher-student interactions in Korean high school science classrooms. *International Journal of Science and Mathematics Education, 1,* 67-85.

Locke. E. A. (1976). The nature and causes of job satisfaction. In M.D. Dunnette (Ed.), *Handbook of Industrial and Organizational Psychology*, Chicago, IL: Rand McNally.

Locke , E. A. Latham , G. P. (1990). *A theory of goal setting and task performance*. Englewood Cliffs, NJ: Prentice Hall.

Mahoney, K. T., Buboltz, W. C., Buckner, J. E., & Doverspike, D. (2011). Emotional labor in American professor. *Journal of Occupational Health Psychology, 16*(4), 406-423.

Maslach, C., & Jackson, S. E. (1986). *Maslach Burnout Inventory Manual* (2nd ed.). Palo Alto, CA: Consulting Psychologists Press.

Maslach, C., Schaufeli, W., & Leiter, M. (2001). Job burnout. *Annual Review of Psychology, 52*, 397-422.

Mayer, J., & Salovey, P. (1997). *Emotional development and emotional intelligence: Implications for educators*. New York, NY: Basic Books.

Ministry of Culture, Sports, and Tourism. (2014). *2013 Sports White Paper*. Seoul: Korean Institute of Sports Science.

Park, Y. M., & Lee, S. M. (2012). A longitudinal analysis of burnout in middle and high School Korean teachers. *Stress and Health, 29*(5), 427–431.

Shin, H., Puig, A., Lee, J., Lee, J., & Lee, S. (2011). Cultural validation of the Maslach Bunout Inventory for Korean students. *Asia Pacific Educational Psychology, 12*, 633-639.

Stevens, J. (1996). *Applied multivariate statistics for the social sciences* (3rd ed.). Mahwah, NJ: Lawrence Erlbaum Associates.

Stuhr, P., Sutherland, S., & Ward, P. (2011). Lived-positive emotionality in elementary physical education. *Pedagogies: An International Journal, 7*(2), 165-181.

Sutton, R. (2005). Teachers' emotions and classroom effectiveness. *The relevance of Educational Psychology to Teacher Education, 78*(5), 229-234.

Taxer, J., & Frenzel, A. (2015). Facets of teachers' emotional lives: A quantitative investigation of teachers' genuine and hidden emotions. *Teaching and Teacher Education, 49*, 78-88.

Tsouloupas, C., Carson, R., Matthews, R., & Barber, L. (2010). Exploring the association between teachers' perceived student misbehavior and emotional exhaustion: the importance of efficacy beliefs and emotion regulation. *Educational Psychology, 30*(2), 173-189.

Tuxford, L., Bradley, G. (2014). Emotional job demands and emotional exhaustion in teachers. *Educational Psychology,* 1-19.

Yin, H. (2015). The effect of teachers' emotional labour on teaching satisfaction: moderation of emotional intelligence. *Teachers and Teaching: theory and practice, 21*(7), 789-810.

Zhang, Q., & Zhu, W. (2008). Exploring emotion in teaching: Emotional labor, burnout, and satisfaction in Chinese higher education. *Communication Education, 57*(1), 105-122.

4

Comparison of Open and Closed Stance Forehand Strokes among Intermediate Tennis Players

Tajul Arifin Muhamad
1Departemant Sport Management, Faculty of Education,
Universiti Kebangsaan Malaysia, Kajang 43600, Malaysia
Email: tajul.a@ukm.edu.my

Fatemeh Golestani (Corresponding author)
1Departemant Sport Management, Faculty of Education,
Universiti Kebangsaan Malaysia, Kajang 43600, Malaysia
2Enghelab Tennis Club, Enghelab Sport Complex, Tehran, Iran
Email: Golestani2015@gmail.com

Mohd Radzani Abd Razak
Departemant Sport Management, Faculty of Education,
Universiti Kebangsaan Malaysia, Kajang 43600, Malaysia
Email: jingga@ukm.edu.my

Abstract

Background: Nowadays tennis is becoming faster and players are able to hit powerful from virtually anywhere on the tennis court. Training programmers and effective planning will help in designing safe, effective, and productive programs designed to help optimize the tennis performance of players. **Objective:** This research examine the effectiveness of open and closed stance forehand strokes in terms of percentage of success, accuracy and also to investigate whether there is a relation between level of accuracy and the choice of forehand strokes used by tennis player. **Method:** Participants were divided into two groups, namely, male and female who learned forehand strokes for one month. The participants were tested by using a two skill test for percentage of success and level of accuracy. **Result:** Founding showed that the closed stance forehand stroke has far better percentage of success and accuracy among the intermediate tennis players, but the difference was not significant. In addition, male players showed more accuracy and success in this research. And also accuracy did not have any influence to choice of forehand stroke among the intermediate tennis players. **Conclusion:** This research could improve the training protocol design for teaching the closed stance and open stance strokes.

Keywords: Forehand stroke, open stance, closed stance, tennis accuracy, percentage of success

1. Introduction

Tennis is a popular sport played throughout the world. It is estimated that about 75 million people play tennis regularly. Tennis is a sport usually played between two players (singles) or between two teams of two players each (doubles)(Ireland, Degens, Maffulli, & Rittweger, 2015). Each player uses a racket that is strung to strike a hollow rubber ball covered with felt over a net and into the opponent's court (Brown & Soulier, 2013). The object of the game is to play the ball in such a way that the opponent is not able to play a good return. Tennis is an Olympic sport and is played at all levels of society at all ages. The sport can be played by anyone who can hold a racket, including people in wheelchairs (Bahamonde & Knudson, 2003; Duane, 1991; Sandamas, 2013).

Forehand strokes is the most important shot in a player's arsenal after the serve, (Matsuzaki, 2004; Roetert & Groppel, 2001). Rotation of both lower body and the upper body has been described as a significant source of power in the forehand stroke. The energy is transferred upward from the legs to the pelvis, through the trunk to the arm and then to the racket. In the kinetic chain of the lower body, the knee joint is regarded as the "critical middle link" in the proximal transfer of force(Whiting & Zernicke, 2008). The rotation of trunk and the pelvis involves torsional forces in the lower body, not only during the forward swing but also during the follow-through in which this rotational energy is being dissipated. Research into the lower limb kinetics of the closed stance (CS) forehand has shown that a leg drive is essential to create high axial hip rotational torques to aid trunk rotation (Iino and Kojima, 2003). In study by Bryant (2011) and Gallwey (2010) stated the recovery time is quicker in the open stance because a player is already facing the net in the ready position after striking the ball, as opposed to the closed stance in which the weight of the body is moving forward from the step in and then must take the extra step back to the ready position. Only sagittal plane knee moments have been described in these prior studies (Fleisig, Nicholls, Elliott, & Escamilla, 2003; Roetert & Groppel, 2001).

1.1 Closed stance forehand

The forehand stroke in tennis has long been qualified and performed as one style. This style is identified by three names: the closed, squared, or sideways stance forehand. The closed stance forehand brings up the situation during and previous to contact with the ball. A stripe sketched from the back foot to the front foot should run equivalent to the planned path of the ball (Elliott, Reid, & Crespo, 2003).

1.2 Open stance forehand

The alternative option to the closed stance forehand is the open stance forehand. This method has become essential because of the absolute power of the game as played today. The situation of the body in the open stance forehand is such that the hips and shoulders are equivalent or "open" to the net (Alizadehkhaiyat & Frostick, 2015). The right foot (for right-hand dominant players) is placed at the back as the player progresses sideways and gets ready for the ball as the shoulders and hips are turned in anticipation of the approaching ball (Gallwey, 2010). The open stance forehand has been explained insufficiently in early literature and has been noted as the incorrect thing to do if described at all. References stated that if the feet are parallel to the net when a player hits the ball, then after that they are in an incorrect position (Roetert & Groppel, 2001). Despite this, there is very little published data concerning three-dimensional tennis biomechanics and almost nothing related to lower limb kinetics of the forehand. This study generally intends to examine and compare the effectiveness of the open and closed stance forehand strokes, and to determine whether there is a relationship between the open and closed stance forehand in terms of percentage of success and accuracy level. This study also specifically aims at measuring and analysing the percentage of success and the level of accuracy using the open and closed stance forehand among tennis players. Some previous research studies in the literature have usually involved investigating the effects of tennis strokes on different parts of the body. Some studies have also examined the analysis of tennis strokes with regard to percentage of success and accuracy level among tennis players. However, there is a lack of studies concerning the relationship between different tennis strokes and stance positions(Roetert & Groppel, 2001).

2. Methodology

The population of the study consisted of all intermediate tennis players ranging from 18 to 25 years old who were learning the sport of tennis in Enghelab Tennis Club located in Tehran, Iran. From the research population, sixty-four players were selected as the sample for this study. The framework for this study is described in Figure 1. The participants consisted of 32 males and 32 females. All the participants were the official members of the Enghelab Tennis Club, Tehran. The participants underwent a training programme for four weeks, three times a week for 90 minutes per session. After the training programme, the participants were divided into two groups, namely an 'open stance forehand group' and a 'closed stance forehand group'. The criterion for this classification was their performance in hitting open and closed stance forehand strokes during the training programme. Each research group consisted of 32 players (Mackie, 2013).

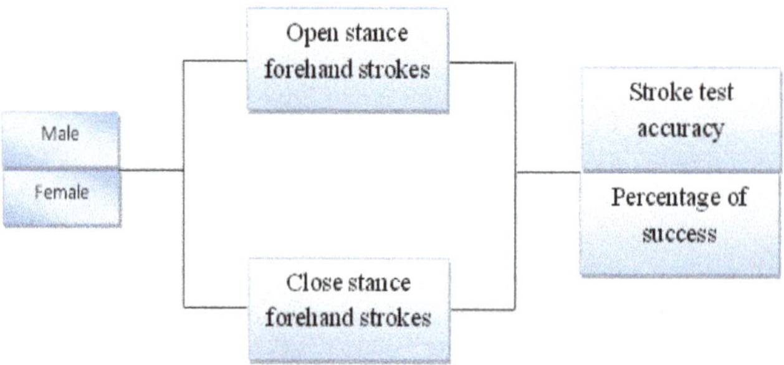

Figure 1. Framework

The tennis players were required to hit AC and DL strokes from the baseline with their preferred technique and to hit balls from the coach (ball feeder). It was important for the coach to master the feeding technique and procedure, so the feeder can provide challenging situations through precise and consistent feeding, and also to provide more repetition of the specific situations for testing the percentage of success and the level of accuracy regarding the open and close stance forehand position. The coach was required to stand exactly at the location required by the situation. The coach could modify this position in order to perform a progression, but progressively move back into the proper position. Basically the coach was feeding the balls at the ground -strike zone. This is the area of the tennis court where nearly all the play takes place in order to win a point. It requires patience, planning, vision and depth. Players need to be patient in this zone. These represent the planning based on the move forward, or for a put-away shot, which should be the player's ultimate goal.

2.1 Testing Procedure

The study investigated differences in the open stance forehand and closed stance forehand strokes when hit and down the line (DL) and across court (AC). Each participant hit (20) open stance or closed stance forehand strokes as if they were playing a real tennis match (powerful and without effect forehand strokes), trying to hit four pre-established targets. The player had been commanded to take just one ball at the same time with the objective of keeping a (5) to (7) second interval between each open stance or closed stance forehand, as it occur in a real matches. Three sessions were designed for each group, namely, open stance, closed stance and stroke and the total score of each player was recorded. According to the difficulty level of task the scoring record of each target was defined, as follows: Three points on the desired target, two points in the intermediate area and 1 point if the third area is hit. Zero points given for not hitting the areas, at the net.

According to Figure 2, each side of the court was split into three parts. Depending on the number of forehand strokes hitting the target (area), participate could score 0 to 3 points. The tennis player had to hit forehand strokes five times for each of the targets. The data was considered as a categorical variable so a test for goodness of fit was performed between an observed sample and theoretical distribution and a contingency test for independence between two or more variables.

Each tennis player from the open stance forehand group and the closed stance forehand had to stand behind the baseline of the tennis court, so they could receive successful shots to their forehand sides. The player hit five forehand strokes at each of the AI, FV, FL, and AV targets. The coach (feeder) who stood on the opposite side of the player side consequently grabbed five balls and could speed up the rhythm and provide a better flow for the test by standing exactly at the location required by the situation. The feeder should preferably use a continental grip to allow any type of feed when creating a specific situation, although the feeder could use the grip necessary to provide the proper shot. The feeder was able to feed from any stroke without looking at the ball, so the feeder could maintain eye contact with the students.

Figure 2. Tennis court

2.2 Data analysis

In order to compare open stance and closed stance strokes among intermediate tennis players using SPSS. The results of the statistical analysis are reported with regard to independent T- tests using SPSS version 21. These included descriptive statistics for age, weight and height of the respondents. The effectiveness of both the open stance and closed stance strokes will be measured in terms of the rate of success and accuracy.

3. Results

According to Table 4-1 in both groups, including open and closed stance, the age of the respondents was between 18 to 25 and the average of age in these two groups was M=21.71 and M=21.34 respectively. The difference between these two groups in terms of age was not statistically different. The average of the height in the open stance group was M=170.97 and in the closed stance group it was 169.19 which was also not significantly different. The minimum respondent age in both groups was same and the average weight in the open group was M=66.97 which was not statistically different from the closed stance group at M=67.72. These results confirmed that both groups were homogenised (Table 1 and Table 2).

Table 1. Descriptive statistics for weight, age and height of tennis players

Learning		N	Minimum	Maximum	Mean	SD
Open stance	Age	32	18	25	21.71	2.565
	Height	32	159	190	170.97	8.926
	Weight	32	44	88	66.97	9.75
Closed stance	Age	32	18	25	21.34	2.404
	Height	32	150	186	169.19	8.682
	Weight	32	44	90	67.72	11.419

Table 2. Difference between open and closed stance for age, weight and height

	t	df	P value	Mean Difference
Age	0.591	64	0.557	0.362
Height	0.822	64	0.414	1.783
Weight	-0.287	64	0.775	-0.748

3.1 Differentiating Between Males and Females

To determine the difference between the males and females in terms of percentage of success and accuracy level in both open and closed stances, an independent t test was applied and the results indicated that there was a significant difference between females and males for success in all tests (Table 3 and Table 4). In the open stance forehand group the average of success for females in the first evaluation was 32.94±6.88 while for males it was 49.31±10.75. In the second evaluation this percentage of success among males increased by 4 %, but the success of females reduced by 1 %. This difference was still significant in the third assessment in which males had a higher percentage of success at 53.0±11.22 compared to females at 36.07±5.30.

For the closed stance forehand group the average of success for females in the first evaluation was 40.104±9.33 while for males it was 53.95±11.25. In the second evaluation this percentage of success among males decreased by 4 % and the female success reduced by 1 %. The difference at this stage was significant. In the last assessment, males had a higher percentage of success at 52.5±10.97 compared to females at 41.14±7.44 (Table 3).

Table 3. Mean comparison between male and female for success in both closed and open stance

		Gender	N	Mean	SD	t	p value
Open stance	success1	Female	16	32.9	6.8	-5.287	<0.05
		Male	16	49.3	10.7		
	success2	Female	16	31.9	9.1	-7.038	<0.05
		Male	16	53.4	8.6		
	success3	Female	16	36.0	5.3	-5.73	<0.05
		Male	16	53.3	11.2		
Closed stance	success1	Female	16	40.10	9.3	-3.79	<0.05
		Male	16	53.9	11.2		
	success2	Female	16	39.6	8.5	-2.988	<0.05
		Male	16	49.4	9.9		
	success3	Female	16	41.1	7.4	-3.425	<0.05
		Male	16	52.5	10.9		

In the open stance forehand group the average accuracy of females in the first appraisal was 11.94±2.13, while males were 14.29±1.961 which was significant at the 0.05 level. The difference between males and females at the next assessment was again significant and males had a higher accuracy than females. This difference was still significant in the third assessment in which males maintained a higher accuracy at 15.12±1.576 compared to females at 12.88±2.315. For the closed stance forehand group the average accuracy of the females in the first evaluation was 12.5±2.633 while for the males it was significantly higher at 15.56±1.548. In the second evaluation, the accuracy among males was higher than the females. The difference at this stage was significant. In the last stage, still the males at 15.75±2.38 showed a higher accuracy than the females at 13.25±2.543 (Table 4).

Table 4. Mean comparison between males and females for accuracy in both open and closed stance forehand

Learning		Gender	N	Mean	SD	t	P value
Open stance	Accuracy1	F	16	11.94	2.135	-3.346	<0.05
		M	16	14.29	1.961		
	Accuracy2	F	16	11.82	3.264	-3.55	<0.05
		M	16	15.12	1.996		
	Accuracy3	F	16	12.88	2.315	-3.29	<0.05
		M	16	15.12	1.576		
Closed stance	Accuracy1	F	16	12.52	2.633	-4.011	<0.05
		M	16	15.56	1.548		
	Accuracy2	F	16	12.63	2.187	-3.468	<0.05
		M	16	14.94	1.526		
	Accuracy3	F	16	13.25	2.543	-2.871	<0.05

F= Female; M= Male; N= Number of players

3.2 Difference Between Open and Closed Stance for Total Success and Accuracy

The total success and total accuracy scores were calculated based on the average of three scores and were applied for comparison between the open and closed stance groups. According to the normal distribution of both variables, an independent sample t test was applied to study the difference between the two groups for total success and total accuracy. The results of the t test revealed that there were no significant differences between open and closed stance forehand for total accuracy and total success as shown in Table 5.

Table 5. Mean comparison between open and closed stance for accuracy

	Learning	N	Mean	SD	t	P value
Total accuracy	Open stance	32	13.5294	2.19445	-1.077	0.286
	Closed stance	32	14.1042	2.13763		
Total success	Open stance	32	42.8431	11.73642	-1.269	0.209
	Closed stance	32	46.25	9.93608		

3.3 Differentiating Between Males and Females

To determine the difference between male and female in terms of percentage of success and accuracy level in both the open and closed stances, an independent t test was applied and the results showed that there was a significant difference between females and males for total success and total accuracy (Table 6). In the open stance, forehand group the average of success for females was 33.66±5.71 while for males it was 52.02±8.50. This difference was significant at the 0.05 level. In the closed stance forehand group a significant difference was also observed for total success among females 40.31±7.10 and males 52.18±8.85. In the closed stance, forehand group the total accuracy for females was 12.21±2.633, which was significantly lower than for males at 14.84±1.30.

Table 6. Mean comparison between gender for total success and accuracy

	Learning	Gender	N	Mean	SD	t	p value
Open stance	Total accuracy	Female	16	12.2157	2.13418	-4.328	<0.05
		Male	16	14.8431	1.30766		
	Total success	Female	16	33.6601	5.71324	-7.394	<0.05
		Male	16	52.0261	8.5005		
Closed stance	Total accuracy	Female	16	12.7917	1.95458	-4.372	<0.05
		Male	16	15.4167	1.39576		
	Total success	Female	16	40.3125	7.10002	-4.185	<0.05
		Male	16	52.1875	8.85519		

4. Discussion

The current research intends to examine and compare the effectiveness of the open and closed stance Tennis forehand strokes, and also determine whether there is a relationship between the open and closed stance forehand in terms of percentage of success and accuracy level. This study also specifically aimed at measuring and analysing the percentage of success and the level of accuracy using the open and closed stance forehand among tennis players. Some previous research studies in the literature have usually involved investigating the effects of tennis strokes on different parts of the body. Some studies have also examined the analysis of tennis strokes with regard to percentage of success and accuracy level among tennis players (Larson & Guggenheimer, 2013; Stare, Žibrat, & Filipčič, 2015; Vaverka & Cernosek, 2013). However, there is a lack of research concerning the relationship between different tennis strokes and stance positions (Erman, Şahan, & Küçükkaya, 2013; Reid, Elliott, & Crespo, 2013)

Muhammad et al in 2011 compares the effectiveness of single and double handed backhand strokes in terms of percentage of success, accuracy, and also to determine whether there is an association between their agility level and the of choice of strokes used. In order to evaluate different 16 tennis players ranging 16- 25 year from National Tennis Centre (NTC) and Bukit Jalil Sports School volunteered to participate in the research. Samples were tested for agility and a two-item skill test for accuracy and percentage of success. They found that double handed backhand have better result and but the difference was not significant and also result shows agility did not have any effectiveness on the choice of backhand strokes (Muhamad, Rashid, Razak, & Salamuddin, 2011).

The first objective of this research was to study the level of accuracy and success of the participants in both the open and closed stance groups in three stages. The methodology of this study included, testing procedure (number of players and group), demographic data (age, weight, height), test of agility (successes and accuracy), and statistical analysis. In this study the participants (ranging from 18 to 25 years old) were 32 males and 32 females. The participants were categorised into two groups, namely 'open stance forehand group' and 'closed stance forehand group'. Then, the mean, the percentage of success, the level of accuracy, and standard deviation of the forehand stroke performance of each player was calculated. The result of three testing steps showed that the closed stance forehand was more accurate than the open stance forehand. This was probably due to the correct forehand techniques used by tennis players in the closed stance forehand group or probably it was an easier method to handle high and fast balls. The level of success was considered between both the closed stance forehand group and the open stance forehand group. Overall, the level of success among the closed stance group was greater than the open stance forehand group. In other words, the closed stance forehand group had a better percentage of success for the intermediate tennis players. The average score for the accuracy and percentage of success for the closed stance forehand group was higher than for the open stance forehand group. This was probably due to the weight and previous experience of the players, which was slightly higher for that group. Therefore, the use of better forehand techniques does not only give more tactical options but also more efficient strokes. The result of this research is similar to previous research conducted by Akram (2011) who considered the one handed backhand and two handed backhand in tennis players (Muhamad et al., 2011).

5. Conclusion

Nowadays tennis is becoming faster and players are able to hit powerful from virtually anywhere on the tennis court. Training programmers and effective planning will help in designing safe, effective, and productive programmes designed to help optimise the tennis performance of players. As a result, players need to train their bodies to meet these increasing demands. Therefore, the researcher feels that future study should examine more strokes and the accuracy level of the tennis players to improve the standard of the game. This information could improve the training protocol design for teaching the closed stance and open stance strokes.

Acknowledgement

The authors are grateful for the assistance and financial support provided by the Universiti Kebangsaan Malaysia.

References

Alizadehkhaiyat, O., & Frostick, S. P. (2015). Electromyographic assessment of forearm muscle function in tennis players with and without Lateral Epicondylitis. *Journal of Electromyography and Kinesiology, 25*(6), 876-886.

Bahamonde, R., & Knudson, D. (2003). Kinetics of the upper extremity in the open and square stance tennis forehand. *Journal of Science and Medicine in Sport, 6*(1), 88-101.

Brown, J., & Soulier, C. (2013). *Tennis: Steps to success*: Human kinetics.

Duane, V. (1991). Factors affecting force loading on the hand in the tennis forehand. *J Sports Med Phys Fitness, 31*, 527-531.

Elliott, B., Reid, M., & Crespo, M. (2003). *ITF biomechanics of advanced tennis*: International Tennis Federation.

Erman, K. A., Şahan, A., & Küçükkaya, A. (2013). The effect of one and two-handed backhand strokes on hand-eye coordination in tennis. *Procedia-Social and Behavioral Sciences, 93*, 1800-1804.

Fleisig, G., Nicholls, R., Elliott, B., & Escamilla, R. (2003). Tennis: Kinematics used by world class tennis players to produce high-velocity serves. *Sports Biomechanics, 2*(1), 51-64.

Gallwey, W. T. (2010). *The inner game of tennis: The classic guide to the mental side of peak performance*. Random House Trade Paperbacks: Random House.

Iino, Y., & Kojima, T. (2003). Role of knee flexion and extension for rotating the trunk in a tennis forehand stroke. *Journal of Human Movement Studies, 45*(2), 133-152.

Ireland, A., Degens, H., Maffulli, N., & Rittweger, J. (2015). Tennis Service Stroke Benefits Humerus Bone: Is Torsion the Cause? *Calcified tissue international*, 1-6.

Larson, E. J., & Guggenheimer, J. D. (2013). The effects of scaling tennis equipment on the forehand groundstroke performance of children. *Journal of sports science & medicine, 12*(2), 323.

Mackie, D. (2013). The Effects of Gender on the Work to Rest Ratio of Elite Level Tennis Players. *Cardiff Metropolitan University, http://hdl.handle.net/10369/5032*.

Matsuzaki, C. (2004). *Tennis fundamentals*: Human Kinetics.

Muhamad, T. A., Rashid, A. A., Razak, M. R. A., & Salamuddin, N. (2011). A comparative study of backhand strokes in tennis among national tennis players in Malaysia. *Procedia-Social and Behavioral Sciences, 15*, 3495-3499.

Reid, M., Elliott, B., & Crespo, M. (2013). Mechanics and learning practices associated with the tennis forehand: a review. *Journal of sports science & medicine, 12*(2), 225.

Roetert, P., & Groppel, J. L. (2001). *World-class tennis technique*: Human Kinetics.

Sandamas, P. (2013). Knee joint loading in the open and square stance tennis forehands. *http://hdl.handle.net/123456789/41756, Master's thesis, University of Jyväskylä*.

Stare, M., Žibrat, U., & Filipčič, A. (2015). STROKE EFFECTIVENESS IN PROFESSIONAL AND JUNIOR TENNIS. *Kinesiologia Slovenica, 21*(2).

Vaverka, F., & Cernosek, M. (2013). Association between body height and serve speed in elite tennis players. *Sports Biomechanics, 12*(1), 30-37.

Whiting, W. C., & Zernicke, R. F. (2008). *Biomechanics of musculoskeletal injury*: Human Kinetics.

5

Movement Characteristics and Heart Rate Profiles Displayed by Female University Ice Hockey Players

Joel Jackson
Faculty of Physical Education and Recreation, University of Alberta, Edmonton T6G 2H9, Canada
E-mail: jkjackso@ualberta.ca

Gary Snydmiller
Augustana Faculty, University of Alberta, Camrose T4V 2R3, Canada
E-mail: gds@ualberta.ca

Alex Game
Faculty of Physical Education and Recreation, University of Alberta, Edmonton T6G 2H9, Canada
E-mail: alex.game@uaberta.ca

Pierre Gervais
Faculty of Physical Education and Recreation, University of Alberta, Edmonton T6G 2H9, Canada
E-mail: pgervais@ualberta.ca

Gordon Bell (Corresponding author)
Faculty of Physical Education and Recreation, University of Alberta, Edmonton T6G 2H9, Canada
E-mail: gordon.bell@ualberta.ca

Abstract

Background: Women's ice hockey is widely popular but the various movement patterns, heart rate responses and work to rest ratios during competitive games has not been adequately investigated. **Objectives:** This study determined the frequency and duration of movements that female players perform in ice hockey games using time-motion analysis. The intensity of the game activities were also assessed by heart rate (HR) responses and work to rest ratios (W:R). **Methods:** Twenty-two university female ice hockey players were filmed performing a number of movements during three regular season league games. **Results:** The following movement patterns were categorized in percent of time performed during the games: forward gliding on ice (36.3 ± 6.2%), forward skating at a moderate intensity (31.2 ± 6.2%), backward glide (9.5 ± 4.1%), standing (7.1 ± 5.9%), struggling (6.3 ± 2.6%), forward skating at maximal intensity (5.3 ± 3.3%), backwards skating at moderate intensity (3.1 ± 3.3%). Defense stood and glided backward more than forwards but skated less at a high or maximal intensity. Positional differences were also observed during different game play situations. The highest HR (□±SD) achieved during shifts was 182 ± 10 and HR averaged 174 ± 9 bpm for the whole duration of the shifts. The shift and game W:R ratios for all players were 1:1.6 and 1: 3.7, respectively. **Conclusions:** The findings of this study indicate that female ice hockey games are played at a low to moderate intensity most of the time (~84% of the time spent) and are interspersed with brief, intermittent high intensity activities that vary according to player position and game play situation. It was also apparent that female players display markedly high HR responses during game-play indicative of a substantial cardiovascular demand in ice hockey.

Keywords: game analysis, work to rest ratios, exercise intensity

1. Introduction

Ice hockey is a popular sport that is played by both genders at a variety of ages and competitive levels (e.g. recreational, representative, professional), including the winter Olympic Games. Hockey is intermittent in nature and requires the players to apply a series of skillful movements on a frozen surface that vary due to the rules, format and strategy of the game (Bloomfield, Polman, O'Donoghue, & McNaughton, 2007b; Bracko, Fellingham, Hall, Fisher, & Cryer, 1998; Cox, Miles, Verde, & Rhodes, 1995). Players in forward and defense positions compete in repeated shifts during three periods lasting twenty minutes each, with stop time and an intermission between the first and second period. The frequency and time spent performing the various movements by players during ice hockey games have been described and documented using video capture devices and time motion analysis techniques (TMA; Green et al., 1976; Seliger et al., 1972; Thoden, & Jette, 1975). As well, heart rate has been recorded during ice hockey games for female (Spiering,

Wilson, Judelson, & Rundell, 2003) and male (Green et al., 1976) players and has been used simultaneously with TMA to further indicate the physiological demands of various activities performed during competition. Furthermore, the physiological demands of this sport also require each player to possess a combination of fitness qualities (e.g. aerobic, anaerobic, strength, power, body composition) to be successful (Geithner, Lee, & Bracko, 2006; Ransdell & Murray, 2011) and various correlates of skating performance have been investigated in male and female ice hockey players (Farlinger, Kruisselbrink, & Fowles, 2007; Gilenstam, Thorsen & Henriksson-Larsen, 2011). However, the majority of TMA research in ice hockey is more than 30 years old (Green et al., 1976; Seliger et al., 1972; Thoden & Jette, 1975). During this time, hockey players have achieved higher levels of physical fitness due to advances in training methodology that has contributed to better performance and likely differences in certain aspects of how the game is played (Montgomery, 2006; Quinney et al., 2008). However, it is important to point out that previous TMA ice hockey research has only investigated male players and there are no published reports for female ice hockey players.

A unique aspect of ice hockey is that due to particular rules of the game, there are periods of time when one or more players of one team may be penalized due to an infraction (i.e. penalty). This results in one team having an additional player or players on the ice providing them with an advantage in trying to score (termed a "power play") while the opposing team has a distinct disadvantage since they have one or more fewer players on the ice ("penalty kill"). This game feature has not been adequately investigated in previous TMA research of ice hockey and is important since these game play situations may change the time spent and types of movements performed. Thus, a novel application of TMA research to ice hockey would be to quantify any differences in movement frequency and time spent during these different gameplay situations. Furthermore, work to rest ratios (W:R) that separate the higher intensity active components to the rest/recovery portions of the game can be calculated from TMA and have been used to further indicate the energetic demands of a sport (Bloomfield, Polman, & O'Donoghue, 2007a; Dobson, & Keogh, 2007). A W:R that approaches 1:1 would indicate that the nature of the activity was of a high intensity whereas a ratio exhibiting more rest or recovery time (e.g. 1:5) would indicate a lower intensity for the activity. Neither TMA of game play situations nor the determination of work to rest ratios has been reported in ice hockey and this knowledge may offer further insight for coaching methodology and conditioning strategies that allow for the design of more sport specific training programs.

Since there have been no published time motion analysis of women's ice hockey that the we know of, the purpose of this study was to investigate the frequency and duration of movement patterns as well as heart rate responses and work to rest ratios during female ice hockey league games and different game play situations. It was hypothesized that there would be significant differences in the frequency and duration of movement patterns during ice hockey games between the first, second and third periods of the game, between the defense and forward positions and the penalty kill and power play game situations. It was also hypothesized that the HR responses and work to rest ratios would differ by position and game play situations.

2. Methods

2.1 Participants

A sample of convenience was used in this study. Twenty-two female hockey players (14 forwards and 8 defense) from the same Canadian Interuniversity Sport (CIS) team volunteered to be in this research study. The participants' mean age, height, and body mass was 22 ± 3 and 22 ± 4 years; 168.7 ± 5.5 and 171.5 ± 6.6 cm; 66.0 ± 5.5 and 72.2 ± 5.6 kg; for forwards and defense, respectively. Note that the defense had a greater body mass than forwards ($P<0.05$), but no other significant differences in demographic data were observed. Prior to all data collection, each participant was required to complete a Physical Activity Readiness Questionnaire (PAR-Q), as well as read and sign an informed consent which was approved by a University Research Ethics Board.

2.2 Experimental Design

This study was descriptive in design and used videotaping and heart rate recordings of players competing in regular season, Canadian Interuniversity Sport (CIS) games that were played against different league rivals. Three games were chosen against different opponents at different times of the regular season (October, November and December). The rationale for this was that these games occurred after the team had competed in six different exhibition games and three regular season games and was done to ensure that the level of competition and how the players performed was representative of a typical CIS ice hockey game. Home games were chosen so that the camera placement and ice arena environment would be identical for all games.

To refine the movement categories chosen for this study, the principal investigator reviewed the available research literature and created a series of movement categories with descriptions for each and distributed this to a panel of 5 individuals with combined expertise in skill analysis, coaching hockey and/or sport science research for review. A subsequent meeting was held during which video clips of CIS games were viewed and a round table discussion occurred to provide feedback and refine the movement categories and their descriptions. As a result of the panel discussion and recommendations made, each description of the different types of movements was finalized. Pilot research was then performed using actual game film and after this preliminary analysis, it was further decided that the TMA would not be separated by whether or not a player was in possession of the puck. This modification was approved by the panel of experts. As well, due to the small number in the goalie position, they were not included in any analysis.

2.3 Exercise Testing and Heart Rate Measurement

Prior to the recording of the first hockey game, each player came to the exercise physiology lab where age was recorded; height was measured in cm using a wall mounted stadiometer (Tanita, Arlington, IL) and weight was measured in kgs using a balance beam scale (HealthoMeter, Bridgeview, IL). A maximum graded exercise test was then conducted to determine peak oxygen consumption (VO2peak) and maximum heart rate (HRmax) on a Monark cycle ergometer (Model 818E, Sweden) using a standardized protocol. Each participant was connected to a calibrated metabolic measurement system (ParvoMedics TrueOne 2400, Utah) with a Rudolph valve mouthpiece and head gear assembly (Hans Rudolph Inc., Kansas) and wore a Polar HR monitor (Polar Canada, Quebec). After a standardized 5 minute warmup at ~70 watts, the graded exercise test began at 110 watts (W) and was increased by 34 W every 2 minutes until ventilatory threshold was observed on the software's graphical display (V-Slope) after which the power output was increased by 34 W every minute until volitional exhaustion. Pedaling rate was maintained at 75 rpm throughout the test. The primary criteria for peak oxygen consumption was a peak and/or plateau in oxygen consumption in combination with a respiratory exchange ratio of > 1.15, achievement of age predicted HR maximum (within 5 b×min-1) or a known HR maximum, and exhaustion (volitional fatigue). This protocol allowed the determination of aerobic fitness as indicted by the peak oxygen consumption as previously reported by our lab (Game, Voaklander, Syrotuik & Bell, 2003).

Eighteen players (11 forwards and 7 defense) agreed to wear Polar® Team Sport HR monitors under their protective equipment during the games and these were pre-set to begin recording 15 minutes prior to each game and store five second HR averages to memory and were downloaded to a computer after each game. The timing of the HR monitors was synchronized with the time displayed on the video cameras. Note that the decision to wear a HR monitor was solely up to each individual player and some players anticipated that they would find wearing the HR monitor distracting during an actual game. The players were allowed to become accustomed to wearing the monitor during practises but 4 players still chose not to wear one. The primary reason cited for this was that these players felt that wearing the HR monitor strap was a distraction and believed that it may interfere with their individual performance.

2.4 Camera Setup and Time Motion Analysis

The video device capture and time motion analysis was based on our previous research of different sports (Forbes, Kennedy and Bell, 2013; Virr, Game, Bell & Syrotuik, 2014). For the present study, two cameras were mounted on opposite sides of the arena, in-line with center ice at an identical height of 20 meters from the ice surface. The positioning and wide angle lens on both digital cameras (GoPro® Hero; 720p, 60fps) allowed for the entire ice surface to be captured. This also allowed for the movement analysis of all players from the same recording vantage point. The video files were stored to SD cards that were later downloaded to a computer.

As a result of the panel discussion and preliminary analysis, the proposed on-ice movement pattern categories are presented in Table 1 below.

Table 1. Movement categories and descriptions

Movement Categories	Description
Standing or very low intensity movements	Stationary or displaying very little motion that would be considered expending a low amount of energy. Most often taking place away from the puck/play. Examples include: a defensive player standing on the offensive blue line, a player standing in front of the net without being engaged with an opposing player, and/or a forward anticipating a play (breakout or regroup) with little movement.
Forward start	Two to three forward strides that are used to accelerate the player from a stationary or near stationary position. The movement is characterized by a strong arm swing and knee drive as well as a pronounced forward lean as the player works to overcome inertia. As the player builds speed (accelerates) the intensity increases exponentially.
Gliding or cruising forward	No or very little skating movement. The exception being easy/low intensity strides used to maintain speed.
Moderate intensity forward skating	Stride frequency is at a moderate rate and speed is above slow, but would not be considered maximal. The player displays purposeful movements to contribute to the offensive rush or to gain defensive positioning. The players arm movements are contributing to their stride, but there is less upper body lean than with a maximal effort.
High or maximal intensity forward skating	The fastest rate of stride frequency which corresponds with; forceful knee drive of the recovery leg; pronounced upper body lean; and deliberate arm movements which add to the strength of the stride. The forward start may also be included in this category if the player continued maximal intensity skating beyond the 2-3 strides of a forward start.
Backward start	Two to three fast backward strides that are used to accelerate the player from a stationary or near stationary position. The movements can be characterized as an effort to overcome inertia. As the player builds speed (accelerates) the intensity increases exponentially.

Gliding or cruising backward	No or very little skating movement. The exception being easy/low intensity strides used to maintain speed.
Moderate intensity backward skating	Stride frequency is at a moderate rate and speed is above slow, but would not be considered maximal. The player displays purposeful movements to maintain position on an opposing player through the neutral zone.
High or maximal intensity backward skating	The player is using fast, powerful pushes or fast, accelerating backwards crossovers in order to match the speed of an attacking opposing player. The backward start may also be included in this category if the player continued maximal intensity skating beyond the 2-3 strides associated with the backward start.
Struggling for position or battling for the puck	The player is using any number of utility movements (lateral crossovers, stops, starts) along with upper body activity to gain/maintain position on an opponent, to protect the puck, or gain possession of the puck. These activities are considered high intensity since there is forceful lower and upper body work. Examples include: corner battles, pins, battles for puck possession, and battles in front of the net.

Dartfish TeamPro 5.0 software (Fribourg, Switzerland) was used to code all ten movement categories within each of the CIS games. Each established movement category was coded to a specific pre-programmed keystroke. A trained observer watched the game while recording each player's movement through selection of the appropriate key assigned to the movement category. The software automatically recorded the number of events and the duration of each event which was then exported to Excel (Microsoft, 2010) for further analysis. The total and mean duration as well as frequency of each activity was measured. The number of shifts, shift time, game work to rest totals, intervals and ratios were determined for each player.

2.5 Work to Rest Ratios

Two separate work to rest ratios were created for the ice hockey players. The first took into account the time spent engaged in demanding and non-demanding movements during a shift and the other used time spent on the ice and on the bench during the periods.

1) Shift work to rest ratio: Ratio of the time spent engaged in high intensity activity to the time spent engaged in low intensity activity. High intensity activities include: forward start, moderate intensity forward skating, high or maximal intensity forward skating, backward start, moderate intensity backward skating, high or maximal intensity backward skating, and struggling for position or battling for the puck. Low intensity activities include: standing or very low intensity activity, gliding or cruising forward, gliding or cruising backward, and stoppages in play where the player remains on the ice.

2) Game work to rest ratio: Ratio of the time spent on the ice during active play to the time spent between stoppages of play on the ice and time on the bench.

2.6 Statistics and video analyses

Mean and standard deviations of time and frequency of each movement category were calculated for all players and averaged across all three games using Microsoft Excel 2010. The data for each player was collapsed across the three CIS hockey games and used in the following analyses.

Separate 2-way analysis of variance (ANOVA) procedures were used to compare the game characteristics, frequency of movement patterns, duration of movement patterns and HR responses between forwards and defense and between the 3 periods, with repeated measures across periods. Separate 2-way ANOVA's procedures were used to compare the frequency of movement patterns, duration of movement patterns and HR responses between both positions, and 3 game-play situations (3). Separate 2-way ANOVA's were used to compare the work to rest ratios between forwards and defense and the 3 game-play situations. Any significant main or interaction effects were further evaluated using a Tukey's HSD multiple comparison test. All statistics were analysed using Statistica 12 (Statsoft, Oklahoma) and significance was set at $P < 0.05$ a priori.

Intra-observer, test-retest reliability was established utilizing the same trained observer that coded all movement patterns during one period from a selected game for ten different players on two different occasions separated by one week. The mean intra-observer intra-class coefficient (ICC) and typical error (TE) were calculated using the spreadsheet created by Hopkins (14) for the frequency and duration of all movement categories was 0.75 and 2.24 and 0.76 and 4.50, respectively. Inter-observer, test-retest reliability was also conducted between two different trained observers coding the same 10 players during the same period and game. The mean inter-observer ICC and TE for frequency and duration of all movement categories was 0.85 and 1.88 and 0.84 and 4.67, respectively.

3. Results

3.1 General characteristic of the ice hockey games

The mean number of shifts per period (6±1 vs. 5±1), mean shift duration (48.0±8.6 vs. 43.4±5.4 s) and total game time on ice (13:59±0:31 vs. 10:16±0:32; min:s) were different between defense and forwards, respectively ($P<0.05$).

3.2 Percentage of game time spent in different movement categories

The mean percentage of time spent in each of the different movement categories for all three periods and games combined is presented in Figure 1. The most time spent during the entire game time was during gliding or cruising and performing moderate intensity skating in the forward direction for all players (P<0.05). As well, the defense stood and glided or skated backward at a moderate intensity more than the forwards, while the forwards glided or skated forward at a moderate and maximal intensity more than the defense did (P<0.05).

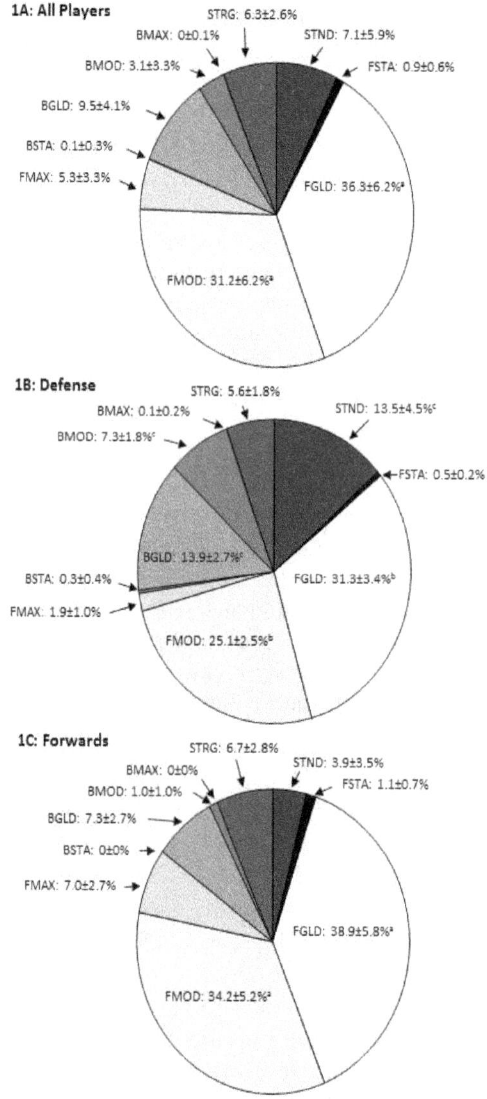

Figure 1. Percentage (%) of time spent in each of the movement categories for all players (A) and positions (B and C) during female ice hockey games

STND=Standing; FSTA=Forward start; FGLD= forward gliding/cruising; FMOD= forward moderate intensity skating; FMAX=forward high/maximal intensity skating; BSTA=backward start; BGLD=backward gliding/cruising; BMOD=backward moderate intensity skating; BMAX=backward high/maximal skating; STRG=struggling. Values are means ± SD.
a = significantly different from all other movement categories; P<0.05.
b = significantly different from all other movements and forwards; P<0.05.
c = significantly different from forwards; P<0.05.

3.3 Movement category frequencies and time

The mean frequency and the duration of time spent in each movement category separated by player position and the 3 periods of game play for all games combined are presented in Table 2. Individuals in the defensive position stood more frequently and for longer periods of time as well as glided and skated backward at a moderate intensity more frequently and longer than forwards in all three periods (P<0.05). Conversely, forwards skated at a high/maximal intensity more frequently and for longer periods of time than defense did (P<0.05). There was also more frequent backward gliding for the defense in the 3rd period compared to the 1st period and this movement was performed for longer periods of time in the 2nd and 3rd period compared to the 1st (P<0.05). It should also be noted that a statistical comparison of the backward start and high intensity backwards skating movement categories could not be performed due to a low number of these movements observed.

Table 2. Mean (±SD) frequency and time spent in each of the movement categories for forwards and defense during female ice hockey games

		Frequency (#)				Duration (s)			
Movement Category	Position	Period 1	Period 2	Period 3	*Game Total*	Period 1	Period 2	Period 3	*Game Total*
STND	D	15 ± 2[a]	13 ± 5[a]	12 ± 4[a]	41 ± 10[a]	48 ± 17[a]	40 ± 21[a]	38 ± 16[a]	125 ± 49[a]
	F	4 ± 2	4 ± 3	3 ± 2	11 ± 6	9 ± 7	8 ± 8	8 ± 7	25 ± 18
FSTA	D	1 ± 1	1 ± 1	1 ± 1	3 ± 1	1 ± 1	2 ± 1	1 ± 1	4 ± 2
	F	1 ± 1	1 ± 1	1 ± 1	4 ± 2	2 ± 2	2 ± 1	2 ± 1	6 ± 3
FGLD	D	34 ± 4	33 ± 7	33 ± 5	100 ± 10	84 ± 13	91 ± 16	89 ± 17	264 ± 33
	F	30 ± 7	28 ± 7	31 ± 8	89 ± 13	85 ± 25	77 ± 21	83 ± 25	245 ± 50
FMOD	D	34 ± 5	32 ± 5	31 ± 4	96 ± 9	71 ± 9	71 ± 20	70 ± 9	213 ± 22
	F	30 ± 6	28 ± 8	30 ± 6	88 ± 13	69 ± 16	68 ± 20	72 ± 14	208 ± 33
FMAX	D	3 ± 1[a]	2 ± 1[a]	3 ± 1[a]	9 ± 3[a]	6 ± 4[a]	4 ± 2[a]	6 ± 3[a]	17 ± 7[a]
	F	7 ± 3	7 ± 2	7 ± 3	21 ± 7	16 ± 6	14 ± 6	14 ± 5	43 ± 15
BSTA	D	0 ± 1	0 ± 0	0 ± 0	1 ± 1	1 ± 1	1 ± 1	1 ± 1	2 ± 2
	F	0 ± 0	0 ± 0	0 ± 0	0 ± 0	0 ± 0	0 ± 0	0 ± 0	0 ± 0
BGLD	D	16 ± 4[a]	19 ± 5[a]	21 ± 4[b]	56 ± 8[a]	31 ± 10[a]	43 ± 12[b]	45± 12[b]	120 ± 24[a]
	F	8 ± 4	7 ± 3	8 ± 2	24 ± 8	14 ± 8	13 ± 6	15 ± 5	43 ± 16
BMOD	D	9 ± 3[a]	9 ± 2[a]	10 ± 2[a]	28 ± 5[a]	19 ± 7[a]	19 ± 4[a]	24 ± 4[a]	61 ± 9[a]
	F	1 ± 1	1 ± 1	1 ± 1	4 ± 3	2 ± 2	2 ± 2	3 ± 2	6 ± 5
BMAX	D	0 ± 0	0 ± 0	0 ± 0	0 ± 0	0 ± 0	0 ± 0	0 ± 1	1 ± 1
	F	0 ± 0	0 ± 0	0 ± 0	0 ± 0	0 ± 0	0 ± 0	0 ± 0	0 ± 0
STRG	D	7 ± 2	7 ± 2	7± 1	21 ± 5	17 ± 7	15 ± 8	13 ± 3	46 ± 15
	F	7 ± 3	7 ± 2	6 ± 3	20 ± 5	15 ± 6	13 ± 6	14 ± 7	42 ± 12

D = defense; F = forwards; STND = Standing; FSTA = Forward start; FGLD = Gliding/cruising forward; FMOD = Moderate intensity forward skating; FMAX = High/maximal intensity forward skating; BGLD = Gliding/cruising backward; BMOD = Moderate intensity backward skating; STRG = Struggling. Game Total = sum of movements for all three periods.
a = significantly different from forwards; P<0.05.
b = significantly different from forwards and from Period 1; P<0.05.

3.4 Game play analysis

The mean (±SD) frequency and duration of the movement categories during game play situations when players were at even strength, or when they were involved in a penalty kill or power play circumstance are found in Table 3. Defense stood more frequently and for longer periods of time during even strength play compared to the forwards in all game play situations (P<0.05). Defense also stood more during the penalty kill compared to forwards during the power play or even strength play and stood less during power plays compared to the penalty kill or even strength situations (P<0.05). All players preformed longer maximum forward starts during the power plays (P<0.05). Further, all players performed forward moderate intensity skating for the longest time during power plays (p>0.05) and significantly less frequently during the penalty kill than both other game play situations and for the least amount of time (p<0.05). Maximum forward skating was performed for longer periods of time for the forwards during the penalty kill compared to the defensemen during even strength and penalty kill situations (P<0.05). Defense glided backward significantly more frequently and longer than forwards during all game play situations and more frequently than forwards during the power play (P<0.05). Defense also skated backwards at a moderate intensity more often and longer than the forwards in all three gameplay situations and longer during even strength play compared to the forwards during the power play (P<0.05). Finally, struggling was greatest during the penalty kill compared to when the team was at even strength or during the power play. Forwards struggled significantly more and for longer times during all gameplay situations compared to the defense during power plays. However, the defense struggled more and longer during the penalty kill than even strength and power play and were different from the forwards during the power play (P<0.05).

Table 3. Mean (±SD) frequency and time spent for forwards and defense during different game-play situations in individual regular season, CIS female ice hockey games

		Frequency (#)			Duration (s)		
MC	Position	Even Strength	Penalty Kill	Power Play	Even Strength	Penalty Kill	Power Play
STND	D	3 ± 0[a]	2 ± 1[b,c]	1 ± 1[e,f]	8.6 ± 2.3[a]	6.6 ± 2.0[b,c]	2.6 ± 2.5[e,f]
	F	1 ± 0	1 ± 1	1 ± 1	2.0 ± 1.2	3.8 ± 3.1	2.0 ± 1.6
FSTA	D	0 ± 0	1 ± 0	2 ± 2	0.3 ± 0.1	0.7 ± 0.4	2.1 ± 2.4[e]
	F	0 ± 0	1 ± 1	1 ± 1	0.6 ± 0.4	1.8 ± 1.7	1.2 ± 1.4[e]
FGLD	D	7 ± 0	8 ± 1	9 ± 4	18.6 ± 1.4	21.7 ± 2.7	23.6 ± 5.0
	F	9 ± 1	10 ± 2	9 ± 1	23.6 ± 3.6	23.5 ± 5.8	23.9 ± 5.3
FMOD	D	7 ± 1[f]	6 ± 0	8 ± 2[f]	15.0 ± 1.0[f]	13.1 ± 2.5	18.1 ± 3.5[e,f]
	F	9 ± 1[f]	7 ± 1	9 ± 1[f]	20.2 ± 2.6[f]	14.7 ± 3.0	21.6 ± 3.9[e,f]
FMAX	D	1 ± 0	1 ± 0	2 ± 2	1.2 ± 0.4[d]	1.3 ± 0.9[d]	3.0 ± 2.7
	F	2 ± 1	2 ± 2	2 ± 2	4.5 ± 1.5	5.6 ± 4.1	3.7 ± 3.1
BSTA	D	0 ± 0	0 ± 0	0 ± 0	0.2 ± 0.2	0.0 ± 0.0	0.0 ± 0.1
	F	0 ± 0	0 ± 0	0 ± 0	0.0 ± 0.0	0.0 ± 0.0	0.0 ± 0.0
BGLD	D	4 ± 1[c]	3 ± 1	3 ± 2	8.4 ± 1.5[a]	7.4 ± 0.7[a]	7.6 ± 5.2[a]
	F	2 ± 1	3 ± 1	2 ± 1	4.2 ± 1.2	5.9 ± 1.8	3.4 ± 1.9
BMOD	D	2 ± 0[a]	1 ± 0[a,e]	1 ± 1[a,e]	4.0 ± 0.6[a,c]	3.2 ± 0.6	3.4 ± 2.2
	F	0 ± 0	0 ± 0	0 ± 0	2.4 ± 0.7	3.2 ± 0.9	2.0 ± 1.1
BMAX	D	0 ± 0	0 ± 0	0 ± 0	0.1 ± 0.1	0.0 ± 0.1	0.0 ± 0.1
	F	0 ± 0	0 ± 0	0 ± 0	0.0 ± 0.0	0.0 ± 0.0	0.0 ± 0.0
STRG	D	2 ± 0	3 ± 0[c,e]	0 ±1[a,f]	3.2 ± 1.0[f]	5.7 ± 1.6[e]	0.7 ± 1.0[a,e,f]
	F	2 ± 0	2 ± 1	2 ± 1	4.3 ± 1.3	3.9 ± 2.2	3.8 ± 2.9[e,f]

MC = Movement category; D = Defense; F = Forwards; STND = Standing; FSTA = Forward start; FGLD = Gliding/cruising forward; FMOD = Moderate intensity forward skating; FMAX = High/maximal intensity forward skating; BGLD = Gliding/cruising backward; BMOD = Moderate intensity backward skating; STRG = Struggling. Game Total = sum of movements for all three periods;
a = significantly different from forwards in all game play situations; $P<0.05$.
b = significantly different from forwards during even strength play; $P<0.05$.
c = significantly different from forwards during power play; $P<0.05$.
d = significantly different from forwards during penalty kill; $P<0.05$.
e = significantly different even strength play; $P<0.05$.
f = significantly different during penalty kill; $P<0.05$.

3.5 Heart rate analysis

All players regardless of position had elevated peak and mean heart rate responses while playing (shifts) compared to the recovery heart rates between the shifts in play when sitting on the bench and the heart rates recorded during the intermissions spent in the dressing room between periods of play (Table 4). The lowest heart rate and the mean heart rate recorded during the first intermission recovery period was different from the second intermission for the forwards but there were no differences observed for the defense. Also, all players displayed significantly lower heart rates during the recovery time between shifts in the first period compared to the second period, but not the third (Figure 2).

Table 4. Mean (±SD) heart rate measures for all players during female ice hockey games

HR Measurement	Defense	Forwards	All Players
Peak Shift HR	184 ± 12[a]	180 ± 7[a]	182 ± 10[a]
Mean Shift HR	176 ± 11[a]	173 ± 7[a]	174 ± 9[a]
Low HR Between Shifts	129 ± 14	132 ± 10	131 ± 12
Mean HR Between Shifts	148 ± 14	148 ± 9	148 ± 11
INT 1 Low HR	103 ± 7	99 ± 8[b]	101 ± 8
INT 1 Mean HR	116 ± 9	112 ± 7[b]	114 ± 8
INT 2 Low HR	101 ± 9	108 ± 10	105 ± 10
INT 2 Mean HR	117 ± 10	123 ± 8	121 ± 9

a = significantly different from all recovery heart rates during shifts and during intermissions.
b = significantly different from peak and mean shift HR and the second intermission HR.

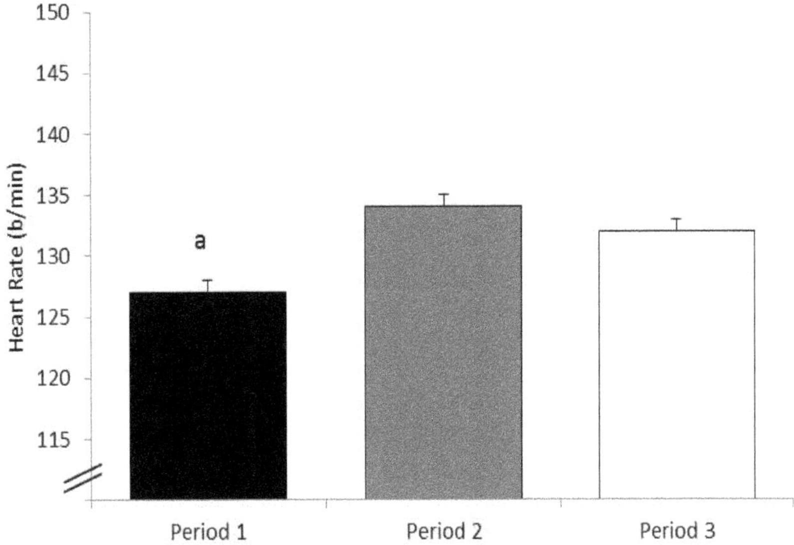

Figure 2. Lowest mean (±SD) recovery heart rate measurements during the three periods for all players during female ice hockey games

a = significantly different from period 2.

3.6 Work to Rest Ratios

Table 5. Mean (±SD) work to rest ratios (W:R) for all players during different game-play situation for female ice hockey games

	Position	Even Strength	Penalty Kill	Power Play
	D	1 to 2.0 ± 0.2	1 to 2.2 ± 0.5	1 to 2.0 ± 0.4
Shift W:R	F	1 to 1.3 ± 0.5	1 to 1.5 ± 0.7	1 to 1.2 ± 0.5
	AP	1 to 1.6 ± 0.5	1 to 1.8 ± 0.7a	1 to 1.5 ± 0.6
	D	1 to 3.1 ± 0.5	1 to 3.7 ± 2.8	1 to 1.3 ± 0.7
Game W:R	F	1 to 4.1 ± 1.1	1 to 6.1 ± 6.5	1 to 2.2 ± 3.1
	AP	1 to 3.7 ± 1.0	1 to 5.1 ± 5.3	1 to 1.8 ± 2.4

D = defense; F = forwards; AP = all players.

a = significantly different from power play, $P<0.05$.

4. Discussion

The popularity of female ice hockey has increased and has experienced a rise in participation of 59% from 2002 to 2013 (Hockey Canada, 2014). However, the sport science research quantifying the movement characteristics and physiological demands has been not been reported in female hockey (Geithner, Lee & Bracko, 2006; Spiering et al., 2003). This type of information can be gleaned from time motion analysis research (Barris & Button, 2008) and has much value in understanding the demands of any sport as well as providing a scientific basis to the design of more effective training programs, sport specific assessments, developing various coaching strategies and document any disparities in the demands of different player positions or game play situations unique to the sport (Dobson & Keogh, 2007; Taylor, 2003). Thus, it was deemed important to investigate the frequency of occurrence and time spent performing different movement patterns using time motion analysis typical of female ice hockey games. A hierarchy of movement patterns was revealed and there were significant differences in frequency and duration of several movement activities between the defense and forward positions. There were also significant differences in the frequency and duration of certain movements during different game-play situations (i.e. even strength vs. power play vs. penalty kill). Heart rate was significantly elevated during game activities and reached near maximum levels in short periods of time during a shift made up of various activities of different intensities. Work to rest ratios supported that the sport of women's ice hockey was intermittent in nature, with the majority of time spent in low to moderate activities interspersed with high intensity, short duration skating that varied depending on the game play situation.

The findings of this study revealed that all players, regardless of position spent the majority of the game time in the forward glide (36.3%) and moderate intensity forward skating (31.2%) movement categories. This was similar to that reported by Bracko et al. (1998) for professional male hockey players that spent 39.0% of their total ice time in a two foot skating glide; 16.2% in a cruise stride; and, 10.0% in a medium intensity stride. This indicated that players devote the majority of their on-ice time engaged in low to moderate intensity movement categories while moving forward regardless of position. As was expected, the present study showed that defense stood and moved backwards more frequently but moved forward less frequently compared to forwards which has also been shown in other research (Lafontaine, Lamontagne & Lockwood, 1998). This can be explained by the contrast in positional demands, where defense are required to skate backwards more frequently (staying between the attacking opposition and their net) and often must remain stationary in certain areas of the ice (e.g. front of the net, blue line) more often than the forwards.

Dillman, Stockholm, and Greer (1984) and Green et al. (1976) found a higher mean skating velocity for forwards compared to defense in male hockey players, but differences in forward sprinting frequency and duration between positions has not been reported for female players. In the present study, the forwards skated at a high and/or maximal intensity more frequently and for longer periods of time than players in the defense position throughout a whole game. This may be partially explained by the fact that the forwards are required to move the puck up the ice for scoring opportunities and may also be related to the aggressive fore-checking nature often required by the forward position in ice hockey games. It was also observed that the defense glided backward more frequently in the 3rd period compared to the 1st and for longer periods of time in the 2nd and 3rd period. This may have been because players in this position adopted a more defensive style of play at this point during the game given that the present team was either tied with the opposition or had more goals at the beginning of the 3rd period. It is difficult to compare these differences in the present study with other research since little TMA research has been conducted in female ice hockey players.

One aspect of ice hockey games that may change how frequent and for how long players spend performing different on-ice activities is during game play situations when a penalty has been assessed and one or more players are removed from the play (penalty kill) resulting in one team having a player advantage (power play) over the other. The strategy and positioning when defending during a penalty and when on the offensive with an extra player is different than when there has been no penalty assessed to either team (even strength) in ice hockey. In a penalty kill situation, a team is trying to keep their opposition in the outside perimeters of the zone created in front of the net to eliminate passing and shooting while the team with the player advantage attempt to move the puck around the defensive perimeter rapidly to create a "good" scoring chance. The present study showed that the defense stood less during the power play when a greater movement of the puck is required and often conceded by the opposing team due to the player advantage. All players skated forward at a moderate intensity less frequently during the penalty kill when establishing position is most important for defending. Defense also stood and skated backward more often and for longer periods of time compared to forwards in all game play situations. Struggling for position or to gain possession of the puck was greatest during the penalty kill game situation for all players likely because this would be a priority for effective defending. However, the defense struggled less than forwards during all gameplay situations but more often during the power play, likely due to attempting to keep the puck in the offensive zone. Lafontaine et al. (1998) reported some differences in skill frequencies between game-play situations in men's ice hockey, but this information was limited. Thus, the movement pattern profile during different game-play situations in ice hockey does vary significantly as dictated by the strategy employed for these situations.

4.1 Heart Rate Reponses

Heart rate monitoring using portable monitors provides continuous feedback of the physiological state of each player that can be attained during actual sport performance (Forbes, Kennedy & Bell, 2013, Spiering et al., 2003; Stanula & Roczniok, 2014; Virr, Game, Bell & Syrotuik, 2014). The heart rate data revealed that there was a high cardiovascular demand placed on the female ice hockey players during games, with average peak and mean shift heart rates measured reaching 96% and 92% of maximum heart rate, respectively. These high heart rate responses are quite remarkable given the short time a player was on the ice during a shift (range of 32 – 54 s) and the intermittent nature of low to high activities performed within the brief time of a single shift. Our data was supported by Spiering and colleagues (2003) whom also reported on-ice mean heart rates of 90% of maximum in female hockey players while Bell et al. (2011) and Green et al. (1976) reported heart rates been 94 to 98% and 87 to 92% of maximum in male hockey players, respectively. There were no significant differences in peak and mean HR during shifts between forwards and defense despite the expectation that forwards would have a greater cardiovascular response due to the anticipated higher intensity activities of playing this position. The present findings were contrary to the difference in peak and mean shift heart rates for defense and forwards in males reported by Bell et al. (2011) and could be due to a difference in shift time and the frequency and duration of activities performed by male and female players. The reason for these high heart rate responses during short, intermittent activities performed by hockey players could be due to several factors including an increase in sympathetic neural activity, elevated catecholamine concentrations, increased chemoreceptor stimulation from circulating ions, increased afferent neural activity from mechano-receptors and/or an increase in aerobic energy demand. Further research would be necessary to determine this.

Few studies have published heart rate measured in between shifts or periods in ice hockey as an indicator of recovery. In the present study, heart rate recovered to between 70 and 80 % of maximum between shifts and between 56 and 64% of maximum in between periods. The recovery heart rates between shifts were significantly lower in the first period compared to the second period but not during the third period for all players. The forwards also displayed significantly higher heart rates during the second intermission compared to the first. Certainly differences in player fatigue and the associated metabolic by-products, thermal stress, possible dehydration during the game and cardiorespiratory fitness level (Linseman, Palmer, Sprenger & Spriet, 2014; Lythe & Kilding, 2011; Matthew & Delextrat, 2009; McInnes, Carlson, Jones & McKenna, 1995) may have influenced recovery heart rate to a greater extent during the second intermission for the forwards. However, despite similar elevated heart rate during activities throughout shifts, the defense showed similar decreases in recovery heart rate during both intermissions. Another factor that could influence recovery heart rate is competition stress. Fernandez-Fernandez et al. (2014) reported that elite female tennis players displayed significantly higher mean HR during matches that they were losing compared to those that they were winning. In this study, the team was not losing during the third period in two games and was tied in the other game where the opposition scoring the winning goal with three minutes left in regulation time. Finally, game play situations were also shown to influence recovery heart rate with higher heart rates observed during the power play compared to even strength play. The reason for this may be that there were less stationary and low intensity activities observed during power plays compared to even strength play. However, no previous research has reported heart rate responses during different game-play situations in female ice hockey.

4.2 Work to Rest Ratios

Work to rest ratios have been reported in TMA studies on team sports especially those that have repeated or intermittent activities and are used to further indicate the demands of a competition or certain parts of the competition by specifying how much time is spent performing activities of moderate-high intensity (work) compared to how much time is spent in low intensity activities and in recovery and depending on the ratio, it may reflect the energy demands of playing a sport (Bloomfield et al., 2007a; Dobson & Keogh, 2007; O'Donoghue, 2008; Rudkin & O'Donoghue, 2008). The shift work (high intensity) to rest (low intensity) ratio refers to on-ice activities; where a work to rest ratio that approaches 1:1 indicates frequent bursts of high intensity activity separated by short rest periods, and a lower work to rest ratio (e.g. 1:5) indicates that bursts of high intensity movement are separated by longer rest periods. The game work to rest ratio refers to the time spent on-ice versus and the time spent sitting on the bench. A work to rest ratio approaching 1:1 would be an indication of a short amount of bench time between shifts, whereas a lower ratio (e.g 1:5) indicates an extended time on the bench between shifts.

The average shift and game work to rest ratio in all players during even strength play was 1:1.6 and 1:3.7, respectively. Bloomfield et al. (2007a) observed a work to rest ratio of 1:1.6 that distinguished purposeful movements from non-purposeful movements in elite male soccer players. Although this ratio was the same as the shift ratio in the present study it is important to point out that the purposeful movements reported by Bloomfield et al. (2007a) included various low intensity activities. In this study, the high intensity movements for the shift work to rest ratio also included moderate intensity backward and forward skating that could also be considered purposeful, however many instances of these movements throughout the games were somewhat low in intensity. The division of purposeful and non-purposeful movements may lead to an overestimation of the contribution of high intensity movements in ice hockey and other sports (Bloomfield et al., 2007a). It is also difficult to directly compare work to rest ratios in other sports such as soccer where players remain in play for the majority of the game versus a sport like ice hockey where players consistently substitute off and have time to recover.

The results of this study also revealed that the shift work to rest ratio for penalty kills was lower than during power plays, but not even strength play. It was expected that both penalty kills and power plays would have lower shift W:R's compared to even strength play indicating a lower intensity compared to even strength play. This contradictory finding may have been due to a more passive style of penalty kill adopted by the team in the current study, characterized by an increase in stationary/low intensity activity with more focus on position in the defensive zone. It may also be because the current team struggled to gain possession of the offensive zone during power plays which resulted in continually trying to regroup and break the puck out of their own zone; a scenario that would be characterized by a significant amount of high intensity forward skating.

4.3 Limitations

The results of this study are based on a convenient sample of female ice hockey players belonging to the same team that competed during a regular CIS season. Three different games against different opponents at various times of the season were analysed in the present study. The scores for all games were within two goals, with two wins and one loss by the present team and the number of shots for and against was 22±4 and 23±2, respectively. These findings indicate that the observed games were similar in play and competitive in nature. Not all players agreed to wear the heart rate monitors during game play as they personally felt it was a distraction even though there was no heart rate feedback provided to participants during the game and the monitor chest straps were not restricting in anyway. The time-motion analysis methods used in this study required an observer to subjectively categorize the movement patterns of female hockey players and although this method has been widely published, the validity and reliability has been criticised (Barris & Button, 2008; Dobson & Keogh, 2007). It is also important to note that some of the backward movement categories chosen (e.g. backward start and backward high intensity skating) were performed too infrequently by any player to be analysed. The analysis in the present study did not distinguish between movement times or frequency when the players were in control of the puck or were not and this may have influenced the performance of some of the movement activities. As well, no attempt in the current analysis was made to determine whether any differences in movement patterns were related to scoring chances, defensive success or game changing outcomes. Finally, differences in coaching strategy applied between games, periods or during game play situations were out of the control of this study but were deemed to be similar according to personal communication with the head coach.

4.4 Practical Applications

The findings from this time motion, heart rate and work to rest ratio analysis of ice hockey contributes to a better understanding of how women's ice hockey is played and the physiological responses of the players during actual league games. As well, the implementation of shift times, recovery times, heart rate responses and the knowledge of work to rest ratios for shifts and the game can contribute to the development of more effective in-season and off-season conditioning programs. Furthermore, knowing the types, frequency and duration of the various movement categories may also aid in the selection of valid and reliable fitness assessments to evaluate players and monitor training; provide support in player selection; evaluate readiness to play after an injury or individualizing conditioning assignments; and, assist with designing game simulation workouts for players that are not selected to play in a league games and can experience a game-like exercise stimulus. Despite the seemingly high intensity, short duration activities and intermittent nature of ice hockey performed, the majority of the time spent and the elevated cardiovascular demand during the game would suggest that cardio-respiratory fitness is important. Recent research has shown a significant relationship between aerobic fitness and repeated shift performance in male ice hockey players (Peterson et al., 2015) that supports the current findings in female ice hockey players despite an earlier study that was unable to find a relationship between aerobic fitness and recovery from intense intermittent skating in female ice hockey players (Carey, Drake, Pliego & Raymond, 2007). Our findings would suggest that female players require a variety of well-developed fitness qualities to perform and compete in ice hockey.

5. Conclusions

In summary, the novel aspect of this study was that it is the first to present the different types and time spent performing various movement patterns during competitive women's ice hockey games. The majority of female ice hockey games involved gliding on the ice and skating in the forward direction at a moderate intensity for all players. Movement activities directly related to the forward and defense positions differed as expected with the forwards performing more moderate intensity gliding and skating in the forward direction and the defense showing more backward gliding and skating during even strength play. Movement activities also varied depending on game play situations and by position. Heart rate reached near maximum levels during relatively short periods of intermittent on ice activity and recovered in between periods. Finally, shift and game work to rest ratios indicate that hockey is a high intensity, intermittent sport and these ratios varied by game play situation. This was the first study to determine the frequency and time spent performing activities specific to the game of ice hockey in female players and how these activities vary by position and game play situations unique to ice hockey.

Acknowledgements

The authors would like to thank Jessie Gill, Ben Davis, Ciaran O'Flynn, the University Hockey Team, Coaching and Training staff. This research was supported by a grant from the Sport Science Association of Alberta.

References

Barris, S. & Button, C. (2008). A review of vision-based motion analysis in sport. Sports Medicine, 38(12), 1025-1043.

Bell, G., Game, A., Bouchard, J., Reid, C., Gervais, P., & Snydmiller, G. (2011). Near maximal heart rate responses during a varsity ice hockey game. Applied Physiology, Nutrition and Metabolism, 36(Suppl.), S2.

Bloomfield, J., Polman, R., & O'Donoghue, P. (2007a). Physical demands of different positions in FA premier league soccer. Journal of Sport Science and Medicine, 6(1), 63-70.

Bloomfield, J., Polman, R., O'Donoghue, P., & McNaughton, L. (2007b). Effective speed and agility conditioning methodology for random intermittent dynamic type sports. Journal of Strength and Conditioning Research, 2(4), 1093-1100.

Bracko, M. R., Fellingham, G. W., Hall, L. T., Fisher, A. G., & Cryer, W. (1998). Performance skating characteristics of professional ice hockey forwards. Sports Medicine, Training and Rehabilitation, 8(3), 251-263.

Carey, D. G., Drake, M. M., Pliego, G. J., & Raymond, R. L. (2007). Do hockey players need aerobic fitness? Relation between VO2max and fatigue during high-intensity intermittent skating. Journal of Strength and Conditioning Research, 21(3), 963-966.

Cox, M. H., Miles, D. S., Verde, T. J., & Rhodes, E. C. (1995). Applied physiology of ice hockey. Sports Medicine, 19(3), 184-201.

Dillman, C. J., Stockholm, A. J., & Greer, N. (1984). Movement of ice hockey players. International Symposium on Biomechanics in Sports, 2, 189-194.

Dobson, B. P. & Keogh, J. W. L. (2007). Methodological issues for the application of time-motion analysis research. Strength and Conditioning Journal, 29(2), 48-55.

Falinger, C. M., Kruisselbrink, L.D., & Fowles, J. R. (2007). Relationships to skating performance in competitive hockey players. Strength and Conditioning Journal, 21(3), 915-922.

Fernandez-Fernandez, J., Boullosa, D.A., Sanz-Rivas, D., Abreu, L., Filaire, E., & Mendez-Villanueva, A. (2014). Psychophysiological stress response during training and competition young female competitive tennis players. International Journal of Sports Medicine, 36(1), 22-28.

Forbes, S. C., Kennedy, M. D., & Bell, G. J. (2013). Time-motion analysis, heart rate, and physiological characteristics of international canoe polo athletes. Journal of Strength and Conditioning Research, 27(10), 2816-2822.

Game, A., Voaklander, D., Syrotuik, D., & Bell, G. (2003). Incidence of exercise-induced bronchospasm and exercise induced hypoxaemia in female varsity hockey players. Research in Sports Medicine, 11: 11-21.

Geithner, C. A., Lee, A. M., & Bracko, M. R. (2006). Physical and performance differences among forwards, defensemen, and goalies in elite women's ice hockey. Journal of Strength and Conditioning Research, 20(3), 500-505.

Gilenstam, K. M., Thorsen, K., & Henriksson-Larsen. (2011). Physiological correlates of skating performance in women's and men's ice hockey. Journal of Strength and Conditioning Research, 25(8), 2133-2142.

Green, H., Bishop, P., Houston, M., McKillop, R., Norman, R., and Stothart, P. Time-motion and physiological assessments of ice hockey performance. Journal of Applied Physiology, 40(2), 159-163.

Hockey Canada. (2014). [Online] Available: http://www.hockeycanada.ca/en-ca/Hockey-Programs/Female/Statistics-History.aspx (January 22, 2014).

Hopkins, W. G. (2014). [Online] Available: http://www.sportsci.org/ (June 30, 2014).

Lafontaine, D., Lamontagne, M., & Lockwood, K. (1998). Time-motion analysis of ice-hockey skills during games. International Symposium on Biomechanics in Sport, 16, 481-484.

Linseman, M. E, Palmer, M. S, Sprenger, H. M, & Spriet, L. L. (2014). Maintaining hydration with a carbohydrate-electrolyte solution improves performance, thermoregulation, and fatigue during an ice hockey scrimmage. Applied Physiology, Nutrition and Metabolism, 39(11), 1214-1221.

Lythe, J. & Kilding, A. E. (2011). Physical demands and physiological responses during elite field hockey. International Journal of Sports Medicine, 32(7), 523-528.

Matthew, D., & Delextrat, A. (2009). Heart rate, blood lactate concentration, and time-motion analysis of female basketball players during competition. Journal of Sports Sciences, 27(8), 813-821.

McInnes, S. E., Carlson, J. S., Jones, C. J., & McKenna, M. J. (1995). The physiological load imposed on basketball players during competition. Journal of Sports Sciences, 13(5), 387-397.

Montgomery, D. L. (2006). Physiological profile of professional hockey players – a longitudinal comparison. Applied Physiology, Nutrition and Metabolism, 31(3), 181-185.

O'Donoghue, P. G. (2008). Time-motion analysis. In M. Hughes & I. M. Franks (Eds.), The Essentials of Performance Analysis: An Introduction (pp. 180-205). New York: Routledge.

Peterson, B. J., Fitzgerald, J. S. Dietz, C. C., Ziegler, K. S., Ingraham, S. J., Baker, S. E., & Snyder, E. M. (2015). Aerobic capacity is associated with improved repeated shift performance in hockey. Journal of Strength and Conditioning Research, 29(6), 1465-1472.

Quinney, H. A., Dewart, R., Game, A., Snydmiller, G., Warburton, D., & Bell, G. (2008). A 26 year physiological description of a National Hockey League team. Applied Physiology, Nutrition and Metabolism, 33(4), 753-760.

Ransdell, L. B. & Murray, T. (2011). A physical profile of elite female ice hockey players from the USA. Journal of Strength and Conditioning Research, 25(9), 2358-2363.

Rudkin, S. T. & O'Donoghue, P. G. (2008). Time-motion analysis of first-class cricket fielding. Journal of Science and Medicine in Sport, 11(6), 604-607.

Seliger, V., Kostka, V., Grusova, D., Kovac, J., Machovcova, J., Pauer, M., & Urbankova, R. (1972). Energy expenditure and physical fitness of ice-hockey players. European Journal of Applied Physiology, 30(4), 283-291.

Spiering, B. A., Wilson, M. H., Judelson, D. A., & Rundell, K. W. (2003). Evaluation of cardiovascular demands of game play and practice in Women's Ice Hockey. Journal of Strength and Conditioning Research, 17(2), 329-333.

Stanula, A. & Roczniok, R. (2014). Game intensity analysis of elite adolescent ice hockey players. Journal of Human Kinetics, 44, 211-221.

Taylor, J. (2003). Basketball: Applying time motion data to conditioning. Strength and Conditioning Journal, 25(2), 57-64.

Thoden, J. S. & Jette, M. (1975). Aerobic and anaerobic activity patterns in junior and professional hockey. Movement (Special Hockey), 2, 145-153.

Virr, J. L., Game, A., Bell, G. J. & Syrotuik, D. (2014). Physiological Demands of women's rugby union time motion analysis and hear rate response. Journal of Sport Sciences, 32(3), 239-247.

6

The Effects of Balance Training on Stability and Proprioception Scores of the Ankle in College Students

Andrew L. Shim (Corresponding author)
Department of Kinesiology & Human Performance, Briar Cliff University
3303 Rebecca Street, Sioux City, IA. USA
E-mail: andrew.shim@briarcliff.edu

Kristin Steffen
Department of Physical Therapy, University of South Dakota
414 Cherry Street, Vermillion, SD. USA
E-mail: kristin.steffen@usd.edu

Patrick Hauer
Department of Physical Therapy, Briar Cliff University
3303 Rebecca Street, Sioux City, IA. USA
E-mail: patrick.hauer@briarcliff.edu

Patrick Cross
Department of Physical Therapy, Briar Cliff University
3303 Rebecca Street, Sioux City, IA. USA
E-mail: patrick.cross@briarcliff.edu

Guido Van Ryssegem
Department of Recreational Sports, Oregon State University
211 Dixon Recreation Center, Corvallis, OR. USA
E-mail: guido.vanryssegem@oregonstate.edu

Abstract

Objective: The purpose of this study was to determine if stability and proprioception scores improved on college-aged students using a slack line device. **Methods:** One group of 20 participants aged 18-23 from a Midwestern university performed a pre-test/post-test on a computerized posturography plate to determine Center of Pressure (CoP) and Limit of Stability (LoS) scores. Participants performed three 20-30 minute sessions per week of balance and proprioceptive training using a Balance Bow for a period of four weeks. Data were analyzed (SPSS 21.0) using a dependent t-test to determine if any changes occurred between pre- and post-test scores after four weeks. **Results:** The analyses found no significance difference in Center of Pressure (CoP), normal stability eyes open (NSEO), normal stability eyes closed (NSEC), perturbed stability eyes open (PSEO), perturbed stability eyes closed (PSEC), or LoS forward (F), backward (B), or right (R) scores in college-aged participants. A significant difference was found in LoS left (L) and a notable trend towards significance was found in LoS R results. **Conclusion:** With the exception of LoS L stability scores, it was concluded that 12 sessions of 20-30 minutes, utilizing a slack line device, over a four week training period did not significantly improve stability and proprioceptive scores of the ankle in college-aged participants.

Keywords: Proprioception, Limit of Stability (LoS), Center of Pressure (CoP), slack line device

1. Introduction

Injuries are common in many sports, activities, and in daily living. They occur in varying degrees and in all areas of the body. Ankle injuries account for 27,000 injuries every day in the United States, making it the most common reported sports injury (Lynch & Renstrom, 1999). Most of these injuries happen in individuals under the age of 35 (Lynch & Renstrom, 1999) probably due to the intensity of the activity as well as levels of competition. Fried (2010) reported that 30% of individuals who sprain their ankle develop chronic ankle instability. Amrinder et al. (2012) identified other components that cause ankle instability, such as mechanical instability, ankle strength deficits, ligament deafferentation, and proprioceptive deficits.

Westcott, Lowes, and Richardson (1997) define postural stability as, "the ability to maintain or control the center of mass (COM) in relation to the base of support (BOS) to prevent falls and complete desired movements". Balance is the process with which we maintain postural stability. Defined further, it is the ability to control postural stability (Alexandra et al., 2000). They are important factors contributing to the proper functioning of the ankle. A person's sense of balance is utilized in daily activities of daily living, but it becomes more important when engaging in activities that are more demanding than one's daily routine, such as playing weekend sports. Poor balance has been shown to increase the risk of ankle injury (Hrysomallis, 2007). Certain types of balance training has been shown to have a positive effect and decrease the risk of ankle injuries (Hrysomallis, 2007).

Postural stability and balance are vital components to the proper functioning of the ankle. However as previously identified by Amrinder et al. (2012), another physiological component that is constantly contributing to one's postural stability and balance is proprioception. Goldscheider was one of the first to systematically quantify the awareness of body segment positions and orientations, later defined as 'proprioceptions' and further explained this definition as a perception not necessarily perceived consciously but contributes to conscious sensations such as muscle sense, total posture, and joint stability (Amrinder et al., 2012). One primary reason for ankle instability, or lack thereof, lies in the functioning of the ankle's proprioceptors and communication with the brain. The central nervous system's (CNS) role is to deliver signals through the afferent neural pathways to produce awareness of limb, trunk, and head position and movement, which contributes to reflexive and cognitive motor skills (Shim et al., 2009). Past injuries due to developmental delays can result in slower synapses through the CNS. Scar tissue due to reoccurring injuries at particular joint sites such as the ankle with or without exostosis formation, and peroneal tendon tears have been shown to delay responses of the central nervous system (Amrinder et al., 2012).

Proprioceptive receptors of the ankle joint complex communicate with the brain, in order to confirm the position and motion of the ankle, and relay the correct motor response to the muscles to correct the perturbed foot in attempt to prevent injury. The application of an external force often occurs at a fast rate, so when this protective neurologic response is slow, an ankle injury may occur (Fried, 2010; Kandel, 2013). If neural adaptations do not occur to improve this response, the risk of re-injury is present (Houglum, 2001).

Effective methods have been found to improve the body's balance and proprioceptive abilities, and, therefore, helping to prevent or reduce the risk of injury (Amrinder et al., 2012; Emery, Cassidy, Klassen, Rosychuk, & Rowe, 2005; Hubscher et al., 2010; Hupperets, Verhagen, & van Mechelen, 2009; Lynch & Renstrom, 1999; Martinez-Amat et al., 2012; Shim et al., 2013). These studies have focused on the effects of various types of balance training, including proprioceptive training, to increase stability and reduce injury risk.

The slack line, a device with a piece of webbing strung between two points of attachment, is one such device. However, there is minimal research indicating its effectiveness in improving balance and proprioception. As slack line devices are becoming more popular for use in gym, fitness, and clinical settings, more research on the effectiveness of these devices is warranted. Therefore, the purpose of this study was to examine the effect of a four week program, utilizing the Balance Bow, on balance in a healthy, college-aged population. It was hypothesized that a four week program would have a positive effect on the balance scores of the participants. A one group pre-test, post-test design was selected to see if the slackline device was an effective tool towards improving proprioception scores on healthy college aged participants. This experimental one group pre-test, post-test design eliminated the use of a control group based on several studies conducted in the past using the Balance Bow (Shim et al., 2009; Shim & Crider, 2011) and demonstrating non-significance from a college aged subject group.

2. Methods

2.1 Subjects

20 participants aged 18-23 years from a Midwestern university were recruited for this study. The population included three males and 17 females (n=20). Five of these participants were Division One athletes compared to the rest of the sample size who were recreational participants. After approval for the study was granted by the Institutional Review Board (IRB), participants were recruited for the study. All participants were asked to sign an informed consent, a health status, and physical activity questionnaire to ensure the safety of the subjects, as well as give a subjective opinion about each participant's ankle stability. Participants were excluded from the study if a person did not attend the slack line training sessions, the pre- or post-test assessments, or 10 of the 12 intervention sessions over a four week period.

2.2 Instruments

A Bertec computerized posturography plate (Columbus, OH) was used to measure physical weight, Center of Pressure (CoP), and Limit of Stability (LoS) scores. The Bertec perturbed surface cover represented an unstable surface. The Balance Bow is a commercial slack line device manufactured by Ironwear Fitness Inc. (Pittsburgh, PA) that was designed to assist with improving balance. Exercises were performed on the Balance Bow with the participant's eyes open and closed in order to promote proprioceptive training. A stopwatch was used to record balance times for each subject.

2.3 Procedure

Each subject performed a pre-test to determine a baseline score on the Bertec balance plate for CoP NSEO, NSEC, PSEO, PSEC, and LoS R, L, F, B. Participants stood on the balance plate with both legs at the appropriate foot markings with arms relaxed and at their sides and were assessed on their normal stability CoP with their eyes open, according to the manufacturer's protocol. The next measurements consisted of the eyes closed, in order to provide information about the individual's proprioception. Participants were also assessed on CoP and LoS scores using a perturbed surface. Each participant was given the same exact instructions during the pre-testing procedure, prior to having data collected. Following the pre-test, each participant took part in a balance training program using the Balance Bow. A four week intervention program was designed to work on balance and proprioception skills, and focused primarily on the ankle joint and lower extremities. During the training session, participants were shown how to properly do each exercise, practiced them before being on the slack line device, and asked any questions they had about the intervention program.

Participants engaged in three specific exercises on the Balance Bow that included the power line, tight rope, and single leg standing drill. The power line exercise involved the participant standing with both feet perpendicular to the slack line and maintaining equilibrium as long as possible. The tight rope involved participants standing and balancing with both feet parallel to the slack line device with one foot in front of the other and also held to maintain equilibrium as long as possible. The front foot was alternated with each exercise to create equal training effects during each session. The single leg exercise involved the participant balancing with one foot perpendicular to the slack line while using the other leg as a counterbalance. Participants attempted to maintain equilibrium in these positions for as long as possible and recorded their balance times in seconds. At least five repetitions of each exercise were attempted per training session.

Two additional repetitions of each exercise were attempted with eyes closed. A spotter was available to prevent the participant from injuring themselves during the drills. Participants were asked to perform these exercises three days a week for four weeks under the supervision of one of the investigators. Training sessions were spaced at least 24 hours apart. Participants resumed their normal daily activity level in addition to performing the balance training sessions.

After the four week balance and proprioceptive training intervention with the Balance Bow, participants performed a post-test using the same exact protocol as the pre-test on the Bertec balance plate. Differences in CoP (NSEO, NSEC, PSEO, PSEC) and LoS (R, L, F, B) scores were assessed using a dependent t-test ($p < .05$). SPSS (version 21.0) was utilized to analyze the results.

Table 1. Descriptive Statistics (n=20)

	Mean	Std. Deviation	Range Lower	Range Upper
Age	19.90	1.6827	18.00	23.00
Body Weight (kg)	70.58	12.60	54.10	92.74
Height (cm)	169.67	1.43	24.40	29.90
CoP				
NSEO	-0.0850	2.9948	-1.4866	1.3166
NSEC	1.1500	4.0283	-0.7353	3.0353
PSEO	0.2300	2.8720	-1.1141	1.5741
PSEC	-1.4850	6.5411	-4.5464	1.5764
LoS				
F	2.7100	24.5737	-8.7909	14.2109
B	-13.2150	36.8037	-30.4396	4.0096
L	-26.3300	41.5803	-45.7902	-6.8698
R	-18.6100	41.4209	-37.9956	0.7756

3. Results

Descriptive statistics are summarized in Table 1. No significant differences were found in CoP NSEO, NSEC, PSEO, PSEC, LoS F, and LoS B. A significant difference was found in LoS L and there was a trend towards significance with LoS R (see Table 2). Figure 2 showed the pre- and post-test means of all scores measured. The LoS L and R scores are significantly higher than all other scores shown. Still, the LoS L scores had the greatest amount improvement. While most of the data did not show significant differences in the change of stability scores at $\alpha < .05$, there were changes in mean differences worth noting. Mean differences increased between the CoP pre-test PSEC (M= 87.740) and post-test PSEC (89.225), as well as LoS pre-test (M= 65.565) and post-test (M= 78.780). While not significant, improvement in balance and stability scores were observed based on the resulting trend seen in Figure 1.

Table 2. Significant Values

	t-value	p-value
CoP		
NSEO	-.127	.900
NSEC	1.277	.217
PSEO	.358	.724
PSEC	-1.015	.323
LoS		
F	.493	.628
B	-1.606	.125
L*	-2.832	.011
R**	-2.009	.059

*Significant at the 0.05 level

**Trending towards significance at the 0.05 level

Additionally, worth noting are the differences between the LoS R and L results. A significant improvement was found between the pre-test and post-test LoS L (p= .011). While not significant, a notable improvement in the mean was found in pre-test R (M= 133.165) and post-test R (M= 151.775). This suggests that balance training performed on the Balance Bow primarily helped improve right and left stability scores. This may be due to the observable differences noted in the single leg balance exercises performed during the balance training intervention. Differences between the first and last sessions in the right and left single leg standing exercise training mean times are shown in Table 3.

Table 3. Training Differences in R and L Means (n=20)

First Session	Mean (sec)	Last Session	Mean (sec)
Right	6.685	Right	14.476
Left	8.566	Left	14.825
Eyes Closed Right	2.33	Eyes Closed Right	2.613
Eyes Closed Left	2.328	Eyes Closed Left	2.655

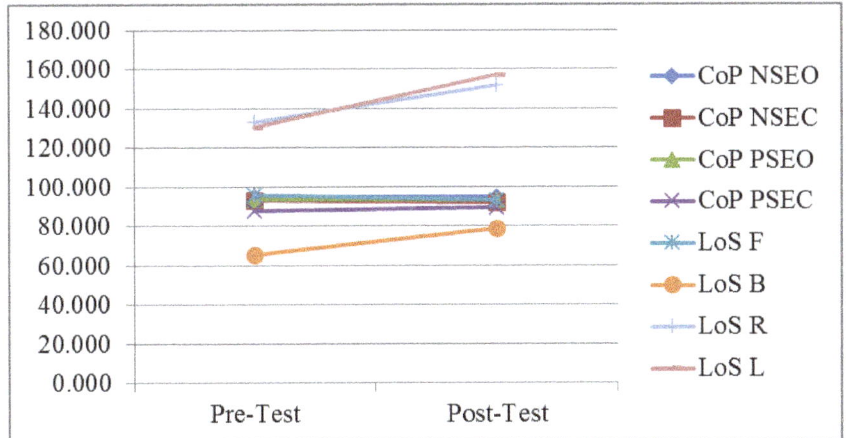

Figure 1. Pre & Post Test Means

4. Discussion

The improvements in single leg stance is important because the majority of ankle injuries are inversion sprains, which often occur in the frontal plane and deal with lateral ankle stability (Lynch & Renstrom, 1999). With improvement in these areas, the risk of ankle injury could be greatly reduced due to the study findings. Changes in the other variables investigated may not have occurred due to a ceiling effect. First of all, five of the subject participants were Division I athletes. The remaining participants were physically active four or more days of the week and/or involved in intramural sports. A minority of the participants, only four of the 20, were inactive or active less than three days of the week. Due to the high involvement of physical activity and training in the majority of subjects, the margin for change and improvement of scores may have been minimal compared to those individuals who were not as physically active as their fellow participants. If significant improvements were made for a few of the non-active individuals in this study, they may have been masked due to the minimal ability for change in the majority of individuals demonstrating higher physical activity involvement.

The training intervention protocol, developed from recommended exercises performed on the Balance Bow by Ironwear Fitness manufacturers, may not have been adequate for noticeable changes to occur. The training intervention consisted of 20 - 30 minute sessions performed three times a week for four weeks on the Balance Bow Previous studies have seen significant changes in balance abilities when the training protocol lasted longer than four weeks (Amrinder, 2012; Emery et al., 2005; Hrysomallis, 2007; Hupperets et al., 2009; Linford et al., 2006). Although Emery et al. (2005) found significant changes in balance abilities by requiring daily training sessions lasting only 20 minutes, other studies, in which significant balance improvement have been noted, required participants to engage in 30 or 40 min sessions (Amrinder et al., 2012; Hupperets et al., 2009; Linford et al., 2006). Therefore, the training protocol in this study may not have been appropriate for significant changes in stability and proprioception to present themselves within this population.

There are many other factors that can affect balance, such as vestibular imbalance, sinus congestion, prior surgeries, injuries, weakness, etc. While we were aware of these components, they were not taken into account in this study. They may or may not have contributed to differences in the hypothesized results. Future studies should investigate the differences in stability scores after a period of balance training on a slack line device between individuals with high physical activity involvement and individuals with low physical activity involvement. Differences found in these studies could be meaningful to determine if certain populations are more susceptible to changes in stability compared to others. Additional studies should also examine populations who often have decreased balance and proprioception due to reduced functionality and a compromised CNS, such as older adults or those who are at risk for ankle injuries or children with delayed movement issues. Furthermore, additional studies should focus on the appropriate modes, duration, frequency, intensity of various slack line exercises in order to create "best practice" protocols for preventing ankle injuries for various populations. While this study did not investigate balance differences in gender, other studies have found that girls have a better sense of balance than boys (Lee & Lin, 2007; Nolan et al., 2005; Odenrink, 1984; Peterson et al., 2006; Seco et al., 2012; Smith et al., 2012). Therefore, training protocols for a slack line device may need to differ based on age, gender, and other variables.

5. Conclusion

A four week period of balance and proprioceptive training on a slack line device was found to have no significant effect on CoP NSEO, NSEC, PSEO, PSEC, or LoS F, B, or R scores in college aged participants. A significant difference was found in LoS L and a notable trend towards significance was found in LoS R results. Due to the fact this is the only known published study that has investigated training effects of balance and proprioception utilizing the Balance Bow, future research is needed to determine the accuracy of these findings. Additional studies, with various populations, examining longer balance training periods, session durations, intensities, or session frequencies could reveal best practice protocols for improving balance and proprioceptive abilities, and, thus, reducing the risk for an ankle injury.

References

Amrinder, S., Deepinder, S., & Singh, S. J. (2012). Effect of proprioceptive exercises on balance and center of pressure in athletes with functional ankle instabilty. *Medicina Sportiva, 8*(3), 1927-1933.

mery, C. A., Cassidy, J. D., Klassen, T. P., Rosychuk, R. J., & Rowe, B. H. (2005). Effectiveness of a home-based balance-training program in reducing sports-related injuries among healthy adolescents: A cluster randomized controlled trial. *CMAJ, 172*(6), 749-754. doi: 10.1503/cmaj.1040805

Fried, S. (2010). Win the sprain game. *Men's Health, 25*(7), 108-110.

Houglum, P. A. (2001). *Therapeutic Exercise For Athletic Injuries*. Champaign: Human Kinetics.

Hrysomallis, C. (2007). Relationship between balance ability, training and sports injury risk. *Sports Med, 37*(6), 547-556.

Hubscher, M., Zech, A., Pfeifer, K., Hansel, F., Vogt, L., & Banzer, W. (2010). Neuromuscular training for sports injury prevention: a systematic review. *Med Sci Sports Exerc, 42*(3), 413-421. doi: 10.1249/MSS.0b013e3181b88d37

Hupperets, M. D., Verhagen, E. A., & van Mechelen, W. (2009). Effect of unsupervised home based proprioceptive training on recurrences of ankle sprain: randomised controlled trial. *BMJ, 339*, b2684. doi: 10.1136/bmj.b2684

Lee, A. J., & Lin, W. H. (2007). The influence of gender and somatotype on single-leg upright standing postural stability in children. *J Appl Biomech, 23*(3), 173-179.

Lephart, S. M., Pincivero, D. M., Giraldo, J. L., & Fu, F. H. (1997). The role of proprioception in the management and rehabilitation of athletic injuries. *Am J Sports Med, 25*(1), 130-137.

Linford, C. W., Hopkins, J. T., Schulthies, S. S., Freland, B., Draper, D. O., & Hunter, I. (2006). Effects of neuromuscular training on the reaction time and electromechanical delay of the peroneus longus muscle. *Arch Phys Med Rehabil, 87*(3), 395-401. doi: 10.1016/j.apmr.2005.10.027

Lynch, S. A., & Renstrom, P. A. (1999). Treatment of acute lateral ankle ligament rupture in the athlete. Conservative versus surgical treatment. *Sports Med, 27*(1), 61-71.

Martinez-Amat, A., Hita-Contreras, F., Lomas-Vega, R., Caballero-Martinez, I., Alvarez, P. J., & Martinez-Lopez, E. (2012). Effects of 12-week proprioception training program on postural stability, gait and balance in older adults: A controlled clinical trial. *J Strength Cond Res*. doi: 10.1519/JSC.0b013e31827da35f

Nolan, L., Grigorenko, A., & Thorstensson, A. (2005). Balance control: sex and age differences in 9- to 16-year-olds. *Dev Med Child Neurol, 47*(7), 449-454.

Odenrink, P. S., P. . (1984). Development of postural sway in the normal child. *Human Neurobiology, 3*(4), 241-244.

Peterson, M. L., Christou, E., & Rosengren, K. S. (2006). Children achieve adult-like sensory integration during stance at 12-years-old. *Gait Posture, 23*(4), 455-463.

Powers, S. K. H., E. T. (2012). *Exercise Physiology: Theory and Application to Fitness and Performance.* 148-151. New York: McGraw Hill.

Seco, J., Abecia, L. C., Echevarria, E., Barbero, I., Torres-Unda, J., Rodriguez, V., & Calvo, J. I. (2012). A long-term physical activity training program increases strength and flexibility and improves balance in older adults. *Rehabilitation Nursing, 38*, 37-47. doi: 10.1002/rnj.64

Shim, A.L., Norman, S.P., Kim, Y.A. (2013). Teaching balance training to improve stability and cognition for children. *Journal of Physical Education, Recreation, and Dance,* 84(9),15-17.

Shim, A.L., Crider, D.A. (2011). Can wobble boards improve proprioception scores in college students? *Research Quarterly*, 82(1) Suppl.

Shim, A. L., Crider, D. A., McDaniel, L. W., Bae, S. W. (2009). Comparison of stability scores on college health and wellness students using commercial balance programs. *Journal of Science and Medicine in Sport*, 12(6) Suppl.

Smith, A. W., Ulmer, F. F., & Wong del, P. (2012). Gender differences in postural stability among children. *J Hum Kinet, 33*, 25-32. doi: 10.2478/v10078-012-0041-5

Westcott, S. L., Lowes, L. P., & Richardson, P. K. (1997). Evaluation of postural stability in children: current theories and assessment tools. *Phys Ther, 77*(6), 629-645.

The Effect of Gradual Increase in Contextual Interference on Acquisition, Retention and Transfer of Volleyball Skills

Fatemeh Pasand (Corresponding author)
Department of physical Education, Shiraz University, Iran
E-mail: pasand@shirazu.ac.ir

Heydar Fooladiyanzadeh
Department of physical Education, Shiraz University, Iran
E-mail: hidar.f68@gmail.com

Gholamhossien Nazemzadegan
Department of physical Education, Shiraz University, Iran
E-mail: ghnazem@yahoo.com

Abstract

Background: A general viewpoint on contextual interference shows that a blocked practice schedule facilitates the acquisition of a skill while a random practice is more useful in the retention and transfer of that skill. **Objective**: The aim of this study was to investigate the effect of gradual increase in contextual interference upon acquisition, retention and transfer of volleyball skills. **Methods**: For this purpose, 45 participants were randomly selected from male students at Shiraz University-Iran. After pre-test, the participants were equally distributed in three experimental groups: blocked (low CI), random (high CI) and percentile gradual increase. After nine training sessions and recording the scores, the students were tested for acquisition, retention and transfer. $p \leq 0.05$ was considered as significance level in all the tests. **Results**: There was significant difference between the groups in acquisition sessions in favor of the blocked group. Retention and transfer test results also showed a significant difference between the groups in favor of random training and gradual increase groups compared to blocked training group .However no significant difference was observed between random with gradual increase training groups. **Conclusion**: According to the findings of this research, it can be concluded that random and gradual increase in contextual interference training methods may increase the performance of subjects in terms of volleyball skills in retention and transfer tests.

Keywords: Gradual Increase of Contextual Interference, Blocked, Random, Volleyball, Acquisition, Retention, Transfer

1. Introduction

Education and training conditions are among the most important topics in learning the motor skills. When planning to teach a number of skills in an education and training session, trainers are faced with the question of succession in training students to develop more effective learning conditions (Schmidt & Lee, 1988). It is very important to organize the trainings to increase their effectiveness. It seems that the exercise of skill is always dependent upon learning; therefore, appropriate training based on principles of motor learning can lead to the storage and retrieval of information in memory, resulting in generation of motor skill according to previously learnt activities (Gallahue & Ozmun, 2002). Multi-skill training in a training session on the one hand, provides a more attractive environment for the learner and saves time on the other hand. It seems that the use of contextual interference is an approach that satisfies these ends (Porter & Saemi, 2010). Highlighting the appropriate training program for the learners is a main research objective in learning the motor skills (Schmidt & lee, 1988). Therefore, one of the primary duties of trainers is to organize the training environment in such a way to improve athletic performance. In this case, two types of training programs in the form of block and random have been proposed. Blocked training is a training stereotype in which the skills are repeated without interference of other activities and all the training efforts of a skill are completed before starting the training of the next skill. In contrast, there is no predefined order of repetitions in random training. Variable training program has been a method for more effective learning of motor skills in recent decades. In planning the variable training, while performing a task, one or several other tasks are also exercised. A method for planning the variable training is taking advantage of a phenomenon known as contextual interference (CI). Contextual interference is a phenomenon whereby interference during learning the skill results in optimal exercise of the skill, which facilitates learning. Blocked and random training methods can bring about different interference levels. Obviously, a combination of blocked and random trainings can be considered as an array of training known as gradual increase. When you are trained in a skill by blocked training method, contextual interference is minimal but there is a high level of contextual interference when several different (but interrelated) skills are trained in a randomized training session (Schmidt & Lee, 1988).

Many studies have indicated that changing random training conditions may lead to poor performance and strong retention and in the same time result in good performance and poor retention in blocked training conditions. It should be noted that in the majority of studies on contextual interference, blocked vs random training has been investigated while there have been few studies on training method of gradual increase in contextual interference and only a few motor skills have been evaluated. In this approach, the training progresses from blocked to random over time with increased comprehensiveness, indicating increased contextual interference. Porter (2008) showed that repeated efforts in the early stages of learning by the learners allows for searching efficient problem-solving strategies, correction of motor errors and development of a basic motor pattern to successfully achieve the planned action. Gradual increase is a new way to provide contextual interference during training sessions in which the training, initially begun with blocked efforts (low contextual interference), is followed by random training (high contextual interference) (Porter, 2008). However, the results of field research in this context are contradictory, so that no effect of contextual interference has been observed in the previous studies in cluding of the study of Meira & Tani (2001) in assessment of dart-throwing skill, Shewokis (2003) in computer games, Jones and French (2007) in volleyball skills as well as Vera, and Varez & Medina (2008) in soccer skills.

The majority of studies on contextual interference have dealt with blocked vs random training while few studies have been conducted on training method of gradual increase in contextual interference, which have evaluated only a few motor skills. In this method, the training progresses from blocked to random over time with increased comprehensiveness, which indicates increased contextual interference. On the other hand, there are a few vague evidences concerning the effect of contextual interference in conditions out of the laboratory. Service, set and forearm pass are important skills in volleyball, which have a decisive impact on the outcome of volleyball tournaments. Because of such importance, a large proportion of training sessions are dedicated to these skills by trainers. For a good service, in addition to good physics and expertise, the athlete must have a good understanding of skills. This understanding can include exact knowledge of exercising the skill, indications of exercise and perhaps more importantly, identifying the skills that require further concentration and attention. In this regard, this study aims to evaluate the effect of gradual increase in contextual interference on acquisition, retention and transfer of volleyball skills in three levels of blocked, random and gradual increase.

2. Methods

2.1 Participants

In this study, 45 male students with mean age of (22.50±1.7) years from Shiraz University in Iran were recruited. They volunteered to participate in the study as well as they had no history of sports activities in volleyball and only received training related to volleyball skills. After pretest the participants were randomly assigned to three groups of 15 subjects, including blocked, random and gradual increase.

2.2 Task

Volleyball skills: The volleyball skills in this study included forearm pass, set and service, each performed with a specific guideline (AAHPERD-2 Test) (Antonius and Travlos, 2010).

Simple service: A simple service in which the player hits under the ball towards specified areas with one hand standing behind the line of 9 meters. Set: The subject knuckles to the six areas in the field with a pass coming from a fellow player. Forearm pass: The subject bumps to the six areas in the field with a pass coming from a fellow player.

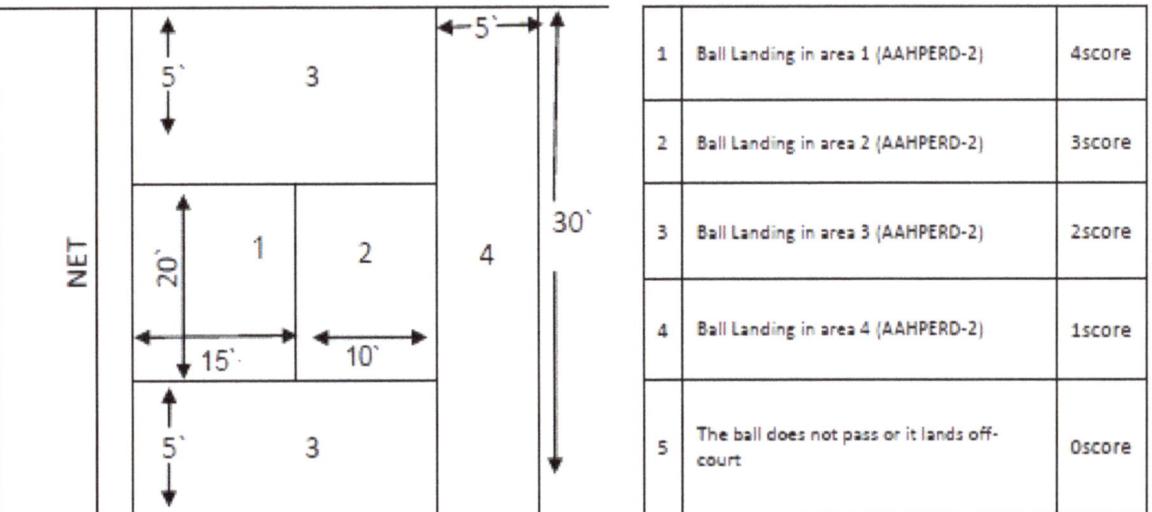

1	Ball Landing in area 1 (AAHPERD-2)	4score
2	Ball Landing in area 2 (AAHPERD-2)	3score
3	Ball Landing in area 3 (AAHPERD-2)	2score
4	Ball Landing in area 4 (AAHPERD-2)	1score
5	The ball does not pass or it lands off-court	0score

Figure 1. Scores of participants' performance and score ranks in volleyball court (AAHERD-2 test)

2.3 exercise procedure

After randomly selecting 45 students as sample from the population, the study steps were first explained for the subjects. After pre-test, they were randomly assigned to three groups of 15 members to match them based on pre-test scores. The groups were trained for skills during three weeks in three sessions per week (nine sessions total).
The first group performed the skills through blocked method. This group was trained for skills in each session using the blocked method hitting 45 trials in each session (15 sets, 15 forearm passes and 15 services).
The second group performed the skills by random method. This group was randomly trained in each session (45 hits per session). In this training method, the participants were trained for set, forearm pass and service skills so that none of skills was performed in duplicate (e.g. set, forearm pass, service/forearm pass, set, service/set, service, forearm pass).
The third group performed the skills by gradual increase method. This group was trained for ball throwing skill in each session through gradual increase in contextual interference method. This means that they performed 40 out of 45 training trials by blocked method (14 services, 13 sets, 13 forearm passes) and five trials by random method (set, forearm pass, service, forearm pass, set) in the first session. They performed 35 out of 45 training efforts by blocked method (11 services, 12 sets, 12 forearm passes) and 10 trials by random method (set, forearm pass, service, forearm pass, set, service, forearm pass, set, service, forearm pass) in the second session. Random efforts were increased by 10% with increasing number of training sessions up to the last session (session 9) until all the skills were randomly performed in the end. The participants were trained for each task during nine sessions (three sessions per week) and three blocks 15 trials for each session (45 trials of all the three skills with a total of 1215 trials).
Acquisition test was performed after the last training session similar to pre-test and training sessions. The scores of skill exercise were recorded after training efforts. Retention test was done 48 hours after the last training session similar to pre-test. Transfer test was done 48 hours after the last training session similar to pre-test with the difference that the transfer test was performed by changing the location of skill exercise. This means that if the participants exercised the skills in the right side of volleyball court during training, they exercised the skills in the left side in the transfer test.

2.4 scoring the performance of participants

By observing the relative threshold of technical matters on the part of subjects, the scoring criterion was recorded for them based on the accuracy of receiving and directing the ball in set and forearm pass as well as landing site of ball in service by the AAHPERD-2 test (Antonius and Travlos, 2010).

2.5 Data Analyses

Analysis of variance with repeated measurements as well as ANOVA was used for data analysis. If the difference between groups was significant, post hoc Tukey test was used. All analyzes were performed using SPSS software, version 16. The significance level was set at 0.05.

3. Results

This experimental study aimed to evaluate the effect of gradual percentile increase in contextual interference on performance and learning of volleyball skills through pre-test, acquisition sessions and post-test, retention and transfer sessions by three training methods (blocked, random and gradual increase). The effect of contextual interference on learning of volleyball skills was designed and developed based on change of skills with different generalized motor program of Magill & Hall (1990), desired skills according to Bortoli et al (1998) as well as French et al(1990), Jones & French (2007).

Table 1. Means and standard deviations for the phases and Groups

Phases	Pre-Test		Acquisition		Retention		Transfer	
Groups	M	SD	M	SD	M	SD	M	SD
Blocked	13	2/10	33/06	1/70	26/40	2/16	22/93	2/93
Random	13/42	2/24	18/35	1/33	34	1/96	35/78	2/91
gradual increase	10/40	2/92	26/40	2/16	34/46	1/95	34/66	1/98

With respect to the effect of gradual increase in contextual interference on acquisition, retention and transfer phases of volleyball skills, analysis of variance results with repeated measures and Post-hoc Tukey test showed a significant difference between the study groups (F=5.18 , p=0.0001). In addition, the Post-hoc Tukey test results showed that the difference was in favor of blocked relative to random (p=0/015). Furthermore, the Tukey test results indicated that gradual increase in contextual interference had no significant effect on acquisition, retention and transfer phases (p=0.77, p=0.069).

In the acquisition phase, there was significant difference in p≤0.05 confidence level between set, forearms pass and service skills in blocked, random and gradual percentile increase groups (F=281.85, p=0.0001). The Post-hoc Tukey test results showed that the difference was in favor of blocked relative to random and gradual increase methods (p=0/0001). However, there was no significant difference between random and gradual increase methods (p=0.62).

In retention phase of volleyball skills, the difference was in favor of random and gradual increase relative to the blocked training group. A comparison of the results of blocked, random and gradual increase training methods showed a significant difference in confidence level of $p \leq 0.05$ in retention phase between set, forearm pass and service skills ($F=73.78$, $P=0.0001$). Moreover, the Post-hoc Tukey test results indicated a significant difference between blocked and gradual increase training methods in retention phase ($p=0.0001$).

The results of comparing blocked, random and gradual increase training methods in transfer phase indicated significant difference in confidence level of $p \leq 0.05$ between set, forearm pass and service skills ($F=107.16$, $P=0.0001$). However, the Post-hoc Tukey test results showed no significant difference between random and gradual increase training methods ($p=0.496$).

4. Discussion

The aim of this study was to investigate the changes in contextual interference on organization of education and training of volleyball skills through three training methods of blocked, random and gradual increase in order to evaluate and compare learning opportunities of 45 students in three phases of acquisition, retention and transfer. The findings of this study in acquisition phase showed significant differences in confidence level of $p \leq 0.05$ in favor of blocked relative to random and gradual increase methods in three skills of set, forearm pass and service. In this way, the results were consistent with the results of Smith et al (2003).

Better performance of blocked group relative to random and gradual increase groups is probably due to the absence of interfering tasks as well as exercise of tasks without requirement of new processing in the blocked group. That is because this group prepared a training schedule, which was immediately used in later efforts using short-term memory and caused improved exercise in this phase. However, in the random and gradual increase groups, according to expansion and reconstruction theory of comprehensive action plan, a new task should be designed due to overlap with other tasks. Proponents of expansion theory argue that the development of a training program with high contextual inference (random training) inserts the image of various tasks into the active memory, which in turn results in complete image rich in tasks through the resulting inter- and intra-task processing operations. Reconstruction theory of action plan suggests that in random training program, the action plan used in previous efforts is forgotten as a result of interference with other efforts. The processing activities required for restructuring a forgotten plan of action creates a strong image of skills, which will in turn enhance learning, as a result of which the exercised is abated. In other words, contextual interference causes poor exercise of random and gradual increase methods in the acquisition phase due to implicating the subject in inter- and intra-task processing. Therefore, these perceptual processes and cognitive efforts during acquisition sessions enhance retention and transfer phases. The results of this study are not consistent with the findings of Menayo, Moreno, Sabido (2010), Dias and Mendes (2010), Ollis, Button & Fairweather (2005), and no effect of contextual interference was observed. These researchers observed no significant difference between the performance of different training groups in various phases of training. Non-compliance of the results of this study can be attributed to difference in field and laboratory tasks as well as differences in the number of training sessions, complexity of the task and expertise level of subjects. On the other hand, Goode & Magill (1986) stated that one of the reasons for insignificant difference between training groups related to scoring less sensitive in the field tasks rather than laboratory.

Part of the results of this study with respect to observing better effect of blocked training method compared with other training methods in acquisition sessions is consistent with results of Guadagnoli & Lee (2004), Smith, Gregory & Davies (2003). In addition, part of these results concerning a significant difference between training groups in retention test was consistent with research conducted by Smith (2002), Saemi, Porter, Ghotbi Varzaneh, Zarghami, & Shafinia (2012), Porter & Saemi (2010), Porter (2008), Kalkhoran & Shariati (2012). Reviewing the literature on contextual interference, Magill & Hall (1990) reported that when the tasks are exercised under different motor programs, a stronger contextual interference effect is observed relative to when motor programs are the same. This hypothesis of Magill & Hall on the difference between motor programs and parameter in generation of interference effect has been supported by numerous laboratory studies. While some studies indicate the impact of contextual interference for parameter estimation in retention tests, such impact has not been observed in generalized motor program (GMP) even if the trained tasks are controlled by the same or different parameters (Giuffrida, Shea & Fairbrother, 2002 and Lai, Shea, Wulf, & Wright, 2000). Shea & Morgan (1979) and Shea & Zimny (1983 and 1988) have suggested that when the training is performed in a random order, there are advantages for learning through interaction between working memory of two or more similar tasks. Increased interference in working memory during training leads to extensive differentiated processing, which eventually facilitates retention. On the other hand, Lee and Magill (1983) and Magill and Hall (1990) argue that interference causes oblivion of action plan in working memory, so these plans are reconstructed in any new effort under random conditions. This reconstruction process causes increased retention and transfer.

While the majority of contextual interference studies have been conducted in laboratory environments, much attention has been recently paid to generalizability of contextual interference results in field environments. The results of field environments are inconsistent and mediocre benefit of high contextual interference has been cited for retention and transfer in laboratory conditions in sports environments because of features such as complexity of skills and expertise level of the learner. In applied research, several skills of various sports activities have been studied and the results are still incompatible with each other. For example, the results of studies with the same tasks controlled by a motor program requiring parameter adjustments are inconsistent. For instance, the results of this study are not consistent with

Chamberlin (1991) jump shot in basketball as well as Hall and Boyle (1993) on shuffleboard skill, which reported no significant difference between training arrangement methods. The results are also inconsistent with those of Meira & Tani (2001) in acquisition of dart -throwing skill. On the other hand, the results of this study in acquisition phase were not consistent with studies conducted by Rouhollahi, Rozan & Mehrotra (2014) and Afsanepurak, Karimiyani, Moradi & Safaei (2012). Landin and Hebert (1997) reported no significant difference between training methods in acquisition of basketball shooting skills.

However, there are limitations in this study that should be considered in future research. For example, positive results can be obtained by increasing the sample size or increasing the efforts related to trainings.

According to the results of this study, it can be generally concluded that contextual interference can lead to learning of motor skills in blocked, random and gradual percentile increase in contextual interference methods. Overall, skill training methods should be designed considering several factors such as age, expertise and experience level of subjects, motor and cognitive abilities, processing capacity of environmental information and several other factors that can affect motor learning, and there should always be an appropriate optimal structure between pervasive expertise level and difficulty of training skills.

5. Conclusion

The results support the claim that training with contextual interference in both aspects of memory power in connection with expansion, differentiation and reconstruction hypothesis of action plan causes progress with respect to forgetting and reconstruction hypothesis. Although it generally seems that random and gradual percentile increase training methods are superior for learning, more research is needed to confirm this matter. Moreover, according to the results obtained with respect to higher impact of gradual increase and random methods relative to blocked method, the application of these training methods is suggested in order to educate motor skills in different age ranges.

Acknowledgments

We are thankful students of Shiraz University for volunteering their time to participate.

References

Afsanepurak, S. A., Karimiyani, N., Moradi, J., & Safaei, M. (2012). The Effect of Blocked, Random, and Systematically Increasing Practice on learning of Different Types of Basketball Passes. *European Journal of Experimental Biology, 2*(6), 2397-2402 .

Antonius, K., Travlos. (2010) (1). "Specificity and variability of practice, and contextual interference in acquisition and transfer of an underhand volleyball serve". Perceptual and Motor Skills. Vol. 110, Issue, pp: 298-312.

Bortoli, L., Robazza, C., Durigon, V., & Carra, C. (1992). Effects of contextual interference on learning technical sports skills. *Perceptual and motor skills, 75*(2), 555-562 .

Chamberlin, C., Rimer, T., & Skaggs, D. (1990). *The ecological validity of the contextual interference effect: A practical application to learning the jump shot in basketball.* Paper presented at the annual meeting of the North American Society for the Psychology of Sport and Physical Activity. Houston, TX, May.

Dias, G., & Mendes, R. (2010). Effects of a contextual interference continuum on golf putting task. *Revista Brasileira de Educação Física e Esporte, 24*(4), 545-553 .

Feghhi, I., Valizadeh, R., Rahimpour, M., Tehrani, M. A., & Karampour, S. (2015). Contextual Interference in Learning Three Table Tennis Services. *Procedia-Social and Behavioral Sciences, 191*, 546-549 .

French, K. E., Rink, J. E., & Werner, P. H. (1990). Effects of contextual interference on retention of three volleyball skills. *Perceptual and motor skills, 71*(1), 179-186 .

Gallahue, D., & Ozmun, J. (2002). Understanding motor development: Infants, children, adolescents, adults with PowerWeb .

Giuffrida, C. G., Shea, J. B., & Fairbrother, J. T. (2002). Differential transfer benefits of increased practice for constant, blocked, and serial practice schedules. *Journal of motor behavior, 34*(4), 353-365 .

Goode, S., & Magill, R. A. (1986). Contextual interference effects in learning three badminton serves. *Research quarterly for exercise and sport, 57*(4), 308-314 .

Guadagnoli, M. A & ,.Lee, T. D. (2004). Challenge point: a framework for conceptualizing the effects of various practice conditions in motor learning. *Journal of motor behavior, 36*(2), 212-224 .

Hall, K., & Boyle, M. (1993). The effects of contextual interference on shuffleboared skill in children. *Research quarterly for exercise and sport, 67*(1), 52-58 .

Jones, L. L., & French, K. E. (2007). Effects of contextual interference on acquisition and retention of three volleyballskills 1. *Perceptual and motor skills, 105*(3), 883-890.

Kalkhoran, A. F., & Shariati, A. (2012). The Effects of Contextual Interference on Learning Volleyball Motor Skills. *Journal of Physical Education and Sport, 12*(4), 550 .

Lai, Q., Shea, C. H., Wulf, G., & Wright, D. L. (2000). Optimizing generalized motor program and parameter learning. *Research quarterly for exercise and sport, 71*(1), 10-24 .

Landin, D., & Hebert, E. P. (1997). A comparison of three practice schedules along the contextual interference continuum. *Research quarterly for exercise and sport, 68*(4), 357-361 .

Lee, T. D., & Magill, R. A. (1983). The locus of contextual interference in motor-skill acquisition. *Journal of Experimental Psychology: Learning, Memory, and Cognition, 9*(4), 730 .

Magill, R. A., & Hall, K. G. (1990). A review of the contextual interference effect in motor skill acquisition. *Human movement science, 9*(3), 241-289 .

Meira Jr, C. M., & Tani, G. (2001). The contextual interference effect in acquisition of dart-throwing skill tested on a transfer test with extended trials. *Perceptual and motor skills, 92*(3), 910-918 .

Menayo, R., Moreno, F., Sabido, R., Fuentes, J., & Garcia, J. (2010). Simultaneous treatment effects in learning four tennis shots in contextual interferenceconditions1, 2. *Perceptual and motor skills, 110*(2), 661-673 .

Ollis, S., Button, C., & Fairweather, M. (2005). The influence of professional expertise and task complexity upon the potency of the contextual interference effect. *Acta Psychologica, 118*(3), 229-244 .

Porter, J. M. (2008). Systematically increasing contextual interference is beneficial for learning novel motor skills .

Porter, J. M., & Saemi, E. (2010). Moderately skilled learners benefit by practicing with systematic increases in contextual interference. *International Journal of Coaching Science, 4*(2), 61-71 .

Rouhollahi,V. Rozan,M. Mehrotra,A.(2014). Effect of Different Practice Schedules on Learning and Performance in Handball Task, *American Journal of Sports Science*. Vol. 2, No. 4, 2014, pp. 71-76.

Saemi, E., Porter, J. M., Ghotbi Varzaneh, A., Zarghami, M., & Shafinia, P. (2012). Practicing along the contextual interference continuum: A comparison of three practice schedules in an elementary physical education setting . *Kineziologija, 44*(2), 191-198 .

Schmidt, R. A., & Lee, T. (1988). Motor control and learning .

Shea, J. B., & Morgan, R. L. (1979). Contextual interference effects on the acquisition, retention, and transfer of a motor skill. *Journal of Experimental Psychology: Human Learning and Memory, 5*(2), 179 .

Shea, J. B., & Zimny, S. T. (1983). Context effects in memory and learning movement information. *Advances in Psychology, 12*, 345-366 .

Shea, J. B., & Zimny, S. T. (1988). Knowledge incorporation in motor representation. *Advances in Psychology, 50*, 289-314 .

Shewokis, P. A. (2003). Memory consolidation and contextual interference effects with computer games. *Perceptual and motor skills, 97*(2), 581-589 .

Smith, P. J. (2002). Applying contextual interference to snowboarding skills. *Perceptual and motor skills, 95*(3), 999-1005 .

Smith, P. J., Gregory, S. K., & Davies, M. (2003). Alternating versus blocked practice in learning a cartwheel. *Perceptual and motor skills, 96*(3c), 1255-1264 .

8

Effect of Kinetic Resistance Training and Technique on Special Strength Level and Effective Kinematic Variables in Instep Kick for Soccer Juniors

Amr Ali Shady
Sport Training Department, Faculty of Sport Education, Mansoura University, Mansoura, Egypt
E-mail: dr_ashady2004@yahoo.com

Abstract

Background: Training with resistance is considered the essential and complementary part of players' preparation period during training season through developing different aspects. **Objective**: This study aims to investigate the Effect of Kinetic resistance training and technique on special power level and effective kinematic variables in instep kick for soccer juniors. **Methodology**: 20 junior soccer players (age: 17.54 ±0.5 years, body mass: 69.05 kg, height: 170 cm, training age=7.7 years) participated in this study were randomly assigned into two groups experimental (n=10) trained with kinetic resistance training program and technique and control (n=10) trained with traditional soccer training program only where, the experimental approach was used. **Results**: The kinetic resistance trainings and technique positively affected the special power level, kicking accuracy and time and effective kinematic variables in instep kick. **Conclusion**: The researcher recommended that coaches should give attention to special strength developing and to be an essential part of the training program through kinetic resistance trainings and technique. Also coaches should depend on the kinematic variables affecting performance for detecting the improvement level in performance as a result of kinetic resistance trainings and technique.

Keywords: kinetic resistance, technique, special strength, kinematic, Instep Kick

1. Introduction

Soccer has been affected by the scientific development in sports and physical education to develop players' abilities and achievements through taking care of special physical preparation devoted to increasing functional efficiency of vital organs and developing physical and skillful characteristics discriminating soccer player. Training with resistance is considered the essential and complementary part of players preparation period during training season through developing different aspects. The scientific researches and studies indicated the improvement in young players physical fitness level following the resistance training programs right instruction and steps (Roberts & Weider, 1994).

Muscular strength in its different shapes including explosive strength, maximum strength and rate of force development plays a major role in enhancing such skills performance (Cabri et al., 1988). And hence for soccer player to perform different shapes of skill performances during the game, some physical abilities should be available. Where these physical abilities type, quantity and timing differentiate based on each skill singularity and type (Keshek & Elbosaty , 2000).

The success in kinetic skill performance depends on player ability in employing physical components especially the muscular strength during skill performance. Different players have high levels of muscular strength that appears in muscular strength tests but couldn't be applied in skill performance as it requires the ability of good kinetic correlation and movement right transmission. The good co-operation of the kinetic transmission process of the exerted strength from the trunk to the thigh then leg then ankle works in an open reaction chain starting from trunk to ankle (Noguchi et, al., 2012). The muscular strength in the upper and lower part of the body moves through a set of muscles groups participating in soccer kicking skill. Thus during the design of soccer players special strength developing training programs especially juniors, central muscles strength working in physical activity should be developed and the exercises should be similar to the performance nature not only the shape but also the speed of each part of the body and in the same muscular working direction(Schmitz,2003).

Through this study the researcher defined the Kinetic Resistance as a resistance based on rubber bands (as shown in Figure 1) where the player exerts muscular contractions with shape and kinetic path similar to the soccer kinetic performances type. The instep kick is one of the most needed skills in soccer, constituting a basic element of the game when a faster and more powerful ball needs to be generated (Inoue et.al., 2012). So the existence of information about the needed characteristics through different skills performance became an essential for coaches where the technological development in motion analysis field has revealed the interlaced relations between body parts motions through performing skills that can be obtained by tracking and analyzing player motion during the performance stages of these skills.

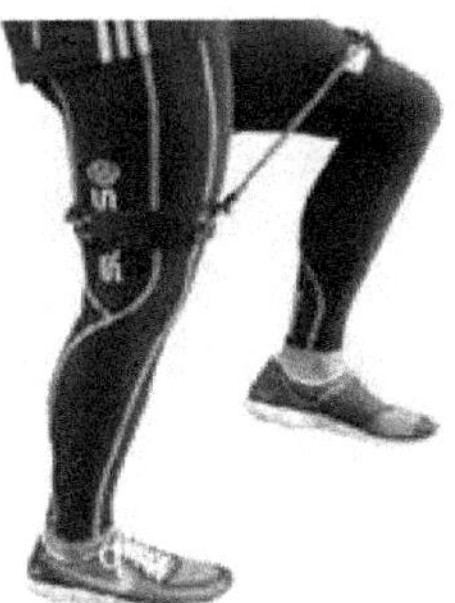
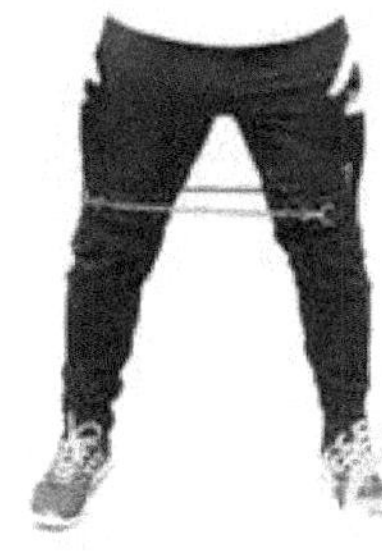
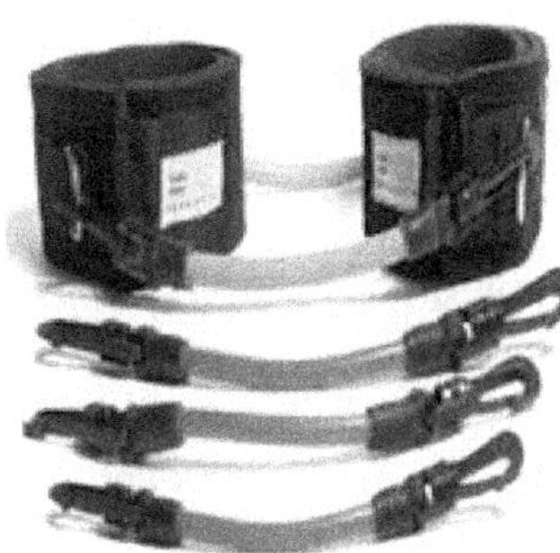

Figure 1. The rubber calibration bands used in the kinetic resistance training program (Resistance Band, 2015)

Kinematic analysis and kinematic variables extraction for the instep kick is one of the most preferred methods for detecting the extent to which players have benefit from the gained strength levels whereas the speed change in leg parts including hip, leg or ankle is a strong indicator to evaluate the player ability to benefit of the gained strength levels he has (Reilly & Williams, 2003).

The researcher indicates that detecting the characteristics of the kinetic performance during training and modifying it according to the skill kinetic performance goal is one of the substantial tasks for the soccer training programs success. Hence the more similarities between exercise and actual kinetic performance, the more peculiarity the exercise and its effectiveness for enhancing skill kinetic performance increases. Selecting the appropriate training method depends on diagnosing and accurately characterizing the skill kinetic performance to determine the role of muscular strength as an essential physical variable in this performance, and since the special strength training style starts from the skill kinetic performance characteristics as a primary base in selecting training method and building exercises to be used in soccer dedicated training.

The researcher noticed that the inability of many players on employing the muscular strength , they have in kinetic performance specially at soccer kicking since most players have high strength levels but cannot employ this strength during kinetic performance. Through the researcher acquaintance on several previous studies and scientific references in sport training as general and soccer field specially, it was clear to him the paucity of these studies that handled the effect of kinetic resistance trainings on kicking skill, however, these studies have clarified the importance of special strength developing on improving kicking skill. Hence appears the importance of this study as one of the experimental studies that proposes a new method for developing soccer juniors kicking skill and providing the necessary information needed by soccer coaches.

From all of the above the researcher in this study aims to investigate the effectiveness of kinetic resistance training and technique on the special strength level , instep kick performance accuracy and time and kinematic variables affecting the instep kick of soccer juniors in the experimental group compared to the control group.

And in order to go through this study the researcher assumed that

i. There are significant differences between the experimental group pre-test and post-test measurements of the special strength, soccer kicking performance level and kinematic variables affecting the soccer juniors instep kick for the post-test.

ii. There are significant differences between the control group pre-test and post-test measurements of the special strength, soccer kicking performance level and kinematic variables affecting the soccer juniors instep kick for the post-test.

iii. There are significant differences between the control and experimental groups in the post test measurement of the special strength, soccer kicking performance level and kinematic variables affecting the soccer juniors instep kick for the experimental group post-test.

In next section the research methodology and sample are described in detail indication the research variables and the training program foundations including training units time and number of repetitions.

2. Methods

2.1 Research Methodology

The researcher utilized the experimental methodology through the experimental design of two groups experimental and control to achieve the aims of research and hypnoses.

2.2 Research Sample

Twenty soccer juniors were selected (age: 17.54 ±0.5 years, body mass: 69.05 kg, height: 170cm, training age=7.7 years) and randomly assigned into two groups experimental (n=10) and control (n=10).

2.3 Research variables

- Special Strength : was evaluated using (three consecutive springs speed – three right hops speed- three left hops speed- vertical jump) tests knowing that speed = distance/ time.
- Instep Kick: was evaluated using (kicking accuracy - kicking time) tests.
- Kinematic variables affecting the instep kick: the following variables were extracted (Angular displacement (θ) - Linear displacement (S^R) - Angular velocity (ω) - Linear velocity (V^R) - Linear acceleration (a^R)).

The researcher utilized high-speed video camera (250 frame / sec.) and the "Motion Track" movement analysis program to extract the kinematic variables though determining the appropriate time moments to detect theses variables that were prepared to be statistically processed.

2.4 The Training Program Foundations

The scientific foundations and regulations of the training program were determined according to (Perrin, 1993; Evans, 1997; Moran & George, 2000) as following:

- Integrated and proper warm up that includes general flexibility
- The exercise should be performed during the full range of the exercise movement.
- The special strength training program should start with the muscular strength establishment using the general and inclusive exercises for all body muscles and that was considered by the researcher through the body weight exercises and the low intensity polymeric exercises for the different muscles sets during the general preparation stage (two weeks long).
- The exercise should be similar to the game skill that tack place during completion and has been trained on.
- The training load components should proportioned (intensity – size – rest) according to what that scientists have reported as following :
  - o Load Intensity: 50-80% of the maximum limit of the individual level.
  - o Load Size: (8-12) repetitions.
  - o Sets count : (3:4) sets
  - o Rest between repetitions: (1-3) from performance time.
  - o Rest between sets: (3-4) minutes.
  - o Number of training units: 3 training units per week.
  - o Duration of the program: 8 weeks
  - o The content of the training program is executed after a good warm up in other words in the main part of the training unit and then the rest of the training unit is continued.
  - o The training duration in each training unit ranges from 35:45 minutes.
  - o Static flexibility exercises are performance during rest.

3. Results

Table (1) indicates the existence of significant difference between the pre-test and post-test in special strength and instep kicking time and accuracy of the experimental group for the post-test.

Table 1. Differences between pre-test and post-test of Special Strength and instep kick of the experimental group

n=10	Measuring Unit	Pre-test		Post test		t-value	Improvement Percentage
Variables		Mean	Std. D	Mean	Std. D		
three consecutive springs speed test	m/sec	2.504	0.05	2.799	0.02	17.75	%11.78
three right hops speed test	m/sec	2.72	0.02	2.985	0.09	8.85	%9.74
three left hops speed test	m/sec	2.702	0.02	3.01	0.07	16.19	%11.40
vertical jump test	c m	47.5	2.64	73.7	2.67	56.14	%55.16
kicking accuracy	Degree	2.77	0.03	4.385	0.02	137.31	%58.30
kicking time	Sec	0.38	0.02	0.28	0.02	16.218	%26.70

T. spreadsheet at 0.05 = 1.833

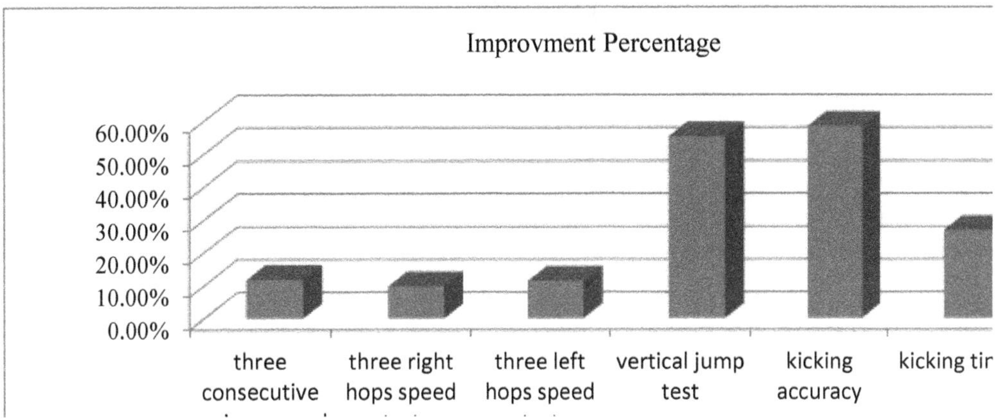

Figure 2. Improving percentage between pre-test and post-test of special strength and instep kick variables of the experimental group

Table 2. Differences between pre-test and post-test of the kinematic variables of the experimental group

n=10	Variables	skill Stages	Pre-test		Post test		t-value	Improvement Percentage
			Mean	Std. D	Mean	Std. D		
Hip Joint	Angular displacement (θ)	backswing	162.5	9.85	175.7	1.34	4.43	%8.12
		Impact	125.06	1.95	131.13	0.74	8.98	%4.85
		Follow-up	116.14	1.32	118.64	0.13	6.36	%2.15
	Linear displacement (S^R)	backswing	0.271	0.02	0.356	0.02	9.60	%31.37
		Impact	0.209	0.02	0.269	0.01	8.78	%28.71
		Follow-up	0.28	0.02	0.371	0.01	11.24	%32.50
	Angular velocity (ω)	backswing	11.81	1.44	18.95	0.01	15.78	%60.42
		Impact	0.411	0.03	0.62	0.01	22.32	%50.85
		Follow-up	7.197	1.30	9.221	0.01	4.93	%28.12
	Linear velocity (V^R)	backswing	1.286	0.06	1.828	0.01	23.52	%42.15
		Impact	1.291	0.06	1.821	0.01	24.13	%41.05
		Follow-up	0.725	0.05	1.109	0.15	9.30	%52.97
	Linear acceleration (a^R)	backswing	12.059	0.47	13.942	0.02	12.25	%15.61
		Impact	10.996	0.84	13.757	0.15	10.02	%25.11
		Follow-up	12.732	1.19	15.8	0.09	8.22	%24.10
Knee Joint	Angular displacement (θ)	backswing	65.9	1.10	68.4	1.07	5.51	%3.79
		Impact	110.6	0.84	112.8	0.79	4.71	%1.99
		Follow-up	171.8	4.10	178.5	1.08	4.63	%3.90
	Linear displacement (S^R)	backswing	0.426	0.03	0.318	0.02	8.26-	%25.35-
		Impact	1.996	0.04	2.03	0.04	2.25	%1.70
		Follow-up	2.625	0.08	2.725	0.02	3.28	%3.81
	Angular velocity (ω)	backswing	1.854	0.03	2.461	0.07	22.14	%32.74
		Impact	14.06	1.07	19.195	0.63	12.06	%36.52
		Follow-up	0.286	0.02	0.347	0.01	9.04	%21.33
	Linear velocity (V^R)	backswing	4.521	0.30	5.638	0.15	9.60	%24.71
		Impact	1.305	0.30	2.638	0.20	11.17	%102.15
		Follow-up	2.75	0.18	3.223	0.03	8.39	%17.20
	Linear acceleration (a^R)	backswing	52.59	1.28	55.505	0.28	6.69	%5.54
		Impact	57.6	0.97	61.1	1.10	8.71	%6.08
		Follow-up	32.7	0.95	35.5	1.43	9.63	%8.56
Ankle Joint	Angular displacement (θ)	backswing	151.6	1.26	152.5	0.97	1.96	%0.59
		Impact	128	1.49	133.6	1.26	7.07	%4.38
		Follow-up	138.9	1.10	139.6	0.84	2.68	%0.50
	Linear displacement (S^R)	backswing	0.384	0.01	0.423	0.01	10.30	%10.16
		Impact	0.414	0.01	0.46	0.02	9.66	%11.11
		Follow-up	0.609	0.01	0.686	0.02	14.88	%12.64
	Angular velocity (ω)	backswing	3.552	0.02	4.527	0.76	4.02	%27.45
		Impact	2.981	0.67	4.693	0.07	7.52	%57.43
		Follow-up	1.527	0.24	1.953	0.02	5.37	%27.90
	Linear velocity (V^R)	backswing	5.263	0.30	6.485	0.18	9.81	%23.22
		Impact	5.831	1.19	8.959	0.02	8.24	%53.64
		Follow-up	2.609	0.28	3.839	0.06	15.02	%47.14
	Linear acceleration (a^R)	backswing	24.085	0.83	28.7	0.82	12.87	%19.16
		Impact	124.8	2.44	130.5	0.71	6.75	%4.57
		Follow-up	52	0.82	54.9	0.88	7.65	%5.58

T. spreadsheet at 0.05 = 1.833

Table (2) indicates the existence of significant difference between the pre-test and post-test in kinematic variables (Angular displacement (θ)-Linear displacement (SR)- Angular velocity (ω)- Linear velocity (VR)-Linear acceleration (aR)) of the experimental group for the post-test.

Table 3. Differences between pre-test and post-test in the Special Strength and instep kick of the control group

n=10	Measuring Unit	Pre-test		Post test		t-value	Improvement Percentage
Variables		Mean	Std. D	Mean	Std. D		
three consecutive springs speed test	m/sec	2.48	0.05	2.65	0.02	7.62	%6.59
three right hops speed test	m/sec	2.70	0.02	2.82	0.03	13.41	%4.36
three left hops speed test	m/sec	2.69	0.01	2.79	0.02	18.22	%4.01
vertical jump test	c m	46	2.40	58.1	5.59	6.448	%26.30
kicking accuracy	Degree	2.78	0.03	3.42	0.20	9.48	%23.31
kicking time	sec	0.37	0.01	0.34	0.01	5.77	%8.47

T. spreadsheet at 0.05 = 1.833

Table (3) indicates the existence of significant difference between the pre-test and post-test in special strength and instep kicking time and accuracy of the control group for the post-test.

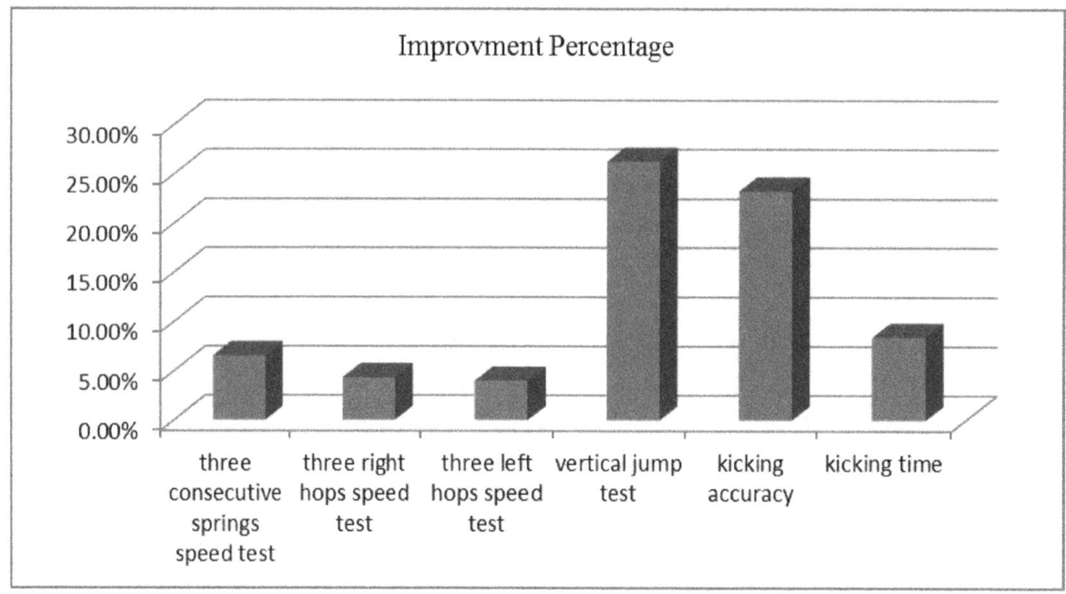

Figure 3. Improving percentage between pre-test and post-test in special strength and instep kick variables of control group

Table 4. Differences between pre-test and post-test of the kinematic variables of the control group

n=10	Variables	skill Stages	Pre-test Mean	Pre-test Std. D	Post test Mean	Post test Std. D	t-value	Improvement Percentage
Hip Joint	Angular displacement (θ)	backswing	161.7	11.67	164.6	3.10	0.888	%1.79
		Impact	126.18	2.25	126.63	2.38	0.387	%0.36
		Follow-up	116.76	0.52	117.02	2.44	0.363	%0.22
	Linear displacement (S^R)	backswing	0.267	0.02	0.278	0.04	0.866	%4.12
		Impact	0.197	0.01	0.231	0.03	3.510	%17.26
		Follow-up	0.274	0.02	0.283	0.02	3.857	%3.28
	Angular velocity (ω)	backswing	11.864	1.47	12.493	1.11	2.994	%5.30
		Impact	0.429	0.02	0.52	0.06	4.021	%21.21
		Follow-up	7.297	1.55	8.387	1.02	2.245	%14.94
	Linear velocity (V^R)	backswing	1.295	0.07	1.333	0.03	1.667	%2.93
		Impact	1.286	0.06	1.478	0.19	2.666	%14.93
		Follow-up	0.73	0.05	0.754	0.03	4.609	%3.29

	Linear acceleration (a^R)	backswing	11.864	0.36	12.13	0.32	3.392	%2.24
		Impact	10.853	0.61	11.55	0.64	2.991	%6.42
		Follow-up	12.18	0.79	12.77	1.09	1.796	%4.84
Knee Joint	Angular displacement (θ)	backswing	65	2.75	66.3	3.43	2.623	%2.00
		Impact	109.5	3.44	110.6	3.10	4.714	%1.00
		Follow-up	170.8	2.94	171.5	2.80	4.582	%0.41
	Linear displacement (S^R)	backswing	0.416	0.02	0.265	0.02	21.37-	%36.30-
		Impact	1.954	0.08	1.982	0.11	1.114	%1.43
		Follow-up	2.588	0.06	2.616	0.36	0.267	%1.08
	Angular velocity (ω)	backswing	1.844	0.03	2.162	0.27	3.807	%17.25
		Impact	14.36	0.82	16.1	2.02	2.904	%12.12
		Follow-up	0.29	0.01	0.318	0.01	9.635	%9.66
	Linear velocity (V^R)	backswing	4.371	0.21	4.96	0.43	4.848	%13.48
		Impact	1.255	0.30	1.62	0.29	7.378	%29.08
		Follow-up	2.64	0.32	2.934	0.25	2.631	%11.14
	Linear acceleration (a^R)	backswing	51.84	0.99	52.575	1.12	2.258	%1.42
		Impact	58	1.05	59.15	0.88	5.437	%1.98
		Follow-up	33	0.67	34	0.67	6.708	%3.03
Ankle Joint	Angular displacement (θ)	backswing	151	1.05	151.55	1.01	1.492	%0.36
		Impact	127.2	1.23	129.4	1.51	8.819	%1.73
		Follow-up	138.3	1.16	138.6	1.07	1.963	%0.22
	Linear displacement (S^R)	backswing	0.38	0.01	0.398	0.01	6.194	%4.74
		Impact	0.421	0.01	0.443	0.01	5.659	%5.23
		Follow-up	0.613	0.01	0.645	0.01	8.231	%5.22
	Angular velocity (ω)	backswing	3.562	0.01	4.016	0.60	2.396	%12.75
		Impact	2.831	0.47	3.389	0.38	6.374	%19.71
		Follow-up	1.499	0.20	1.692	0.14	5.505	%12.88
	Linear velocity (V^R)	backswing	5.14	0.17	5.63	0.26	6.133	%9.53
		Impact	5.631	1.14	6.14	0.73	3.324	%9.04
		Follow-up	2.709	0.21	3.202	0.28	10.400	%18.20
	Linear acceleration (a^R)	backswing	23.885	0.82	25.8	1.01	12.165	%8.02
		Impact	125.3	1.77	127.5	1.18	7.570	%1.76
		Follow-up	52.2	0.79	53.7	1.06	5.581	%2.87

T. spreadsheet at 0.05 = 1.833

Table (4) indicates the existence of significant difference between the pre-test and post-test in kinematic variables (Angular displacement (θ)-Linear displacement (SR)- Angular velocity (ω)- Linear velocity (VR)-Linear acceleration (aR)) of the control group for the post-test.

Table 5. Differences between post-test of the experimental group and post-test of the control group in Special Strength and instep kick

n1=n2=10	Measuring Unit	Post test		Post test		t-value
Variables		Mean	Std. D	Mean	Std. D	
three consecutive springs speed test	m/sec	2.799	0.02	2.65	0.02	13.66
three right hops speed test	m/sec	2.985	0.09	2.82	0.03	4.93
three left hops speed test	m/sec	3.01	0.07	2.79	0.02	8.06
vertical jump test	c m	73.7	2.67	64.3	2.31	8.33
kicking accuracy	Degree	4.385	0.02	3.42	0.20	15.47
kicking time	sec	0.28	0.02	0.34	0.01	7.57

T. spreadsheet at 0.05 = 1.833

Table (5) indicates the existence of significant difference between post-test of the experimental group and post-test of the control group in special strength and instep kicking time and accuracy for the post-test of the experimental group.

Table 6. Differences between post-tests of experimental group and control group in kinematic variables

n1=n2=10	Variables	skill Stages	experimental group		control group		t-value
			Mean	Std. D	Mean	Std. D	
Hip Joint	Angular displacement (θ)	backswing	175.7	1.34	164.6	3.10	12.008
		Impact	131.13	0.74	126.63	2.38	5.708
		Follow-up	118.64	0.13	117.02	2.44	2.143
	Linear displacement (S^R)	backswing	0.356	0.02	0.278	0.04	6.049
		Impact	0.269	0.01	0.231	0.03	5.338
		Follow-up	0.371	0.01	0.283	0.02	12.943
	Angular velocity (ω)	backswing	18.95	0.01	12.493	1.11	18.503
		Impact	0.62	0.01	0.52	0.06	4.74342
		Follow-up	9.221	0.01	8.387	1.02	2.569
	Linear velocity (V^R)	backswing	1.828	0.01	1.333	0.03	46.842
		Impact	1.821	0.01	1.478	0.19	5.585
		Follow-up	1.109	0.15	0.754	0.03	8.244
	Linear acceleration (a^R)	backswing	13.942	0.02	12.13	0.32	17.831
		Impact	13.757	0.15	11.55	0.64	11.875
		Follow-up	15.8	0.09	12.77	1.09	8.498
Knee Joint	Angular displacement (θ)	backswing	68.4	1.07	66.3	3.43	2.214
		Impact	112.8	0.79	110.6	3.10	2.369
		Follow-up	178.5	1.08	171.5	2.80	7.333
	Linear displacement (S^R)	backswing	0.318	0.02	0.265	0.02	4.791
		Impact	2.03	0.04	1.982	0.11	1.841
		Follow-up	2.725	0.02	2.616	0.36	1
	Angular velocity (ω)	backswing	2.461	0.07	2.162	0.27	3.542
		Impact	19.195	0.63	16.1	2.02	3.895
		Follow-up	0.347	0.01	0.318	0.01	5.513
	Linear velocity (V^R)	backswing	5.638	0.15	4.96	0.43	6.137
		Impact	2.638	0.20	1.62	0.29	12.501
		Follow-up	3.223	0.03	2.934	0.25	3.610
	Linear acceleration (a^R)	backswing	55.505	0.28	52.575	1.12	7.824
		Impact	61.1	1.10	59.15	0.88	6.090
		Follow-up	35.5	1.43	34	0.67	3.737
Ankle Joint	Angular displacement (θ)	backswing	152.5	0.97	151.55	1.01	2.69
		Impact	133.6	1.26	129.4	1.51	7.875
		Follow-up	139.6	0.84	138.6	1.07	3.354
	Linear displacement (S^R)	backswing	0.423	0.01	0.398	0.01	6.228
		Impact	0.46	0.02	0.443	0.01	2.939
		Follow-up	0.686	0.02	0.645	0.01	9.461
	Angular velocity (ω)	backswing	4.527	0.76	4.016	0.60	3.812
		Impact	4.693	0.07	3.389	0.38	9.887
		Follow-up	1.953	0.02	1.692	0.14	5.591
	Linear velocity (V^R)	backswing	6.485	0.18	5.63	0.26	11.409
		Impact	8.959	0.02	6.14	0.73	12.178
		Follow-up	3.839	0.06	3.202	0.28	7.455
	Linear acceleration (a^R)	backswing	28.7	0.82	25.8	1.01	7.010
		Impact	130.5	0.71	127.5	1.18	7.115
		Follow-up	54.9	0.88	53.7	1.06	4.129

T. spreadsheet at 0.05 = 1.833

Table (6) indicates the existence of significant difference between post-test of the experimental group and post-test of the control group in kinematic variables (Angular displacement (θ)-Linear displacement (SR)- Angular velocity (ω)- Linear velocity (VR)-Linear acceleration (aR)) for the post-test of the experimental group.

4. Discussion

As table (1) indicated the existence of significant differences between the pre-test and the post-test of the experimental group at (0.05) level for the post-test in the special strength variables including (three consecutive springs speed – three right hops speed- three left hops speed- vertical jump) tests. The highest rate of change was for the vertical jump test with 16% percentage while, the lowest rate of change was for the three right hops speed test with 9.74% percentage.

In the instep kick level including (kicking accuracy – kicking time), the highest rate of change was for the kicking accuracy test with 58.30% percentage while , the least rate of change was for the kicking time test with 26.70% percentage that indicates the significant improvement in these variable in the post-test. This improvement is due to the training program containing special exercises to develop the special strength , clarifying that selecting the proper exercises allows coaches to develop the players physical and skill characteristics as well as these exercises took into account the correlation between the physical and skill sides considering the performance nature in soccer.

This agree with what (Burnett ,2004; Chek , 2001 ; Comana , 2004 ; Gaines ,2003 ; Jones ,2007; Schmitz , 2003 ; González, et. al. ,2012) have mentioned clarifying that the special strength development had contributed in significantly increasing hip and legs muscles strength. The researcher also believes that the instep kick requires a certain amount of strength to perform the kinetic performance of the kicking process besides organizing, guiding and distributing strength to produce the needed kinetic energy and successful kinetic performance.

According to the researcher this improvement in the instep kick represented by kicking accuracy and kicking time, is due to players ability on employing the gained strength in lower limb muscles participating in the instep kick in performing good kinetic transmission of the gained strength from leg to ankle to generate large quantity of movement in the instep to transmit to the soccer. Where, the kinetic resistance exercises associated with the performance shape and applied on the experimental group to improve the power and kinetic transmission for the muscular function to the muscular groups working in the instep kick.

The results in table (2) indicated the existence of significant differences between the pre-test and post-test of the experimental group at (0.05) level for the post-test in the kinematic variables including linear and angular displacement of the hip joint , angular velocity, Linear velocity and Linear acceleration. This improvement is significantly obvious during the movement preliminary stage which allows the player to increase the scale of the leg back swing and thus generate greater strength during primary of the instep kick. There is also an obvious improvement in the post-test over the pre-test in linear and angular displacement, Linear and angular velocity and Linear acceleration of the hip joint which indicates the transmission of large quantity of energy from hip to knee.

The linear and angular displacement, Linear and angular velocity and Linear acceleration of the ankle also showed an obvious improvement whereas, the largest angular displacement was during the preliminary stage while the largest Linear velocity was during the primary stage having the ankle speed greater than the hip and knee speed which indicate the transmission of the kinetic energy from hip to the knee to ankle which is considered the fastest point with larger linear acceleration than the hip and knee during this stage.

The researcher due the existence of significant differences for the post test to the training program that involves different exercises to develop the lower limb special strength and the instep kick performance level. These exercises concentrated on binding the physical characteristics with the performance nature through the speed and the accuracy needed by the performance. These results agrees with what (De Proft et, al., 1988 & Manolopoulos et. al.,2013) have mentioned clarifying that the speed of knee flexion and expansion is one of the major factors that influence soccer kicking skill.

As table (3) indicated the existence of significant differences between the pre-test and the post-test of the control group at (0.05) level for the post-test in the special strength variables. The highest rate of change was for the vertical jump test with 26.30 % percentage while, the lowest rate of change was for the three right hops speed test with 4.01 % percentage. In the instep kick level, the highest rate of change was for the kicking accuracy test with 23.31 % percentage while , the lowest rate of change was for the kicking time test with %8.47percentage that indicates a significant improvement in these variable in the post-test.

The results in table (4) indicated the existence of significant differences between the pre-test and post-test of the control group at (0.05) level for the post-test in the kinematic variables including angular displacement of the hip joint , angular velocity, linear velocity and linear acceleration. There is also an obvious significantly improvement for the post-test in the linear and angular displacement, Linear and angular velocity and Linear acceleration of the knee joint which , indicates the transmission of large quantity of energy from hip to knee. Also there is also an obvious significantly improvement for the post-test in the linear and angular displacement, Linear and angular velocity and Linear acceleration of the ankle joint.

The researcher due this improvement to the traditional training program that utilized the training methods and steps on the physical and skill characteristics, assuring that any scientifically rated training program must lead to an improvement in the physical and skill performance level except that the amount of improvement is the criterion between the two programs.

Table (5) indicated the existence of significant differences between the post-test of the experimental group and the post-test of the control group at (0.05) level for the post-test of the experimental group in the special strength variables. The highest rate of change was for the three consecutive springs speed test with %13.26 percentage while, the lowest rate of change was for the three right hops speed test with %4.93 percentage.

In the instep kick level, the highest rate of change was for the kicking accuracy test with %15.47 percentage while , the lowest rate of change was for the kicking time test with %7.57 percentage that indicates the obvious significant improvement in these variable in the post-test. This improvement in the kicking accuracy and time is due to the training program containing special exercises to develop the special strength, taking into account the correlation between the physical and skill sides considering the performance nature in soccer.

The researcher believes that through executing the kinetic resistance training program, exercises is performed with the maximum speed to commensurate with the special action of the soccer kinetic performance , which agree with what (Haghighi et.al., 2012; Harries et.al., 2012; Brown , 2000 ; Manolopoulos et. al., 2015 & Schmitz, 2003) have mentioned clarifying that most actions dedicated to the kinetic performance are performed at high speed and increasing the strength at high speed of the movement should lead to sportive performance increasing. The strength also should be organized, guided and distributed to produce the needed kinetic energy and have the successful kinetic performance.

The results in table (6) indicated the existence of significant differences between the post-test of the experimental group and the post-test of the control group at (0.05) level for the post-test of the experimental group in the kinematic variables under consideration. There is an obvious significantly improvement for the post-test in the linear and angular displacement, Linear and angular velocity and Linear acceleration of the hip joint, which is obvious during the preliminary stage and allows the player to increase the scale of the leg back swing and thus generate greater strength during the primary stage. There is also an obvious improvement in the post-test over the pre-test in linear and angular displacement, Linear and angular velocity and Linear acceleration of the hip joint achieving the highest and angular displacement and angular velocity of the hip joint in the primary stage. While, the linear velocity of the knee joint was greater than the Linear velocity of the hip joint of the experimental group indicating the transmission of large quantity of energy from hip to knee.

The experimental group has achieved significant superiority over the control group in linear and angular displacement, Linear velocity and Linear acceleration of the ankle. The highest angular displacement was in the preliminary stage and the highest linear velocity was in the primary stage whereas the ankle speed was greater than the hip and knee during this stage indicating the transmission of kinetic energy from hip to knee to ankle to be the fastest point during the primary stage. The ankle also gained the highest linear acceleration during the primary stage a lot more exceeding the hip and knee.

Table (6) indicates that linear velocity outcome average during performance stages of the instep, the highest speed outcome was at the moment of impact with the ball and the lowest speed outcome was at the maximal back swing. Considering the knee, the the highest speed outcome was at the maximal back swing and the lowest speed outcome was at the moment of impact with the ball and finally for the hip, the the highest speed outcome was at the maximal back swing and the lowest speed outcome was at the maximal forward swing.

These previous results agree with what (Masuda et.al., 2005 & Manolopoulos et.al.,2006) have mentioned clarifying that the instep kick is one of the open kinetic chain skills that requires good kinetic transmission to produce the largest possible quantity of speed and strength though the movement of the chain parts to the end of the chain.

This also agrees with what (Barfield ,1998 & Manolopoulos et.al., 2013) have reached clarifying that the muscles activities levels was higher during the kicking whereas the maximum hip and knee muscles activities happened through the final stage which increase one more time before the moment of impact with the ball.

5. Conclusions

Believing of the important role and impact of kinetic resistance trainings on enhancing soccer players abilities specially soccer juniors concerning the special strength and effective kinematic variables in instep kick, the researcher have introduced this research. Through this research, the researcher investigated the effect of kinetic resistance trainings and technique on special strength level and effective kinematic variables in instep kick for soccer juniors. The experiment results indicated that the kinetic resistance training and technique have achieved positive change in the special strength level, in the instep kick accuracy and time and kinematic variables affecting the instep kick of soccer juniors. From these results the researcher strongly recommended that coaches need to pay attention to developing special strength through having kinetic resistance exercises and good technique as an essential part of soccer juniors special strength training programs. The researcher also recommended to depend on kinematic variables affecting performance to recognize the improvement amount in performance as a result of kinetic resistance exercises and technique.

References

Barfield, B. (1998). The Kinetic of Kicking in Soccer. *Clinicsin Sports Medicine*,17(4),711-728.

Brown, L. (2000). *Isokinetics In Human Performance*. (1st ed.). Human Kinetics, USA.

Burnett, A. (2004). The Biomechanics of Jumping. [Online] Available: www.coachsinfo.com. (October, 15,2015).

Cabri, J., De Proft, E., Dufour, W. & Clarys, J. (1988). The Relation between Muscular Strength and Kick Performance. *Science and Football. Eds: Reilly, T., Lees, A., Davids, K. and Murphy, W. London: E & FN Spon*. 186-193.

Chek, P. (2001). Big Bang Exercise. IDEA Fitness Edge, 8-10. [Online] Available: http://www.ideafit.com/fitness-products/big-bang-exercises. (October, 1, 2015).

Comana, F. (2004). *Function Training For Sports*. (1st ed.). Human Kinetics. Champaign IL, England.

De Proft, E., Cabri, J, Dufour, W, Clarys, J. (1988). Strength Training and Kick Performance in Soccer Players. *Reilly T, Lees A, Davids K, Murphy WJ, eds. Science and football. London: E & FN Spon*, 109 –113.

El-Berawe, E. & Shady. A. (2013). Effectiveness of Special Strength Training on Some Physical and Kinetic Parameters Affecting Instep Kick For Soccer Juniors. *Theories & Applications the International Edition*, 3(2), 146-155.

Evans, M. (1997). *Endurance Athlete'S Edge*. Human Kinetics, USA.

Gaines, S. (2003). *Benefits and Limitations of Quality Exercise, Vertex Fitness* . NESTA , USA.

Ghigiarelli, J., Nagle, E., Gross, F., Robertson, R. , Irrgang, J. , & Myslinski, T. (2009). The effects of a 7-week heavy elastic band and weight chain program on upper-body strength and upper-body power in a sample of division 1-AA football players. *The Journal of Strength & Conditioning Research, 23*(3), 756-764.

González-Badillo, J. J., Pareja-Blanco, F., Rodríguez-Rosell, D., Abad-Herencia, J. L., del Ojo-López, J. J., & Sánchez-Medina, L. (2015). Effects of Velocity-Based Resistance Training on Young Soccer Players of Different Ages. *The Journal of Strength & Conditioning Research*, 29(5), 1329-1338.

Haghighi, A., Moghadasi, M., Nikseresht, A., Torkfar, A &Haghighi, M. (2012). Effects Of Plyometric Versus Resistance Training On Sprint And Skill Performance In Young Soccer Players. *European Journal of Experimental Biology*, 2 (6),2348-235.

Harries, S., Lubans, D. & Callister, R. (2012). Resistance Training To Improve Power And Sports Performance In Adolescent Athletes: A Systematic Review And Meta-Analysis. *Journal of Science and Medicine in Sport* ,15, 532–540.

Inoue, K. , Nunome, H. , Sterzing, T., Shinkai, H. & Ikegami, Y. (2012). Kinetic Analysis of the Support Leg in Soccer Instep Kicking. *30th Annual Conference of Biomechanics in Sports, Melbourne*, 1(1).

Jones, R. (2007). Functional Training. Introduction. Reebo Santana, Jose Carlos Uni. USA, 9-15. [Online] Available: http://ronjones.org/Handouts/FT1-Intro&Assessment.pdf

Keshk, M. & Elbosaty, A. (2000). *Skill and Tactic Preparation Foundations In Soccer (Juniors-Adults)*. (1st ed.). *Mansoura*.

Manolopoulos, E., Gissis, I, Galazoulas, C., Manolopoulos, E., Patikas, D., Gollhofer, A. &Kotzamanidis, C. (2016). The Effect of Combined Sensorimotor-Resistance Training On Strength, Balance and Jumping Performance of Soccer Players. *In Journal of Strength & Conditioning Research*. 30 (1): 53-9.

Manolopoulos, E., Katis, A., Manolopoulos, K., Kalapotharakos, V. & Kellis, E. (2013). Effects of a 10-Week Resistance Exercise Program on Soccer Kick Biomechanics and Muscle Strength. *Journal of Strength & Conditioning Research*, 27(12), 3391–3401.

Manolopoulos, E., Papadopoulos, C. & Kellis, E. (2006). Effects of Combined Strength And Kick Coordination Training On Soccer Kick Kinetic in Amateur Players. *Scandinavian Journal of Medicine & Science in Sports*.16(2), 102-110.

Masuda, K., Kikuhara, N., Demura, S., Katsuta, S. & Yamanaka, K. (2005). Relationship between Muscle Strength In Various Isokinetic Movements And Kick Performance Among Soccer Players. *J. sports med. Phys. Fitness*, 45, 44-52.

Moran, G. & Glynn, G. (2000). *Dynamics Of Strength Trining And Conditioning*. (3rd ed.). Wcb Mc Grow, Hill, New York, USA.

Noguchi, T., Demura, S. & Nagasawa, Y. (2012). Relationship between Ball Kick Velocity and Leg Strength: A Comparison between Soccer Players and Other Athletes. *SciRes* 2(3),95-98.

Perrin, D. (1993).*Isokinetic Exercise and assessment* . (1st ed.). Human Kinetics , USA.

Reilly, T. & Williams, A. (2003). *Science and Soccer*. (2nd ed.). Taylor & Francis e-Library.

Roberts, S. & Weider, B. (1994). *Strength and Weight Training For Young Athletes Contemporary*, (1st ed.). Book 5 Inc Publisher, Chicago USA.

Schmitz, D. (2003). *Quality Training Pyramids*. New Truer High School, Kinetic Wellness Department, USA.

Resistance Bands. [Online] Available:http://myosource.com/kinetic-bands-leg-resistance-exercise-bands/.(October, 2, 2015).

Caffeine Alters Blood Potassium and Catecholamine Concentrations but not the Perception of Pain and Fatigue with a 1 km Cycling Sprint

Dean M. Cordingley (Corresponding author)
Pan Am Clinic Foundation, 75 Poseidon Bay, Winnipeg R3M 3E4, Canada
E-mail: dcordingley@panamclinic.com

Gordon J. Bell
Faculty of Physical Education & Recreation, University of Alberta, Edmonton T6G 2H9, Canada
E-mail: Gordon.bell@ualberta.ca

Daniel G. Syrotuik
Faculty of Physical Education & Recreation, University of Alberta, Edmonton T6G 2H9, Canada
E-mail: dan.syrotuik@ualberta.ca

Abstract

Background: Caffeine has been used by some athletes to improve short-term high-intensity exercise performance; however, the literature is equivocal. **Objectives:** The objective of this study was to investigate the effects of caffeine on plasma potassium and catecholamine concentrations, pain and fatigue perception, to determine whether potassium ion handling and altered perception related to the central nervous system are associated with enhanced performance during a 1 km cycling time trial. **Methods:** Thirteen well trained men with a mean age of 27 ± 6 yrs (body mass: 76.4 ± 6.4 kg, height: 180 ± 7 cm, and $\dot{V}O_2$ max: 57.5 ± 4.6 $ml \cdot kg^{-1} \cdot min^{-1}$) were recruited. Participants were randomized to a caffeine (5 $mg \cdot kg^{-1}$) or a placebo condition using a double blind, cross over design. **Results:** Caffeine had no significant effects on the 1 km time-trial performance indicators of time (82.1 ± 2.4 vs. 81.9 ± 3.9s), peak (633.0 ± 83.6 vs. 638.7 ± 110.1 watts) or average power (466.0 ± 37.3 vs. 467.5 ± 59.9 watts; caffeine and placebo conditions respectively). In addition, caffeine had no significant effect on oxygen consumption ($\dot{V}O_2$) (4.11 ± 0.24 vs 4.06 ± 0.29 L), the perception of pain (5.6 ± 2.4 vs. 5.5 ± 2.6) or fatigue (7.1 ± 1.8 vs.7.1 ± 1.8: caffeine and placebo conditions respectively). There was a significantly greater increase in post-exercise blood lactate ($p<0.05$) and catecholamines ($p<0.05$) as well as a lower pre-exercise blood potassium concentration ($p<0.05$) in the caffeine condition. **Conclusions:** The results suggest that caffeine can enhance certain metabolic parameters, but these changes were unable to augment short-distance (1km), high-intensity cycling performance.

Keywords: ergogenic, anaerobic exercise, performance, oxygen consumption

1. Introduction

1.1 Review of Literature

Caffeine has been used as a supplement to improve exercise performance of various durations and intensities. Caffeine is ergogenic for aerobic (Bridge & Jones, 2006; Cox et al., 2002; Graham et al., 1998; Ivy et al., 2009) and anaerobic events (Anderson et al., 2000; Anselme et al., 1992; Wiles et al., 2006; Wiles et al, 1992). The two most widely accepted hypotheses supporting the purported ergogenic properties of caffeine have been associated with changes in peripheral potassium ion handling and an altered central nervous system perception (Davis & Green, 2009; Doherty, Smith, Davison, & Hughes, 2002; Greer, McLean, & Graham, 1998). A decrease in plasma potassium during aerobic exercise has been used to indirectly indicate maintenance of the sodium/potassium electrochemical gradient in skeletal muscle, permitting the muscle to maintain the force of contraction better under fatiguing conditions (Davis & Green, 2009; Lindinger et al, 1993; Spriet & Howlett, 2000). However, little research has investigated the effects of caffeine on plasma potassium levels after short-term high-intensity exercise (Davis & Green, 2009).

Caffeine also influences the central nervous system via an increase in catecholamines (Berkowitz et al., 1970) that were greater during high intensity anaerobic exercise compared to placebo (Bell et al., 2001; Doherty et al., 2002; Greer et al., 1998). Caffeine also inhibits adenosine receptors in smooth and skeletal muscle (Lynge & Hellsten, 2000; Smith, 2003) which can reduce the perception of exercise-induced pain (Davis & Green, 2009; Spriet & Howlett, 2000).

Previous work by Wiles et al. (2006) showed that pre-race caffeine consumption can improve 1 km cycling time trial performance, but did not attempt to elicit the mechanism by which caffeine acts. The combination of decreased plasma potassium coupled with diminished perceived pain and fatigue with increases in plasma catecholamines and caffeine's antagonistic effect on adenosine receptors may contribute to enhanced short-term high-intensity exercise performance.

1.2 Purpose of the Study

The purpose of this study was to investigate the effects of caffeine on pain and fatigue perception, plasma catecholamine and potassium concentrations to determine whether altered central nervous system perception and/or potassium ion handling were associated with any changes in performance during a 1 km cycling time trial in trained cyclists. It was hypothesized that caffeine supplementation would produce a faster 1 km time-trial in conjunction with both a lower pain and fatigue ratings coupled with an increase in plasma catecholamines and attenuated increases in plasma potassium compared to placebo.

2. Methods

2.1 Participants

Thirteen trained males (age: 27 ± 6 yrs, body mass: 76.4 ± 6.4 kg, height: 180 ± 7 cm, and $\dot{V}O_2$ max: 57.5 ± 4.6 $ml \cdot kg^{-1} \cdot min^{-1}$) with cycling experience were recruited from a University student population and various local cycling clubs. All participants were habituated caffeine users. Each participant was screened using the Physical Activity Readiness Questionnaire (PAR-Q), a participant information letter and an orientation meeting where all study procedures were verbally explained. Written consent was obtained at pre-screening and all procedures were approved by a University Research Ethics Board.

2.2 Experimental Design

A randomized double-blind, crossover design was utilized requiring all participants to complete both placebo and experimental (caffeine) conditions on separate days after a washout period. The data was collected over three separate visits to the laboratory, with a minimum seven days recovery between each visit.

2.3 Procedures

During session 1, the participants arrived at the lab to familiarize themselves with the procedures of the study. Following this, a graded exercise test (GXT) was performed on a Velotron stationary cycle (Racer Mate, Seattle, WA, U.S.A.) to determine maximal oxygen consumption ($\dot{V}O_{2\ max}$). The GXT was done to determine a power output equivalent to 20% of the participant's $\dot{V}O_{2\ max}$ which was used to prescribe the intensity of the recovery exercise following the 1 km cycling time trial. The GXT began at a power output of 100 watts which was increased by 25 watts every minute until volitional exhaustion (Elliott & Grace, 2010). Expired gases were collected and analyzed for O_2 and CO_2 with a metabolic cart (Parvo Medics TrueOne 2400, Utah) that was previously calibrated for volume of air as well as before and after each test with known gas concentrations. Heart rate was recorded every minute from a heart rate monitor (Polar Electro, Finland). $\dot{V}O_{2\ max}$ was determined as the point at which there was a peak and plateau in oxygen uptake (< 100mL/min) with increasing power output or duration of exercise that was also associated with secondary criteria including a respiratory exchange ratio (RER) greater than 1.1, a heart rate ≥ age-predicted maximum and volitional exhaustion (Howley et al., 1995). Each participant was fitted to the Velotron cycle by adjusting the vertical and horizontal position of the seat and handle bars to mimic their own racing bicycle and cycling shoes/pedal combination. These measurements were recorded for replication during the subsequent experimental trials. Each participant was instructed on the same basic strategy for performing the 1 kilometer time-trial and completed one practice time-trial. On departure from the familiarization session, subjects were instructed to avoid all forms of caffeine, alcohol and intense physical activity for 24 hours prior to the experimental trials. The subjects were asked to record and subsequently consume the same meals the day prior to both experimental sessions.

Sessions 2 and 3 were separated by 7 to 10 days to allow for appropriate wash-out with subjects arriving at the lab between 7 and 10am. A blood sample of 10 mL was taken via venipuncture at rest, by an individual trained in this procedure. Each subject then consumed a randomly assigned treatment of either a flavored, non-caloric placebo drink (500 ml of water with Crystal Light, Kraft Canada) or caffeine (Life Brand, Shoppers Drug Mart, Canada) at a serving of 5 $mg \cdot kg^{-1}$ body mass (Graham, 2001) dissolved in 500 ml of the same flavored drink as the placebo. Following consumption of the drink, each subject rested 1 hour, which has been previously shown to be an effective duration for caffeine absorption into the blood stream (Wiles et al., 2006). The cycle ergometer was set-up according to the previously determined measurements and preferred riding position for each participant. Twenty five minutes before the 1 km time trial began, an intravenous catheter was inserted into a forearm vein by a registered nurse. The site was kept patent with 0.5 ml of sterile saline (0.9% NaCl) and prior to every blood sample, a small (2-3 ml) blood sample was drawn and discarded to ensure that any saline was removed. A 10 ml blood sample was then drawn prior to the 10 minute warm-up consisting of a self-selected sub-maximal intensity but with three prescribed, 5 second sprint intervals included at specific time points. This warm-up protocol was followed by a 5 minute period for the subjects to perform light dynamic stretching and recover with an additional 5 minute period for set up and preparation of the metabolic cart. The warm-up was monitored and remained the same for both experimental trials. Subsequently, another blood sample of 10 ml was taken immediately before the 1 km time-trial.

During both 1 km time-trials, participants were provided with consistent verbal encouragement to provide an all-out effort that would mimic a "race". Subjects were also provided with a visual marker on a computer monitor indicating the distance through the 1 km time-trial. The participants were not provided with the time of performance at any point throughout or following the 1 km time-trial. The selected cycle gear ratio was 48/14, which elicited a speed of 40 kilometers per hour at 90 rpm on the Velotron similar to that reported by Wiles et al. (2006). Expired gases were collected during and for 5 minutes after the time trials and analyzed for O_2 and CO_2 with the same calibrated metabolic cart. Following the 1km time trial, 10 ml blood samples were taken immediately after or as soon as feasibly possible, and at 5, 10 and 15 minutes of recovery. The subjects completed a standardized recovery that consisted of cycling at an intensity equivalent to 20% of the individual's $\dot{V}O_{2\,max}$ for 5 minutes followed by a passive recovery sitting on a chair. Following the 5 minute active recovery, the subjects completed the categorical Pain Perception Scale (Cook et al., 1998) and visual analogue fatigue scales (Egerton et al., 2009) while seated.

2.3.1 Blood procedures & Assays

The blood samples were collected in 10 ml syringes and a few drops of blood were immediately placed in an EG7+ cartridge for an Abbot Point of Care i-STAT hand held analyzer (Abbott Laboratories, New Jersey) for the determination of pH and electrolyte analysis. Also, 0.25 ml of whole blood was immediately pipetted into a disposable culture tube containing 8% perchloric acid and vortexed for 30 seconds for deproteinization. The remaining blood was placed in a test-tube coated in ethylenediaminetetraacetic acid (EDTA). The deproteinized and EDTA treated blood tubes were subsequently centrifuged for 10 minutes at 1500 xg in a refrigerated centrifuge (4°C) and then aliquoted into microcentrifuge tubes and frozen immediately at -20°C and then transferred to a -80°C ultra-low freezer until the lab analyses were performed. Blood lactate concentration was determined from the mean of duplicate samples using a standard spectrophotometric assay (Gutmann & Wahlefeld, 1974). Epinephrine and norepinephrine were determined in duplicate using an enzyme-linked immunosorbent assay kit (ELISA) (Rocky Mountain Diagnostics Inc, Colorado Springs, CO).

2.3.2 Data and Statistical Analysis

Sample size was calculated a priori using the primary outcome of performance time. An effect size of 0.82 was calculated (Wiles et al., 2006) with $\alpha = 0.05$ and power set at 80%, requiring a minimum of 12 participants per group. Data from the 2 experimental trials were compared using a two-way ANOVA with repeated measures on both factors (experimental condition by time). A paired t-test was performed to test for mean differences between the 1 km performance time, power output, fatigue and pain. If a significant F-ratio was determined, a Newman-Keuls multiple comparison procedure was performed. Results were considered significant at $P \leq 0.05$ for all statistical analyses. All data are means ± standard deviation unless otherwise noted. Statistica, version 8.0 (StatsSoft Inc., Tulsa, OK) was used to perform all statistical analyses. Four subjects had missing data points for potassium and pH concentrations due to instrument and/or user error and were removed from the statistical analyses of these variables.

3. Results

3.1 Performance Measures

Caffeine ingestion did not improve time (caffeine vs. placebo: 82.1 ± 2.4 vs. 81.9 ± 3.9 seconds), peak power output (caffeine vs. placebo: 633.0 ± 83.6 vs. 638.7 ± 110.1 watts) or average power output (caffeine vs. placebo: 466.0 ± 37.3 vs. 467.5 ± 59.9 watts) during the 1 km cycling time trial.

3.2 Perceived Pain and Fatigue:

The numerical pain scale revealed that caffeine did not reduce perceived pain immediately following a 1 km cycling time-trial (caffeine vs. placebo: 5.6 ± 2.4 vs. 5.5 ± 2.6). The fatigue visual analogue scales revealed that caffeine ingestion did not attenuate leg fatigue (caffeine vs. placebo: 7.1 ± 1.4 vs. 7.4 ± 2.0) or overall fatigue (caffeine vs. placebo: 7.1 ± 1.8 vs. 7.1 ± 1.8) compared to the placebo condition.

3.3 Blood Variables

Blood lactate concentrations were significantly increased post exercise in both the caffeine and placebo condition when compared to pre-1 km cycling time-trial concentrations. Caffeine ingestion caused a greater increase ($p<0.05$; Figure 1) in blood lactate concentrations 0, 5 and 15 minutes post-1 km cycling time-trial compared to the placebo condition.

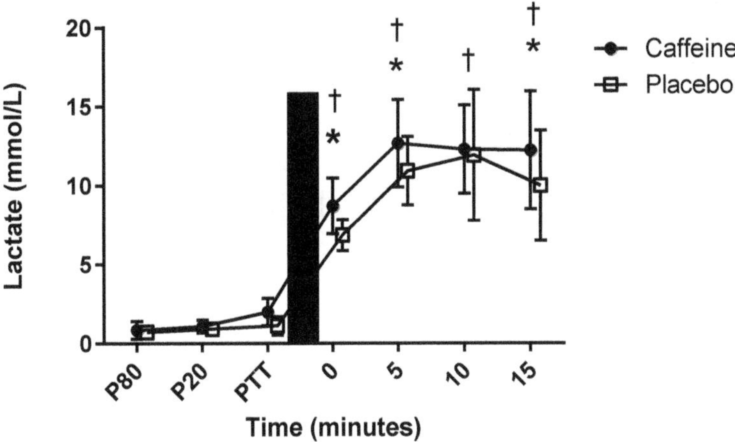

Figure 1. Blood lactate responses (mean ± SD; n=13) prior to and during recovery from cycling 1 km after consuming caffeine or placebo. P80 = 80 minutes pre-time trial; P20 = 20 minutes pre-time trial; PTT=immediate pre-time trial; TT= 1 km time trial. * Significant difference between caffeine condition and placebo, $p<0.05$. †both caffeine and placebo conditions are significantly different from all pre time trial measures.

Caffeine significantly attenuated blood potassium concentrations immediately prior to the 1 km cycling time-trial compared to the placebo condition (Figure 2). Blood potassium levels were elevated ($p<0.05$) immediately following the 1 km cycling time-trial in both the caffeine and placebo conditions compared to pre-exercise levels.

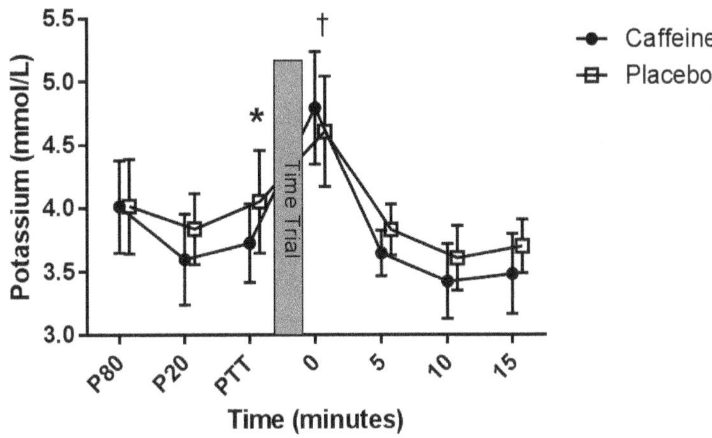

Figure 2. Blood potassium responses (mean ± SD; n=9) prior to and during recovery from cycling 1 km after consuming caffeine or placebo. P80 = 80 minutes pre-time trial; P20 = 20 minutes pre-time trial; PTT=immediate pre-time trial; TT= 1 km time trial. * Significant difference between caffeine condition and placebo, $p<0.05$. † Significant difference from all other time points.

Blood pH was significantly higher pre-exercise compared to all time points post-exercise in both the caffeine and placebo conditions. Caffeine consumption did not differentially alter pH levels at any time point when compared with the placebo condition (Figure 3).

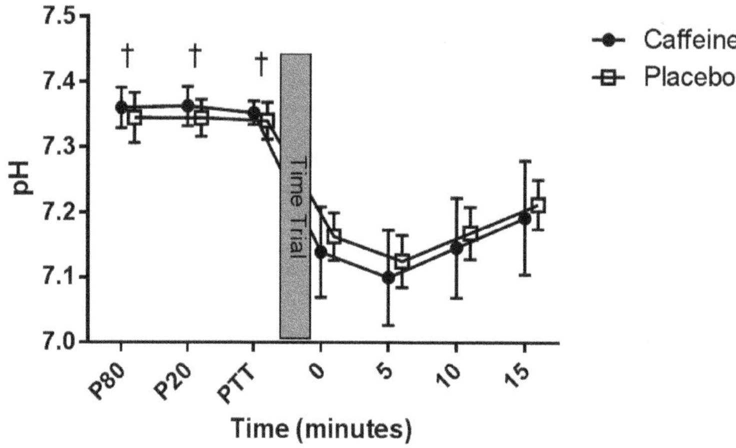

Figure 3. Blood pH responses (mean ± SD; n=9) prior to and during recovery from cycling 1 km after consuming caffeine or placebo. P80 = 80 minutes pre-time trial; P20 = 20 minutes pre-time trial; PTT=immediate pre-time trial; TT= 1 km time trial. † both caffeine and placebo conditions are significantly different from all post time trial measures.

Epinephrine concentration in the blood was significantly increased immediately post-exercise as well as 5 minutes post-exercise compared to all pre-exercise time points, the 10 minute post-exercise and the 15 minute post-exercise time points in both placebo and caffeine conditions. Epinephrine concentration was significantly higher in the caffeine trial immediately following the 1 km cycling time-trial as well as 5 minutes post-exercise when compared to the placebo condition (Figure 4).

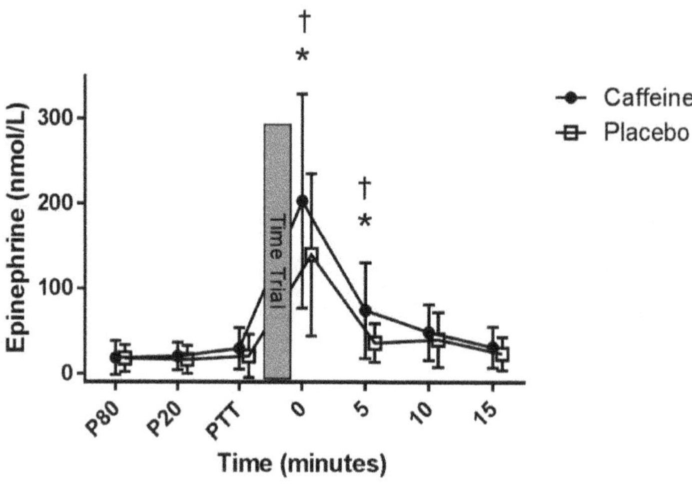

Figure 4. Blood epinephrine (Epi) responses (mean ± SD; n=13) prior to and during recovery from cycling 1 km after consuming caffeine or placebo. P80 = 80 minutes pre-time trial; P20 = 20 minutes pre-time trial; PTT=immediate pre-time trial; TT= 1 km time trial. * Significant difference between caffeine condition and placebo, $p<0.05$. † significantly different than all other time points.

Immediately post-exercise, as well as 5 minutes and 10 minutes post-exercise, norepinephrine concentrations were increased in the blood when compared to all pre-exercise time points in both the caffeine and placebo conditions ($p<0.05$). Caffeine consumption increased norepinephrine concentrations immediately following the 1 km cycling time-trial as well as 5 minutes post-exercise greater than the placebo condition (Figure 5).

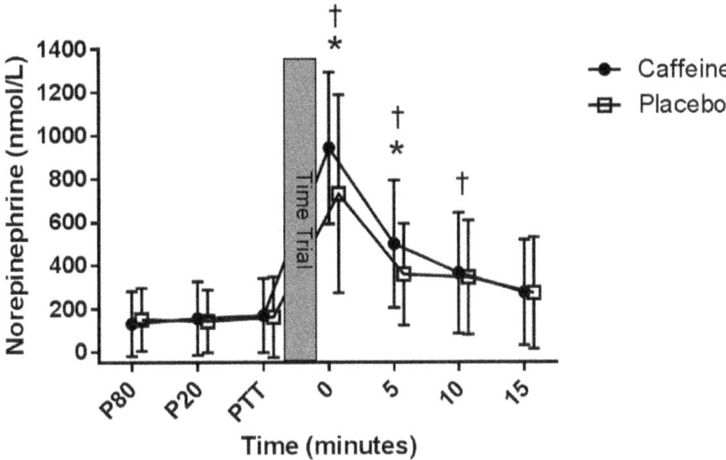

Figure 5. Blood norepinephrine (Nor) responses (mean ± SD; n=13) prior to and during recovery from cycling 1 km after consuming caffeine or placebo. P80 = 80 minutes pre-time trial; P20 = 20 minutes pre-time trial; PTT=immediate pre-time trial; TT= 1 km time trial. * Significant difference between caffeine condition and placebo, p<0.05. † both caffeine and placebo conditions significantly different from pre time trial measure.

3.4 Oxygen Consumption

There was a significant increase in VO_2 during the time trial, peaking at 53.1 and 52.2 $ml \cdot kg^{1} \cdot min^{1}$ for caffeine and placebo conditions representing 92% and 91% of $VO_{2\ max}$, respectively. Caffeine had no significant effect on VO_2 prior to or during the time trial, and despite VO_2 being slightly higher during recovery in the caffeine condition, the response was not significant (Table 1).

Table 1. Oxygen uptake (VO_2; L) before, during and throughout recovery from the 1 km time trial (TT). Values are mean ± SD.

Condition	VO_2 (L) 1 min before the 1 km TT	Total VO_2 (L) during the 1 km TT	5 min total recovery VO_2 (L)
Caffeine	0.49 ± 0.12	4.11 ± 0.24*	10.09 ± 1.26**
Placebo	0.49 ±0.09	4.06 ± 0.29*	9.86 ± 1.33**

* significantly higher than before the 1 km TT, P<0.05.

** significantly higher than before and during the 1km TT, P<0.05.

4. Discussion

Athletes in a variety of sports consume caffeine and products containing caffeine to enhance their exercise performance (Burke, 2008; Spriet, 2014). Caffeine's ability to improve longer duration aerobic activities (i.e., > 5 minutes) is well established while caffeine's effects on short-term high-intensity activities are less conclusive (Davis & Green, 2009). This study examined whether caffeine supplementation would produce a faster 1 km time trial in conjunction with both a lower perceived pain and fatigue rating coupled with an increase in plasma catecholamine concentrations and attenuated increases in plasma potassium concentrations, when compared to a placebo condition. The findings of this study demonstrated that caffeine ingestion, at a dose of 5 $mg \cdot kg^{-1}$ body mass, did not elicit improved performance time, peak power or average power output during a 1 km cycling time-trial. These findings corroborate previous research which also found no performance improvements in short term high intensity exercise combined with caffeine supplementation (Buck et al., 2015; Crowe et al., 2006; Greer et al., 1998). However, Sokmen et al. (2008) has reported that caffeine has ergogenic benefits for repeated bouts of high-intensity exercise ranging in duration from 15 seconds to 3 minutes.

The present study contradicts Wiles et al. (2006) which found a 3% greater improvement in 1 km cycling time-trial performance following 5 $mg \cdot kg^{-1}$ caffeine ingestion. It is important to note that the performance times reported by this latter study (average caffeine time = 71.1 seconds; average placebo time = 73.4 seconds) were much faster than in the present study (82.1 ± 2.4 vs. 81.9 ± 3.9 seconds for the caffeine and placebo conditions, respectively), which might suggest that the improvement in performance times noted by Wiles et al. (2006) might be due to a higher fitness levels of their participants. In support of this contention, Collomp et al. (1992) reported significantly greater sprint swim performance in trained but not recreational swimmers after the ingestion of 250 mg of caffeine. Therefore, the ergogenic benefits of caffeine may be partially dependent on fitness level. Despite this, the participants in the present study were well trained and it remains to be determined whether the fitness status of the individual and previous experience with sprint cycling interacts with the beneficial effects of caffeine on exercise performance. Furthermore, whether or not there is a particular physiological profile of trained muscle that promotes an ergogenic effect during high-intensity short-term exercise with caffeine consumption is unknown, warranting further investigation.

There was no difference in the rating of perceived pain between caffeine and placebo conditions. These findings corroborate Astorino et al. (2011), which used the same pain scale as the current study and found that caffeine did not decrease the perception of pain during a high intensity, knee extension exercise protocol. As well, overall fatigue and fatigue localized to the legs were unaltered with caffeine supplementation in the current study. A possible explanation for this lack of apparent change in perceived pain or fatigue with the caffeine may have been related to waiting 5 minutes after the cycling time trial to complete the pain and fatigue scales. This delay was for logistical reasons since the participants were still attached to the metabolic measurement system for the 5 minute active recovery portion of the experiment. As a result, any effect of caffeine on the perception of pain and fatigue that the subjects experienced during or at the very end of the 1 km time-trial may have been missed.

Caffeine ingestion caused a significant elevation of blood lactate concentration after exercise compared to placebo, which is consistent with previous findings (Bridge & Jones, 2006; Glaister et al., 2012). Lactate concentrations were significantly increased immediately after and 5 and 15 minutes post-exercise with caffeine ingestion compared to placebo. These results support previous studies, which found caffeine to increase post-exercise lactate concentrations greater than placebo (Anselme et al., 1992; Bridge & Jones, 2006; Collomp et al., 1992; Cox et al., 2002; Davis & Green, 2009; Graham, 2001; Graham et al., 1998; Greer et al., 1998; Ivy et al., 2009). The increase in blood lactate may be due to caffeine inhibiting lactate clearance (Graham, 2001), or catecholamines stimulating glycolysis (Cheetham et al., 1986) which might help explain the observed increase in blood lactate without increased performance in the present study.

The findings of the present study confirmed that plasma potassium levels increase with high intensity exercise with the greatest increases occurring immediately following the 1 km simulated cycling time-trial. In the present study, caffeine consumption elicited a significantly attenuated plasma potassium concentration compared to the placebo condition following the 10 minute warm up which may have been due to caffeine's ability to accelerate muscle potassium handling (Mohr et al., 2011). Mohr et al. (2011) suggested that caffeine may stimulate the Na^+-K^+ pump indirectly through increased catecholamine response and increased glucose concentrations, or directly in muscle and this may occur even in anticipation of exercise. The ability to maintain forceful muscle contractions at a high frequency is partly dependent on the cycling of potassium from the interstitial space back into the muscle cell following a muscle contraction (Green, 1997). The initial attenuation of potassium efflux with caffeine supplementation may allow for increased cellular concentrations during the early stages of exercise potentially improving sprint performance; however, performance was not altered in the present study.

In the present study high intensity exercise elicited a plasma catecholamine response immediately following and 5 minutes after the 1 km simulated cycling time-trial and, in addition, norepinephrine was still increased 10 minutes following the time-trial. These findings were consistent with the results of (Zouhal et al., 2008), who reported an increase in catecholamine concentrations with exercise that were closely related to intensity. Caffeine supplementation significantly increased both epinephrine and norepinephrine concentrations immediately following as well as 5 minutes subsequent to the 1 km simulated cycling time-trial, to a greater extent than in the placebo condition. These findings support previous research following high intensity anaerobic exercise (Bell et al., 2001; Doherty et al., 2002; Greer et al., 1998). The increase in both epinephrine and norepinephrine plasma concentrations with caffeine supplementation may suggest a greater stimulus to the central nervous system. However, it is difficult to discern whether the increased epinephrine and norepinephrine concentrations in blood were due to caffeine directly stimulating the adrenal gland, thus enhancing catecholamine production (Berkowitz et al., 1970), or from the suggested blocking mechanism of the adenosine receptors (Smith, 2003). Furthermore, although catecholamines increased with acute caffeine supplementation, there was no associated elevation in VO_2 during the time trial or excess post-exercise oxygen consumption (EPOC) following the time trial.

4.1 Limitations

There are some limitations to the present study worth noting. Although there were some significant differential effects of caffeine compared to placebo on several variables, there was no ergogenic benefit to a 1 km lab based cycling time trial. One aforementioned reason for this may have been due to the fitness level and/or experience of the participants with the 1 km time trials. In addition, although participants had orientations for familiarization to the 1 km simulated cycling time-trial and were instructed to perform an all-out effort, a different or a change in pacing strategy may have confounded the results of this study (Glaister et al., 2012). A change in pacing strategy may have masked the ergogenic effects of caffeine. However, the experimental trials were randomly ordered and an order effect analysis revealed that there was not a significant difference between 1 km finish times between experimental sessions. Although the group mean for the 1 km cycling performance time was not significantly improved, there may have been a person-by-treatment effect for caffeine ingestion since 8 of the 13 (62%) participants in the present study performed a faster 1 km sprint under the caffeine condition (1.1 ± 1.0 seconds). This novel result is also supported by Astorino et al. (2011), who reported meaningful increases in total load lifted in four sets of 70-80% of 1RM during 3 upper and 1 lower body resistance training exercise to failure after the consumption of 6 mg•kg^{-1} of caffeine in 9 of 14 of their participants. Certainly additional research is required to confirm this responder phenomenon and variability between individuals.

5. Conclusion

The results of this study suggest that caffeine ingestion at a dose of 5 $mg \cdot kg^{-1}$ body mass did not improve a lab-based 1 km cycling time-trial performance. Consumption of caffeine prior to a 1 km simulated cycling time-trial did, however, attenuate potassium levels in plasma prior to the sprint performance and increased post-exercise blood catecholamine and lactate levels compared to a placebo condition. These metabolic changes were not reflected in an improved 1 km performance or change in oxygen consumption. Despite the lack of statistical significance for 1 km performance times between the caffeine and placebo conditions, there did appear to be a person-by-treatment effect, with 8 out of 13 subjects improving their performance times. This information is important for sprint cyclists who may supplement with caffeine expecting performance enhancements as some may benefit from its ingestion and others may not. However, based on the group mean performance times, caffeine consumption prior to a 1 km simulated cycling time-trial did not produce an ergogenic effect.

Acknowledgments

This study was designed by DC, GB and DS; data collection was performed by DC, GB and DS; data analyses and interpretation was completed by DC and GB; manuscript preparation was completed by DC, GB and DS. The authors would like to thank Dr. Scott Forbes for his assistance with data collection and manuscript preparation, and Andrea Faid for her phlebotomy skills. Funding for this research was provided by the Sport Science Association of Alberta (SSAA) through the Alberta Sport, Recreation, Parks and Wildlife Foundation.

References

Anderson, M. E., Bruce, C. R., Fraser, S. F., Stepto, N. K., Hopkins, W. G., & Hawley, J. A. (2000). Improved 2000-meter rowing performance in competitive oarswomen after caffeine ingestion. *International Journal of Sport Nutrition & Exercise Metabolism, 10*(4), 464–475.

Anselme, F., Collomp, K., Mercier, B., Ahmaidi, S., & Prefaut, C. (1992). Caffeine increases maximal anaerobic power and blood lactate concentration. *European Journal of Applied Physiology*, *65*(2), 188–191.

Astorino, T. A., Martin, B. J., Schachtsiek, L., Wong, K., & Karno, N. (2011). Minimal effect of acute caffeine ingestion on intense resistance training performance. *Journal of Strength and Conditioning Research*, *25*(6), 1752–1758.

Astorino, T. A., Terzi, M. N., Roberson, D. W., & Burnett, T. R. (2011). Effect of Caffeine Intake on Pain Perception During High-Intensity Exercise. *International Journal of Sport Nutrition & Exercise Metabolism*, *21*(1), 27–32.

Bell, D. G., Jacobs, I., & Ellerington, K. (2001). Effect of caffeine and ephedrine ingestion on anaerobic exercise performance. *Medicine & Science in Sports & Exercise*, *33*(8), 1399–1403.

Berkowitz, B. A., Tarver, J. H., & Spector, S. (1970). Release of Norepinephrine in the Central Nervous System by Theophylline and Caffeine. *European Journal of Pharmacology*, *10*, 64–71.

Bridge, C. A., & Jones, M. A. (2006). The effect of caffeine ingestion on 8 km run performance in a field setting. *Journal of Sports Sciences*, *24*(4), 433–439. http://doi.org/10.1080/02640410500231496

Buck, C., Guelfi, K., Dawson, B., McNaughton, L., & Wallman, K. (2015). Effects of sodium phosphate and caffeine loading on repeated-sprint ability. *Journal of Sports Sciences*, *33*(19), 1971–1979. http://doi.org/10.1080/02640414.2015.1025235

Burke, L. M. (2008). Caffeine and sports performance. *Applied Physiology, Nutrition, and Metabolism*, *33*(6), 1319–1334. http://doi.org/10.1139/H08-130

Cheetham, M. E., Boobis, L. H., Broks, S., & Williams, C. (1986). Human muscle metabolism during sprint running. *Journal of Applied Physiology*, *61*(1), 54–60.

Collomp, K., Ahmaidi, S., Chatard, J. C., Audran, M., & Prefaut, C. (1992). Benefits of caffeine ingestion on sprint performance in trained and untrained swimmers. *European Journal of Applied Physiology*, *64*(4), 377–380.

Cook, D. B., O'Connor, P. J., Oliver, S. E., & Lee, Y. (1998). Sex differences in naturally occurring leg muscle pain and exertion during maximal cycle ergometry. *The International Journal of Neuroscience*, *95*(3-4), 183–202.

Cox, G. R., Desbrow, B., Montgomery, P. G., Anderson, M. E., Bruce, C. R., Macrides, T. A., … Burke, L. M. (2002). Effect of different protocols of caffeine intake on metabolism and endurance performance. *Journal of Applied Physiology*, *93*, 990–999.

Crowe, M. J., Leicht, A. S., & Sprinks, W. L. (2006). Physiological and Cognitive Responses to Caffeine During Repeated, High-Intensity Exercise. *International Journal of Sport Nutrition & Exercise Metabolism*, *16*(5), 528–544.

Davis, J. K., & Green, J. M. (2009). Caffeine and Anaerobic Performance: Ergogenic Value and Mechanisms of Action. *Sports Medicine*, *39*(10), 813–832.

Doherty, M., Smith, P. M., Davison, R. C., & Hughes, M. G. (2002). Caffeine is ergogenic after supplementation of oral creatine monohydrate. *Medicine & Science in Sports & Exercise*, *34*(11), 1785–1792.

Egerton, T., Brauer, S. G., & Cresswell, A. G. (2009). Fatigue After Physical Activity in Healthy and Balance-Impaired Elderly. *Journal of Aging and Physical Activity*, *17*(1), 89–105.

Elliott, A. D., & Grace, F. (2010). An examination of exercise mode on ventilatory patterns during incremental exercise. *European Journal of Applied Physiology*, *110*(3), 557–562. http://doi.org/10.1007/s00421-010-1541-4

Glaister, M., Patterson, S. D., Foley, P., Pedlar, C. R., Pattison, J. R., & McInnes, G. (2012). Caffeine and Sprinting Performance: Dose Responses and Efficacy. *Journal of Strength and Conditioning Research*, *26*(4), 1001–1005.

Graham, T. E. (2001). Caffeine and Exercise: Metabolism, Endurance and Performance. *Sports Medicine*, *31*(11), 785–807.

Graham, T. E., Battram, D. S., Dela, F., El-Sohemy, A., & Thong, F. L. (2008). Does Caffeine Alter Muscle Carbohydrate and Fat Metabolism During Exercise? *Applied Physiology, Nutrition & Metabolism*, *33*(6), 1311–1318.

Graham, T. E., Hibbert, E., & Sathasivam, P. (1998). Metabolic and exercise endurance effects of coffee and caffeine ingestion. *Journal of Applied Physiology*, *85*(3), 883–889.

Green, H. J. (1997). Mechanisms of muscle fatigue in intense exercise. *Journal of Sports Sciences*, *15*(3), 247–256. http://doi.org/10.1080/026404197367254

Greer, F., McLean, C., & Graham, T. E. (1998). Caffeine, performance, and metabolism during repeated Wingate exercise tests. *Journal of Applied Physiology*, *85*(4), 1502–1508.

Gutmann, I., & Wahlefeld, A. W. (1974). Lactate: Determination with lactate dehydrogenase and NAD. In *Methods of Enzymatic Analysis* (H.U. Bergmeyer, pp. 1464–1468). New York and London: Verlag Chemie, Weinheim/Academic Press, Inc.

Howley, E. T., Bassett Jr., D. R., & Welch, H. G. (1995). Criteria for maximal oxygen uptake: review and commentary. *Medicine & Science in Sports & Exercise*, *27*(9), 1292–1301.

Ivy, J., Kammer, L., Zhenping, D., Bei, W., Bernard, J., Yi-Hung, L., & Hwang, J. (2009). Improved Cycling Time-Trial Performance After Ingestion of a Caffeine Energy Drink. *International Journal of Sport Nutrition & Exercise Metabolism*, *19*(1), 61–78.

Lee, K. A., Hicks, G., & Nino-Murcia, G. (1991). Validity and Reliability of a Scale to Assess Fatigue. *Psychiatry Research*, *36*(3), 291–298.

Leung, A. W. S., Chan, C. C. H., Lee, A. H. S., & Lam, K. W. H. (2004). Visual Analogue Scale Correlates of Musculoskeletal Fatigue. *Perceptual and Motor Skills*, *99*(1), 235–246.

Lindinger, M. I., Graham, T. E., & Spriet, L. L. (1993). Caffeine attenuates the exercise-induce increase in plasma K+ in humans. *Journal of Applied Physiology*, *74*(3), 1149–1155.

Lynge, J., & Hellsten, Y. (2000). Distribution of adenosine A1, A2A and A2B receptors in human skeletal muscle. *Acta Physiologica Scandinavica*, *169*(4), 283–290.

Mohr, M., Nielsen, J. J., & Bangsbo, J. (2011). Caffeine intake improves intense intermittent exercise performance and reduces muscle interstitial potassium accumulation. *Journal of Applied Physiology*, *111*(5), 1372–1379. http://doi.org/10.1152/japplphysiol.01028.2010

Smith, A. (2003). Caffeine and Central Noradrenaline: Effects on Mood, Cognitive Performance, Eye Movements and Cardiovascular Function. *Journal of Psychopharmacology*, *17*(3), 283–292. http://doi.org/10.1177/02698811030173010

Sokmen, B., Armstrong, L. E., Kraemer, W. J., Casa, D. J., Dias, J. C., Judelson, D. A., & Maresh, C. M. (2008). Caffeine Use in Sports: Considerations for the Athlete. *Journal of Strength and Conditioning Research*, *22*(3), 978–986.

Spriet, L. L. (2014). Exercise and Sport Performance with Low Doses of Caffeine. *Sports Medicine*, *44*(S2), 175–184. http://doi.org/10.1007/s40279-014-0257-8

Spriet, L. L., & Howlett, R. A. (2000). Caffeine. In *Nutrition in Sport* (pp. 379–392). Oxford; Malden, Mass.: Blackwell Science Ltd.

Wiles, J., Coleman, D., Tegerdine, M., & Swaine, I. (2006). The effects of caffeine ingestion on performance time, speed and power during a laboratory-base 1 km cycling time-trial. *Journal of Sports Sciences*, *24*(11), 1165–1171.

Wiles, J. D., Bird, S. R., Hopkins, J., & Riley, M. (1992). Effect of caffeinated coffee on running speed, respiratory factors, blood lactate and perceived exertion during 1500-m treadmill running. *British Journal of Sports Medicine*, *26*(2), 116–120.

Zouhal, H., Jacob, C., Delamarche, P., & Gratas-Delamarche, A. (2008). Catecholamines and the Effects of Exercise, Training and Gender. *Sports Medicine*, *38*(5), 401–423.

10

Activation of Selected Core Muscles during Pressing

Thomas W. Nesser (Corresponding author)
Kinesiology, Recreation, and Sport, Indiana State University 401 N. 4th Street, Terre Haute, IN 47809 USA
E-mail: tom.nesser@indstate.edu

Neil Fleming
Kinesiology, Recreation, and Sport, Indiana State University 401 N. 4th Street, Terre Haute, IN 47809 USA
E-mail: neil.fleming@indstate.edu

Matthew J. Gage
Department of Health Professions, Liberty University 1971 University Blvd, Lynchburg, VA 24515 USA
E-mail: mjgage@liberty.edu

Abstract

Introduction: Unstable surface training is often used to activate core musculature during resistance training. Unfortunately, unstable surface training is risky and leads to detraining. **Purpose:** The purpose of this study was to determine core muscle activation during stable surface ground-based lifts. **Methods:** Fourteen recreational trained and former NCAA DI athletes (weight 84.2 ± 13.3 kg; height 176.0 ± 9.5 cm; age 20.9 ± 2.0 years) volunteered for participation. Subjects completed two ground-based lifts: overhead press and push-press. Surface EMG was recorded from 4 muscles on the right side of the body (Rectus Abdominus (RA), External Oblique (EO), Transverse Abdominus (TA), and Erector Spinae (ES). **Results:** Paired sample T-tests identified significant muscle activation differences between the overhead press and the push-press included ES and EO. Average and peak EMG for ES was significantly greater in push-press ($P<0.01$). Anterior displacement of COP was significantly greater in push-press compared to overhead press during the eccentric phase. **Conclusion:** The push-press was identified as superior in core muscle activation when compared to the overhead pressing exercise.

Keywords: torso, stability, weight lifting, resistance training

1. Introduction

1.1 Introduce the Problem

The use of core training in the conditioning of both athletes and non-athletes has increased in the last decade (Gamble, 2007). Core training is defined as any exercise which utilizes motor control and muscular capacity of the lumbo-pelvic complex (Leetun, 2004; Gamble, 2007). The muscles of the core typically include the rectus abdominus, external and internal obliques, transverse abdominus, and erector spinae (McGill et al. 2003). The popularity of core training is based on the belief that a strong core allows greater spine stability and more effective transfer of forces from the lower body to the upper body with minimal dissipation of energy (Bompa, 1999; McGill, 2009) leading to an improvement in athletic performance such as higher jumps and faster sprints (Akuthota, 2004; Kibler,2006; King, 2000; Mayhew, 2005; McGill 1999), and reduced risk of lower limb injury (Leetun et al., 2004).

1.2 Explore Importance of the Problem

A current challenge is how best to train the muscles of the core. Basic core exercises include floor planks which require the maintenance of a prone position balanced on the elbows and toes. Floor planks activate core muscle but from a sport performance perspective, they are static and have little transfer to the sports arena (Parkhouse & Ball, 2011). To step up the training intensity, planks have been completed on an unstable surface with increased EMG core muscle activation (Byrne et al. 2014; Snarr & Esco, 2014), though the lack of sport specificity still applies. To train the core in a more sport specific manner, free weight exercises have been completed on an unstable surface. For example, completing a bench press while lying on a Swiss ball or standing on a foam pad during an overhead press. Training on an unstable surface does require more balance, unfortunately, unstable surface training is not ideal.

1.3 Relevant Scholarship

Several Electromyography (EMG) studies have been completed to confirm unstable training can increased core muscle activation (Anderson & Behm, 2005, Norwood et al, 2007, Marshall & Murphy, 2006) though not all core muscle EMG studies agree. Some identified greater core muscle activation on a stable vs. an unstable surface (Willardson et al., 2009, Kohler et al.,2010, Hamlyn et al., 2007), while others identified no difference between stable and unstable conditions (Gullett et al., 2009), Uribe et al., 2010, Saeterbalken & Fimland, 2013). Likewise, Saeterbalken & Fimland, (2013),

Willardson, (2007), Behm et al. (2010), and Hamlyn et al.(2007), identified reduced force output when training on an unstable surface which can lead to detraining.

Along with the possibility of detraining, unstable surface training is not practical. As identified by Kohler et al. (2010), most athletes compete on a "stable surface" (i.e. the ground). Thus the use of an unstable environment is not sport specific reducing the transfer of training to the field. Ground based lifts are most specific to sport due to the stabilization of an external load (barbell or dumbbell) on a stable surface (the ground) much like an athlete stabilizing an implement or opponent.

For practical and sport specific purposes, Behm et al. (2010) suggest the use of "ground-based lifts" such as "Olympic lifts, squats, and dead lifts" as a means to train the muscles of the core. Ground-based lifts are defined as lifts completed while in a standing position requiring the transfer of forces from the ground to the body.

Hamlyn et al. (2007) did just that by examining muscle activity of the upper lumbar erector spinae (UES), lumbar-sacral erector spinae (LES), lower abdominals (LA), and external obliques (EO) during two ground-based lifts, the back squat and the deadlift, with 80% 1-RM, plus three non-ground-based lifts: a bodyweight squat (no external load), a superman and a sidebridge. The two ground-based lifts generated greater UES and LES activity and similar LA and EO activity when compared to the other exercises suggesting ground-based lifts are more effective at core muscle activation than non-ground-based exercises.

1.4 Hypotheses and Research Design

Based on the results of the research identified, ground-based lifts are not only ideal but recommended for core muscle training. However, core muscle activation has not been compared between various ground-based lifts. Therefore, the first purpose of this study was to determine the magnitude of core muscle activation generated during commonly performed ground-based lifts such as the overhead press and push-press, and the second purpose was to determine if one exercise variation generated greater core muscle activation than the other. The push-press was hypothesized to generate greater muscle activation of all muscles measured with a forward shift in the center of pressure when compared to the overhead press due to the increased dynamics of the push-press.

2. Methods

2.1 Experimental Approach

This study was designed to compare core specific muscle activation between various multi-joint resistance training exercises. The dependent variables included activation of the right side rectus abdominus, external oblique, transverse abdominus, and erector spinae.

2.2 Participants

Fourteen recreational trained and former NCAA DI athletes (weight 84.2 ± 13.3 kg; height 176.0 ± 9.5 cm; age 20.9 ± 2.0 years) volunteered for participation. Sample size was based on previous EMG studies (Anderson et al., 2004; Barnett et al., 1995; Gullett et al., 2009; Marshall & Murphy, 2006; Norwood et al., 2007). All participants were free of injury at the time of data collection. All participants signed informed consent forms prior to participation. The university institutional review board approved this study.

2.3 Procedures

All subjects were individually scheduled for data collection. The press exercises were completed random order. All subjects were educated on the procedures and expectations of the research study. Prior to data collection all subjects practiced each exercise with minimal resistance to avoid fatigue. Each data collection session was completed within one hour.

2.4 Overhead Press

Subjects removed a weighted barbell from a squat rack and position it across the anterior deltoids with a closed pronated grip. Upon command, the subjects pressed the weight overhead with no movement of the lower body. Once the elbows were fully extended the bar was returned to the shoulders and repeated two more times. Subjects completed one set of three repetitions with 50 percent body mass.

2.5 Push-press

Subjects removed a weighted barbell from a squat rack and position it across the anterior deltoids with a pronated grip similar to the overhead press. Upon command, the subjects dipped down by slightly flexing the knees and then forcefully extended the knees just prior to pressing the weight overhead to generate momentum. Once the elbows were fully extended the bar was returned to the shoulders and repeated two more times. Subjects completed one set of three repetitions with 50 percent body mass.

2.6 Surface Electromyography

Surface EMG data were recorded from 4 core muscles on the right side of the body; Erector Spinae (ES), Rectus Abdominus (RA), External Oblique (EO), and Transverse Abdominus (TA). Data were collected using a Trigno wireless EMG data acquisition system (Delsys, Boston, MA, USA). Surface electrodes had a single differential configuration, inter-electrode distance of 10 mm, 4-bar formation, bandwidth of 20–450 Hz and 99.9% silver contact material. All efforts were made to conform to the recommendations of SENIAM with regard to preparation and acquisition of EMG signals (Hermens et al., 2000). The skin sites were shaved and cleaned with isopropyl alcohol in order to minimize skin impedance. Data sampling rate was 2,000 Hz throughout all trials. The electrodes for RA were placed 1 cm above the umbilicus and 2 cm lateral to the midline. For EO, electrodes were placed below the ribcage, along a line between the most inferior point of the costal margin and the contra-lateral pubic tubercle. ES electrodes were placed 5 cm lateral to the level of the T9 spinous process. TA electrodes were placed 2 cm medial and inferior to the anterior superior iliac spine (ASIS). This site is below the EO fibers, thus reducing risk of cross-talk for this muscle.

Maximal voluntary isometric contractions (MVIC) were performed in order to normalize EMG data to a maximal reference for each muscle. MVIC procedures for RA, EO and TA, involved subjects lying supine on a table with legs fixed in place. A resisted sit-up from this position was performed for RA. Subjects were instructed to raise their torso off the table with maximal force while investigators held both shoulders in place. A resisted transverse sit-up was performed for EO normalization. Subjects were instructed to raise their right shoulder off the table towards their left hip, while investigators held the right shoulder in place. To measure MVIC for the TA, subjects were instructed to maximally pull their stomach in toward the spine. For ES normalization, subjects lay in a prone position and were instructed to raise their torso off the table with maximal force while the investigators held both shoulders in place.

Synchronous measurements of right knee, hip and elbow joint angle were made using electrogoniometers (Biometrics Ltd. 2000 Hz recording frequency) during all exercises. Data were collected in order to identify the onset of each movement cycle and differentiate the concentric and eccentric phases of the movement. Onset of overhead press and push-press were defined as first extension of the elbow or first flexion of the knee (in the case of push-press).

Following synchronization of EMG with the movement cycle, the root mean square (RMS) values of the raw data were calculated (50 ms window, 0 overlap). For each movement cycle, mean activity for the concentric phase, eccentric phase and overall movement cycle were calculated. These data were then averaged over 3 cycles and expressed as a percentage of MVIC.

2.7 Center of Pressure Data

Center of pressure data were measured during all lifts using a Tekscan HR mat (Tekscan, Boston, MA) in order to assess anterior displacement of the subject's center of pressure (COP) during each movement. The Tekscan HR mat has a surface area of 2323 cm^2 (dimensions: 48.7 x 47.7 cm), a sensor resolution of 4 sensels/cm^2 and a pressure range up to 862 kPa. Subjects were instructed to position themselves directly on the mat with their feet a comfortable distance apart for each lift. Pressure data were recorded at 100 Hz and a 5 V square wave pulse facilitated synchronous collection of EMG, goniometry and planter pressure data.

2.8 Statistical Analysis

Descriptive statistics were performed on all data. Paired samples T-tests were used for data analysis to measure differences in paired muscle activation between the two lifts as well as Cohen's d to determine effect size. Statistical significance was set at $P \leq 0.05$. SPSS 20.0 software (SPSS Inc., Chicago, IL) was used for all analyses.

3. Results

3.1 Electromyography

Group means (SD) average and peak EMG data for each lift are presented in figure 1 and table 1, respectively. Paired sample T-tests identified significant muscle activation differences between the overhead press and the push-press included ES and EO. Average and peak EMG for ES was significantly greater in push-press compared to overhead press. These differences were observed in the overall movement ($P<0.001$), and during both eccentric ($P<0.001$) and concentric phases of the movement ($P<0.01$). Additionally, during the eccentric phase, peak activity in EO was greater in push-press compared to overhead press ($P<0.05$).

Table 1. Average EMG data across the full range of movement, eccentric and concentric phases. Data are expressed as group mean (SD), normalized to percentage of MVIC (mV).

	Push-press	**Overhead Press**	**Effect Size (Cohen's *d*)**
Overall			
RA	5.7 (4.5)	4.5 (3.5)	0.30
TA	13.9 (9.1)	12.5 (16.2)	0.11
EO	18.4 (6.8)	16.4 (8.3)	0.26
ES	32.2 (11.5)***	11.4 (9.1)	2.0
Eccentric			
RA	3.7 (3.4)	5.3 (3.7)	0.45
TA	10.1 (6.9)	13.2 (9.8)	0.37
EO	14.7 (6.3)	19.2 (9.8)	0.55
ES	30.3 (12.9)***	11.7 (8.8)	1.68
Concentric			
RA	6.5 (6.3)	3.7 (3.6)	0.54
TA	16.7 (12.3)	11.9 (8.1)	0.46
EO	21.1 (9.5)*	13.9 (7.6)	0.83
ES	32.0 (13.6)***	11.1 (9.6)	1.78

significant differences between push and overhead press ($P<0.05$; ***$P<0.001$).

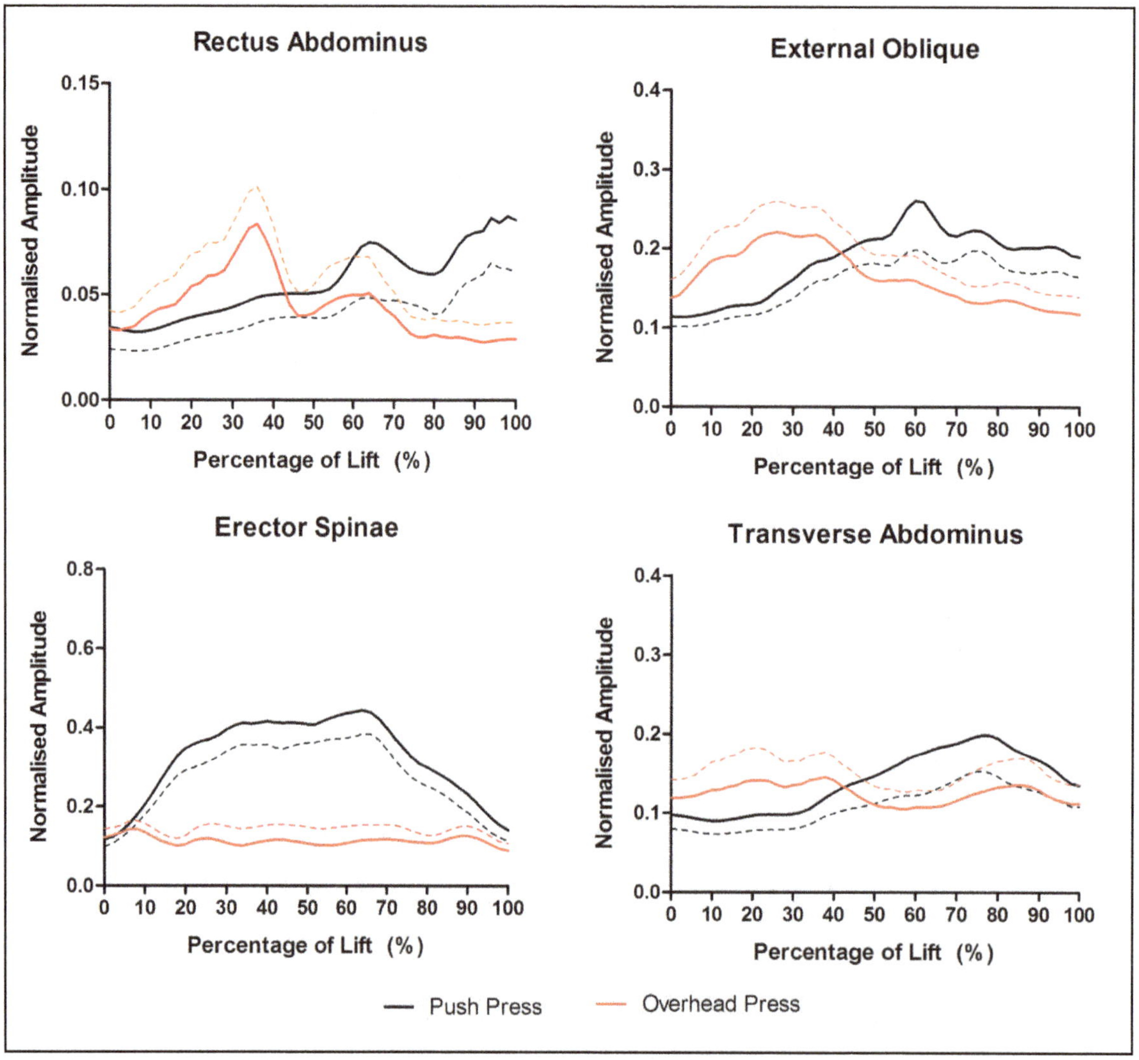

Figure 1. Group mean EMG ensembles for RF, EO, ES and TA during overhead press (red) and push-press (black) movements. Solid lines denote mean while dashed lines denote SEM.

3.2 Center of Pressure

Anterior displacement of COP was also not significantly different between push-press and overhead press for the overall movement (21.8 ± 6.4 vs. 21.2 ± 5.8 cm), or during the concentric phase (21.6 ± 7.9 vs. 24.7 ± 7.7 cm) (figure 2). However, during the eccentric phase, anterior displacement of COP was significantly greater in push-press compared to overhead press (22.1 ± 5.5 vs. 17.5 ± 4.8 cm, $P<0.05$).

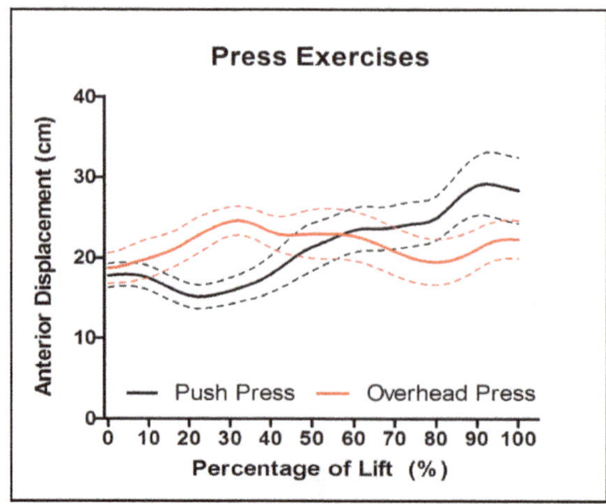

Figure 2. Group mean anterior displacement of COP data during press exercises. Solid lines denote mean while dashed lines denote SEM.

4. Discussions

4.1 Discussion overview

Development of the core has become very popular in the training of both athletes and non-athletes. In the process of doing so, the use of unstable training has gained popularity based on research that identified increased core muscle activation during various free weight exercises (Anderson & Behm, 2005, Norwood et al, 2007, Marshall & Murphy, 2006). At the same time, commonly performed ground based exercises on a stable surface had been overlooked for their capacity to activate the muscles of the core. The purposes of this study was to determine the magnitude of core muscle activation generated during commonly performed ground-based lifts such as the overhead press and the push-press, and determine if one exercise variation generated greater core muscle activation than the other. An unstable surface is not necessary for activation of the core muscles when performing ground- based lifts (Hamlyn et al. 2007).

4.2 EMG comparison

Average EMG for all examined muscles was higher for the push-press compared to the overhead press. However, the greatest difference was seen with the ES for both peak EMG and average EMG during both the concentric and eccentric phases of the lift. The enhanced muscle activation of the ES is likely due to the greater dynamics of the push-press itself and the transfer of energy from the lower extremities to the upper extremities and the need to statically stabilize the spine as identified by Shinkle et al. (2012). The push-press also resulted in significantly greater anterior displacement of COP during the eccentric phase of the lift, despite identical resistance and the eccentric phases being relatively similar in movement between the two lifts. It is likely that adjustments in COP are required in the eccentric phase of the push-press in order to compensate for differing lower limb kinematics in the initial concentric phase. Push-press EO EMG was also identified as superior when compared to the overhead press though only for peak EMG during the eccentric phase and not average EMG for the entire lift.

Willardson et al. (2009) also measured EMG activity on the RA, EO, TA, and ES during the overhead press while performed on a stable surface with 50% and 75% 1-RM and on a BOSU ball with 50% 1-RM. Significantly greater RA and EO activation was observed in the stable condition with 75% 1-RM when compared to the stable condition at 50% 1-RM and 50% 1-RM on the BOSU ball. TA activity in the stable condition with 75% 1-RM was significantly greater than the 50% BOSU ball condition only. No differences were identified with the ES between conditions. Kohler et al. (2010) compared EMG between RA, ES (lower and upper), and EO during the seated overhead press on a stable surface and unstable surface (Swiss ball) with both a barbell and dumbbells. Uribe et al. (2010) basically did the same thing but only observed the RA (of the core muscles) and only used dumbbells. Kohler et al. (2010) identified significant differences between the RA and lower ES during the unstable condition with a barbell when compared to the other conditions while Uribe found no differences in the RA between conditions. None of the above studies tested the push-press thus further comparison with the current data is not possible.

5. Conclusions and Practical Application

Both of the ground-based exercises completed generated core muscle activation without the need of an unstable surface. However, the push-press was identified as superior in core muscle activation when compared to the overhead press. The average EMG of all 4 muscles was higher in push-press compared to overhead press, with the load being equal in both exercises. The push-press appears to be more effective at training the core musculature than the overhead press.

Acknowledgements

No funding was received for this study.

References

Akuthota, V, and Nadler, SF. (2004) Core strengthening. *Archives of Physical Medicine and Rehabilitation,* 85(3 suppl):S86-92.

Anderson, KG, and Behm, DG. (2004) Maintenance of EMG Activity and Loss of Force Output with Instability. *Journal of Strength and Conditioning Research,* 18, 637-640.

Anderson, K, and Behm, DG. (2005) Trunk muscle activity increases with unstable squat movements. *Canadian Journal of Applied Physiology,* 30:33-45.

Barnett, C. Kippers, V. Turner, P. (1995) Effects of Variations of the Bench Press Exercise on the EMG Activity of Five Shoulder Muscles. *Journal of Strength and Conditioning Research,* 9, 222-227.

Behm, DG, Drinkwater, EJ, Willardson, JM, and Cowley, PM. (2010) Canadian Society for Exercise Physiology position stand: The use of instability to train the core in athletic and nonathletic conditioning. *Applied Physiology, Nutrition*, and *Metabolism,* 35:109-112.

Bompa, TO. (1999) *Periodization Training for Sports*. Champaign, IL: Human Kinetics.

Byrne, JM, Bishop, NS, Caines, AM, Crane, KA, Feaver, AM, and Pearcey, GEP. (2014) Effect of using s suspension training system on muscle activation during the performance of a front plack exercise. *Journal of Strength and Conditioning Research,* 28:3049-3055.

Gullett, JC, Tillman, MD, Gutierrez, GM, and Chow, JW. (2009) A biomechanical comparison of back and front squats in healthy trained individuals. *Journal of Strength and Conditioning Research,* 23, 284-292.

Gamble, P. An integrated approach to training core stability. (2007) *Strength and Conditioning Journal,* 29, 58-68.

Hermens, H, Freriks, B, Disselhorst-Klug, C, Rau, G. (2000) Development of recommendations for SEMG sensors and sensor placement procedures. *Journal of Electromyography* and *Kinesiology,* 10: 361-374.

Kibler, BW, Press, J, Sciascia. (2006). The role of core stability in athletic function. *Sports Medicine,* 36(3):189-198.

Kohler, JM, Flanagan, SP, and Whiting, WC. (2010) Muscle activation patterns while lifting stable and unstable loads on stable and unstable surfaces. *Journal of Strength and Conditioning Research,* 24, 313-321.

Leetun, DT, Ireland, ML, Willson, JD, Ballantyne, BT, and Davis, IM. (2004) Core stability measures as risk factors for lower extremity injury in athletes. *Medicine and Science in Sport and Exercise,* 36, 926-934.

Marshall, PWM, and Murphy, BA. (2006) Increased deltoid and abdominal muscle activity during swiss ball bench press. *Journal of Strength and Conditioning Research,* 20: 745-750.

Mayhew, JL, Bird, M, Cole, ML, Koch, AJ, Jacques, JA, Ware, JS, Buford, BN, and Fletcher, KM. (2005) Comparison of the backward overhead medicine ball throw to power production in college football players. *Journal of Strength and Conditioning Research,* 19: 514-518.

McGill, SM. (2009) *Ultimate Back Fitness and Performance*. (4th ed.). Waterloo, Ontario, Canada: Wabuno Publishers.

McGill, SM, Grenier, S, Kavcic, N, Cholewicki, J. (2003) Coordination of muscle activity to assure stability of the lumbar spine. *Journal of Electromyography* and *Kinesiology*, 13:353-359.

Norwood, JI, Anderson, GS, Gaetz, MB, and Twist, PW. (2007) Electromyographic activity of the trunk stabilizers during stable and unstable bench press. *Journal of Strength and Conditioning Research,* 21:343-347.

Parkhouse, KL. and Ball, N. (2011) Influence of dynamic versus static core exercises on performance in field based fitness tests. *Journal of Bodywork and Movement Therapies,* 15:517-524.

Saeterbakken, AH, and Fimland, MS. (2013) Muscle force output and electromyographic activity in squats with various unstable surfaces. *Journal of Strength and Conditioning Research,*27:130-136.

Shinkle, J, Nesser, TW, Demchak, TM, and McMannus, DM. (2012) Effect of Core Strength on the Measure of Power in the Extremities. *Journal of Strength and Conditioning Research,*25:373-380.

Snarr, RL and Esco, MR. (2014) Electromyographical comparison of plank variations performed with and without instability devices. *Journal of Strength and Conditioning Research,* 28:3298-3305.

Uribe, BP, Coburn, JW, Brown, LE, Judelson, DA, Khamoui, AV, and Nguyen, D. (2010) Muscle activation when performing the chest press and shoulder press on a stable bench vs. a Swiss ball. *Journal of Strength and Conditioning Research,* 24, 1028-1033.

Willardson, J. Core stability training: applications to sports conditioning programs. *(2007) Journal of Strength and Conditioning Research,* 21:979-985.

Willardson, J, Fontana, FE, Bressel, E. (2009) Effect of surface stability on core muscle activity for dynamic resistance exercises. *International Journal of Sports Physiology Performance,* 4:97-109.

11

Effects of Plyometric Training on Rock'n'Roll Performance

Nico Nitzsche (Corresponding author)
Chemnitz University of Technology, Department of Human Movement Science and Health
Thüringer Weg 11, 09130 Chemnitz, Germany
E-mail: nico.nitzsche@s2007.tu-chemnitz.de

Norman Stutzig (Corresponding author)
University of Stuttgart, Department of Sport and Motion Science
Allmandring 28, 70569 Stuttgart, Germany

Achim Walther
University Hospital Carl Gustav Carus Dresden, Department of Sports medicine
Fetcherstraße 74, 01307 Dresden, Germany

Tobias Siebert
University of Stuttgart, Department of Sport and Motion Science
Allmandring 28, 70569 Stuttgart, Germany

Abstract

Objectives: The aim of the study was to analyse if plyometric training increases the sport specific performance in rock'n'roll dancers. **Design:** Fifteen semi-professional rock'n'roll dancers participated in a plyometric training study. Pre- and posttests were conducted to document alterations of sport specific performance, reactive strength as well as maximal isokinetic torque. **Method:** The participants (n=15) accomplished two training sessions weekly for a training period of 6 weeks. The training program consisted of different of jumps. Pre- and posttests included a rock'n'roll specific performance test examining the maximal number of kicks within 30 s. Moreover, jumping height and ground contact time (GCT) during drop jump were determined to calculate reactive strength (RSI). Maximal dynamic torque and work were determined during maximal isokinetic contractions of the plantar flexors. **Results:** The number of kicks increased from 46.5 ± 2.6 to 49.4 ± 2.7 ($p=0.00$, $d_Z=1.83$).The RSI increased significantly from 2.57 ± 0.29 to 2.72 ± 0.44 ($p=0.05$, $d_Z=0.55$). The gains of RSI are based on increases in jumping height (pretest: 24.6 ± 4.0 cm, posttest 26.5 ± 4.7 cm, $p=0.01$, $d_Z=0.71$), whereas the GCT remained unaltered ($p=0.53$). The work during maximal isokinetic plantar flexions increased significantly in both legs (jumping leg: $p = 0.04$, $d_Z=0.58$; kicking leg: $p=0.05$, $d_Z=0.55$). **Conclusions:** Plyometric training increases the kicking frequency during rock'n'roll dance. This might be attributed to the observed increase in reactive strength. Training induced changes in muscle activity or structure were discussed. It is suggested to implement plyometric training into the training program of rock'n'roll dancers.

Keywords: Rock'n'roll, plyometric training, reactive strength, plantar flexors

1. Introduction

Physical abilities as strength and power contribute to the complex performance in many sports (Baechle & Earle, 2008). The significance of their contribution depends on the performance system of the competition (Matveev, 1981). The strength efforts in high performance rock'n'roll dancing are mainly short ground contacts during hopping and jumps. A main performance criterion is the dancing velocity regarding to the number of kicks per minute. High performance athletes have to perform kicking frequencies of more than 100 kicks per minute (Kirch, 1995; WRRC, 2012). As the frequency of kicks is equal to the frequency of hops, rock'n'roll dancers perform hops at a frequency of more than 100 per minute. The frequency of kicks or rather hops per minute depends on the reactive strength of the athletes. Reactive strength is the ability to reverse eccentric into concentric muscle actions (Gamble, 2010; Young & Farrow, 2006). Zemkova et al. (2001; 2005) showed that reactive strength and explosive power is higher in rock'n'roll dancers compared to other populations.

The aim of plyometric training is to maximize the reactive strength and power. Reactive strength can be measured using the reactive strength index (RSI). The RSI is the ratio between jumping height and time of touch down (GCT) within a stretch-shortening-cycle (for example during a drop jump). The index can be maximized by increasing jumping height while the GCT remained unaltered or by reducing the GCT while the jumping height is constant. In both cases the force during the ground contact needs to be increased. In literature it is reported that plyometric exercises are effective to develop reactive strength (Lloyd, Oliver, Hughes, & Williams, 2012) and power (Bobbert, 1990; Bobbert, Huijing, & van Ingen Schenau, 1987a, 1987b; Malisoux, Francaux, Nielens, & Theisen, 2006). Plyometric exercise is defined as a quick powerful movement that involves the stretch-shortening cycle (Baechle & Earle, 2008; Komi, 1984, 2003). It was shown that plyometric training increases the jump performance (Markovic, 2007; Matavulj, Kukolj, Ugarkovic, Tihanyi, & Jaric, 2001), RSI as well as sprint abilities (Ronnestad, Kvamme, Sunde, & Raastad, 2008). Increasing the RSI may increase the number of hops in a given time and may lead to increase the number of kicks in rock'n'roll. So far, it is unknown if plyometric training has a benefit effect on number of kicks in rock'n'roll. The aim of the study is to increase the number of kicks in young athletes by a sport specific plyometric training in rock'n'roll. It is hypothesised that plyometric training increases the RSI and the number of kicks in rock'n'roll.

2. Methods

Fifteen semi-professional rock'n'roll dancers (sex: 3 male, 12 female, age: 17.1 ± 3.0 year, weight: 58.8 ± 7.4 kg, height: 167 ± 5 cm, BMI: 17.8 ± 1.9 kg/m^2) participated in the study. All athletes trained at least three times per week. All participants that suffered on a leg injury in the past six months before the study started were excluded from the study. The participants were informed about the aims and risks of the study and gave their written consent before the study started. The study was approved by the local ethical committee of the university hospital of Dresden and conducted in accordance with the latest declaration of Helsinki.

Participants were examined before and after the plyometric training intervention regarding to reactive strength, maximum strength and a sport specific performance test. The training was conducted two times per week with at least one day rest between the training sessions. The training intervention lasted for 6 weeks and was integrated into regular dance training (Brown, Wells, Schade, Smith, & P.C., 2007). All participants completed the training phase.

Each training session started with a general warm-up containing running with moderate intensity followed by dynamic stretching of the leg muscles. Subsequently simple jumping exercises with moderate intensities were performed.

The training program started with 6 repetitions of jumping exercises. Three sets were performed. There was a 3 min rest between the sets. The participants were motivated to perform the jumping exercises with maximal power. According to the recommendations of the American College of Sports Medicine the volume was increased progressively from 42 jumps in the first week to 81 jumps in the last week (Ratamess et al., 2009). Moreover, different jumping exercises as squat jumps, tuck jumps, hurdle jumps and lateral jumps were chosen (Bosco, 1999). Hence, the kind of jumping exercise was also increased progressively in order to the intensity. Therefore, participants started with squat jumps at the beginning and performed multiple hurdle jumps with maximal explosive power in the last week. The overall design of the training program is shown in table 1.

Table 1. Training program performed by rock'n'roll dancers

Week	Repetition	Sets		Jumps total
1	6	3	Squat Jumps	42
	8	3	Lateral Jumps	
2	8	3	Squat Jumps	54
	10	3	Lateral Jumps	
3	10	3	Squat Jumps	66
	12	3	Lateral Jumps	
4	8	3	Tuck Jumps	51
	3x3	3	Hurdle Jumps	
5	10	3	Tuck Jumps	66
	4x3	3	Hurdle Jumps	
6	12	3	Tuck Jumps	81
	5x3	3	Hurdle Jumps	

2.1 Pretest / Posttest

All participants were tested before and after the end of the training intervention. After a standardized warm-up different functional tests were performed.

To assess the effect of training on dancing performance a rock'n'roll specific performance test was conducted. This sport specific motor test is a main criterion for rock'n'roll dancers and closely related to the dance performance (Kirch,

1995). The aim of the test was to complete as many as possible rock'n'roll kicks within 30 seconds. Participants executed the test two times with 5 min rest between the trials. The mean number of kicks of the two trials was used for further analyses.

Maximal dynamic torque (MVDC) during plantar flexion was determined using an isokinetic diagnostic system (ISOMED2000, D&R Ferstl GmbH, Hemau, Germany) (Stutzig & Siebert, 2015). Participants lie supine in the ISOMED2000 with one foot attached to a pedal. The hip and knee angle were completely straight and fixed with straps. The range of motion of the ankle amounted 55°. The dynamic plantar flexion was carried out at an angular velocity of 240 °/s. One set consisting of seven repetitions was conducted. The maximum torque and work were calculated for each repetition. For further analyses the data of the third until the seventh repetition were averaged.

The reactive strength (Young & Farrow, 2006) within a stretch-shortening cycle (Komi, 2000) was assessed using drop jump exercises (Fleck & Kraemer, 2004). Participants stood on a box (height: 30 cm) until jump off (Flanagan, Ebben, & Jensen, 2008). They were asked to touch down and jump off as fast as possible and hence, to jump as high as possible (Taube, Leukel, Lauber, & Gollhofer, 2011). The GCT and the flight time (t_{flight}) were assessed using a force plate (Kistler© Typ 9281EA). The data were recorded by a sample rate of 1000Hz and stored on a computer. The jumping height (H) was calculated based on the flight time:

$$H = \frac{1}{8} * g * t_{flight}^2$$

where g is the gravitational acceleration and t_{flight} is the flight time. Furthermore, a reactive strength index (RSI) was calculated as follows (Abramov, Kuporosov, & Matwejew, 1980; Bruhn, Kullmann, & Gollhofer, 2004; Flanagan et al., 2008):

$$RSI = \frac{H}{t_{gc}}$$

where t_{gc} is the ground contact time. Five single drop jumps were conducted with 30 s rest between the trials. The data of the jump with the best RSI was used for further analyses.

2.2 Statistics

The data are presented as mean and standard deviation. Moreover, data were proved for normal distribution using the Shapiro-Wilk test. A student t-test was used to detect differences between pre and posttests. The effect size (d_Z) was calculated as mean of the differences divided by the standard deviation of the differences (Cohen, 1988). The significant level was set at p=0.05.

3. Results

The number of kicks increased significantly from 46.5 ± 2.6 kicks to 49.4 ± 2.7 ($p=0.00$, $d_Z=1.83$) kicks due to the specific power training (fig. 1).

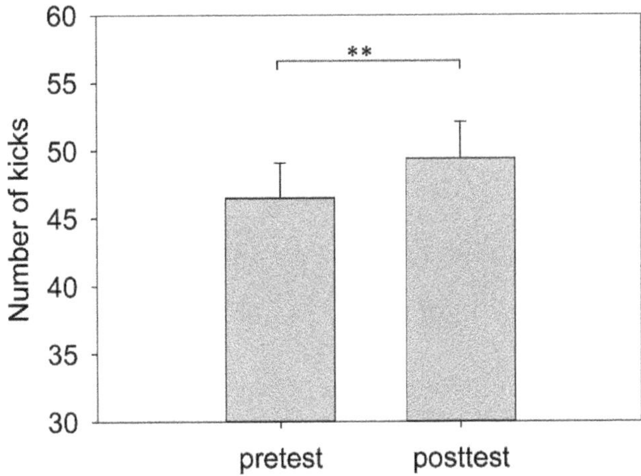

Figure 1. Mean and standard deviation of the number of kicks during the rock'n'roll specific performance test. The left bar shows the results of the test before the training intervention (pretest) and the right bar after the training intervention (posttest). ** Significant between pretest and posttest at p<0.01.

The peak torque during MVDC of the jumping leg increased significantly (p = 0.02, d_Z =0.65) from 41.3 ± 10.9 Nm to 49.9 ± 8.1 Nm. However, the peak torque of the kicking leg did not increase significantly (p = 0.10) (fig.2).

The work during the MVDC increased in both jumping leg (p = 0.04, d_Z =0.58, pre: 27.1 ± 7.4, post: 31.2 ± 5.1) and kicking leg (p = 0.05, d_Z=0.55 pre: 28.3 ± 8.7, post: 32.5 ± 6.6) (fig.3).

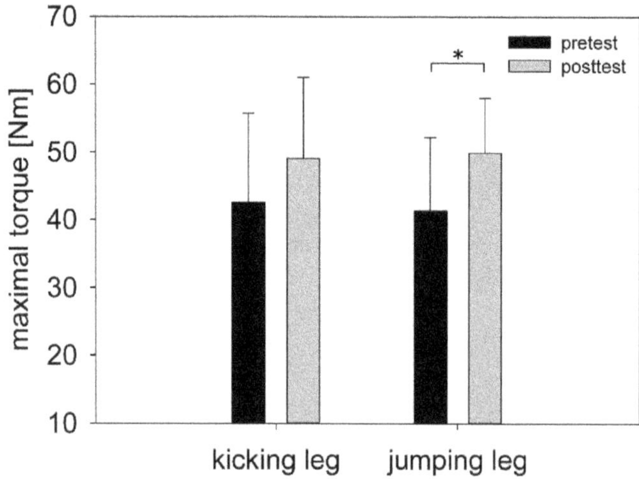

Figure 2. Mean and standard deviation of the maximal torque during the isokinetic plantar flexions of the kicking leg and jumping leg. The black and the grey bars show the results of the test before (pretest) and after (posttest) the training intervention, respectively. * Significant between pretest and posttest at p<0.05.

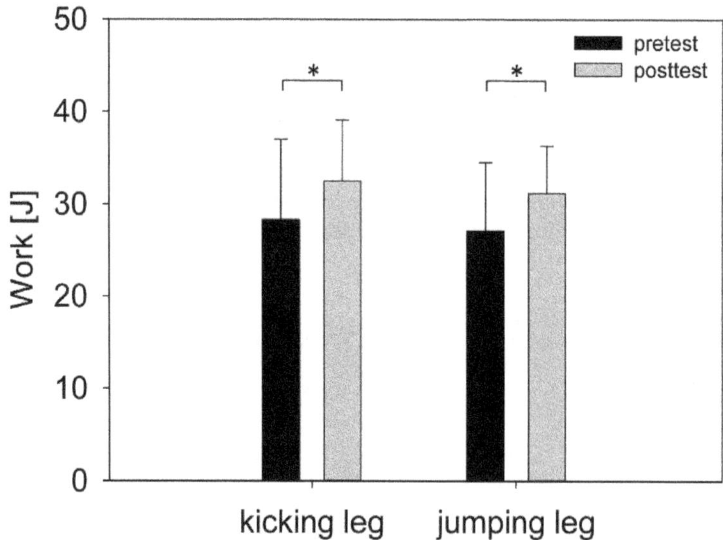

Figure 3. Mean and standard deviation of physical work during the isokinetic plantar flexions of the kicking leg and jumping leg. The black and the grey bars show the results of the test before (pretest) and after (posttest) the training intervention, respectively. * Significant between pretest and posttest at p<0.05.

The GCT during drop jump remained unaltered (p=0.53, d_Z=0.17) throughout the training intervention. The jumping height increased significantly (p=0.01, d_Z=0.71) from 24.6 ± 4.0 cm to 26.5 ± 4.7 cm. Moreover, the RSI increased significantly (p=0.05, d_Z=0.55) from 2.57 ± 0.29 to 2.72 ± 0.44, too (tab.2).

Table 2. Mean, standard deviation (SD) and level of significance (p) of the Drop Jump during pretest and posttest

Test	Parameter	Pretest	Posttest	p
	Ground contact time [s]	0.173 ± 0.015	0.170 ± 0.018	0.53
Drop Jump	Jumping height [cm]	24.6 ± 4.0	26.5 ± 4.7	0.01
	Reactive strength index	2.57 ± 0.29	2.72 ± 0.44	0.05

4. Discussion

This study demonstrates, that a plyometric training improves the sport specific performance of rock'n'roll dancers, e.g. by increasing the number of kicks. The athletes increased their speed from 46.5 to 49.4 kick (in 30 sec). The number of kicks corresponds to an increase of kicking frequency from 93 to 98.8 kicks per minute. According to the international rules of rock'n'roll (WRRC, 2012) the speed of music amounts 50-52 bars per minute for international tournaments. One basic step contains three kicks and lasts 1.5 bars. At a music speed of 51 bars per minute 34 basic steps need to be performed. That means high performance athletes perform a kicking frequency of 102 kicks per minute.

One possible reason for the increased number of kicks may be the observed improvement in the reactive strength index (RSI). This was reported in other plyometric studies too (Lloyd et al., 2012; Markovic, Jukic, Milanovic, & Metikos, 2007). RSI depends on GCT and jumping height (Abramov et al., 1980; Flanagan et al., 2008; Markovic, 2007). Markovic et al. (2007) conducted a plyometric training program 3 times weekly for 10 weeks. Before and after the training intervention the participants (n=30) performed maximal drop jumps. In our study the RSI increased, too. However, in the study of Markovic et al. (2007) the GCT decreased while the jumping height remained unaltered. We observed gains in jumping height and unaltered GCT. The discrepancies might be explained by the different populations participating in the two studies. In our study semi- professional dancers which were experienced in jumping were examined while Markovic et al. (2007) analyzed physical educational students who had no specific jump experience. On the other hand Kyrolainen et al. (2005) accomplished a training program for 10 weeks with recreational man. According to our and other studies (Kubo et al., 2007) they observed gains in jumping height while the GCT remained unaltered. Further, another training study with intermediate or advanced ballet or modern dancers (Brown et al., 2007) found an increase in standing vertical jumping height of 8.3% after 6 weeks of plyometric training.

An increase in jumping height is based on an increase in force impact equaling the impulse (momentum). As the observed GCT of the drop jump is constant, the increase in the impulse is attributable to an increase in the mean force. This is in accordance with increased forces measured during maximal voluntary plantar flexions. In these measurements the increased work (Fig. 3) results from an increased force, too, as the angular velocity as well as the angular range of motion were given by the isokinetic diagnostic system during the plantar flexions. Furthermore, the peak torque was increased significantly for the jumping leg and tends to increase for the kicking leg (Fig. 2). An increase in maximum force (isometric and dynamic) after plyometric training was reported by a series of studies (Kubo et al., 2007; Wilkerson et al., 2004), too. The increases of maximal force can be induced either by an increase of neuromuscular activation or changes in the muscle properties (Duchateau & Baudry, 2011).

It is documented that a time course exist between adaptations of neural and muscle factors (Sale, 1988). In early stages of strength training the neuromuscular performance increase followed by gains in the cross sectional area (Moritani & deVries, 1979).

Increased muscle activity after plyometric training was found using surface electromyography (Gollhofer & Kyrolainen, 1991; Toumi, Best, Martin, F'Guyer, & Poumarat, 2004). Kyrolainen et al. (2005) conducted a plyometric training over 15 weeks with 2 training sessions weekly. They found increased muscle activity in the plantar flexors accompanied by increased MVC force after 10 weeks of training. The changes of muscle activity of the gastrocnemius muscle and MVC force correlated well ($r=0.77$, $p<0.01$). Unfortunately, with the used methods it is not possible to distinguish if the gain in muscle activity is based on increased motor unit recruitment or increased firing rate (Duchateau & Baudry, 2011). The muscle activity can be modulated on supraspinal and spinal level. In this context increased spinal reflex activity was found after plyometric training (Voigt, Chelli, & Frigo, 1998). It was assumed that the increased muscle activity during a stretch-shortening cycle (as in drop jump) after plyometric training is based on changes in the spinal reflex activity (Voigt et al., 1998). It is not reported in literature if supraspinal adaptations occur due to plyometric training.

Moreover, improved neuromuscular performance may also caused by enhanced muscle coordination. Kyrolainen et al. (1998) observed decreased antagonistic activity during plyometric training of the upper limb muscles in untrained women. In our study jumping experienced dancers were trained. So we do not believe that improved muscle coordination is the main source of the increased jumping height and force gains. However, Kubo et al. (2007) compared weight training and plyometric training with regard to muscle activation and jump performance during drop jump. They found increased muscle activation in both training groups but the jumping height increased in the plyometric group only. Kubo et al. (2007) concluded that the improvements in jumping height are attributed to changes in the mechanical properties of the muscle-tendon complex, rather than muscle activation strategies.

First muscle strength may increase due to hypertrophy, namely the increase in the cross sectional area of individual muscle fibers. This was reported by (Andersen & Aagaard, 2000; Hortobagyi et al., 1996; LaStayo, Pierotti, Pifer, Hoppeler, & Lindstedt, 2000; Malisoux et al., 2006). However, there are some studies concluding that plyometric training does not lead to higher isometric strength or muscle hypertrophy (Hakkinen et al., 1990; Prilutsky, 2005).

Changes in muscle fiber type ratio, which could further influence muscle force (Bottinelli, Schiaffino, & Reggiani, 1991; Malisoux, Francaux, & Theisen, 2007), may have little influence, as Kyrolainen et al. (2005) found no changes in the muscle fibertype distribution after a 15 week plyometric training intervention.

In general plyometric training results in an increase in muscle-tendon stiffness (Benn et al., 1998; Lindstedt, LaStayo, & Reich, 2001; Lindstedt, Reich, Keim, & LaStayo, 2002; Pousson, Van Hoecke, & Goubel, 1990; Reich, Lindstedt, LaStayo, & Pierotti, 2000). This may be attributed to an increase of tendon stiffness, muscle stiffness, or both.

Results regarding tendon stiffness after eccentric or plyometric training are ambiguous. In humans, tendon stiffness was reported to increase after training, whether it was eccentric training (Buchanan , Almdale, Lewis, & Rymer, 1986; Duclay, Robbe, Pousson, & Martin, 2009), endurance training (Buchanan & Marsh, 2001) or strength training (Kubo, Kanehisa, Kawakami, & Fukunaga, 2001). This increase may enhance the performance during stretch-shortening cycles by favoring the release of potential energy (Bosco, Komi, & Ito, 1981; Duchateau & Baudry, 2011). However, Kubo et al. (2007) found no change in tendon stiffness but in joint stiffness after plyometric training. Thus, they suggested that greatest adaptations in muscle-tendon stiffness may be located in the muscle.

Performing an 8 week eccentric training program with rats it could be demonstrated, that the stiffness of the muscle increased by 40% significantly (Reich et al., 2000), whereas muscle mass and isometric muscle force remained unchanged. The authors concluded that the 8 week training period is sufficient to induce structural adaptations in the muscle. They suggest that the increase in active muscle stiffness may be attributed to changes in the molecular spring titin. Rode et al. (2009) suggested a physiologically motivated muscle model which explains enhanced muscle stiffness by activation dependent titin-actin interaction. The giant protein titin is a structural part of myosin with a free part acting as a molecular spring connecting myosin to the Z-disc near the actin filament. The structure of its free part is very complex (Linke, Ivemeyer, Mundel, Stockmeier, & Kolmerer, 1998). Different muscles exhibit different titin isoforms with different elastic properties (Prado et al., 2005). It is very interesting, if these isoforms are exclusively determined by the genotype, or may adapt dependent on muscle function or specific training programs as suspected by (Lindstedt et al., 2002; McBride, Triplett-McBride, Davie, Abernethy, & Newton, 2003). A differential expression of titin protein bands in competitive athletes with increased levels of strength and power in comparison to untrained non-athletic individuals was observed by McBride et al. (2003). However, Kyrolainen et al. (2005) found no changes in the titin isoforms isolated from muscle biopsies after 15 weeks plyometric training. So far, further studies are needed to analyse modifications in the fine structure of the contractile and elastic components to find true mechanistic explanations due to plyometric training.

A limitation of this exercise study is that no control group was available. It takes the next step, a homogeneous comparison group of rock and roll dancers to be consulted, which is difficult to implement due to the availability in the rule.

5. Conclusion

In conclusion plyometric training leads to an increased number of rock'n'roll kicks. This increase might be attributed to gains in reactive strength as we found in our study. Despite considerable improvements in jumping performance, in dynamic peak torque as well as work during maximal concentric contractions, the results from this investigation do not reveal any further information about possible adaptations in muscle structure or neural drive of the plantar flexors. However, we suggest the implementation of plyometric training to improve the sport specific performance in rock'n'roll dancing.

References

Abramov, E., Kuporosov, B., & Matwejew, V. (1980). Trenirovka bystroty ottalkivanija. *Legkaja atletika*(1), 20.

Andersen, J. L., & Aagaard, P. (2000). Myosin heavy chain IIX overshoot in human skeletal muscle. *Muscle Nerve, 23*(7), 1095-1104.

Baechle, T. R., & Earle, R. W. (2008). *Essentials of strength training and conditioning* (3. ed.). Champaign, IL: Human Kinetics.

Benn, C., Forman, K., Mathewson, D., Tapply, M., Tiskus, S., Whang, K., & Blanpied, P. (1998). The effects of serial stretch loading on stretch work and stretch-shorten cycle performance in the knee musculature. *Journal of Orthopaedic & Sports Physical Therapy, 27*(6), 412-422.

Bobbert, M. F. (1990). Drop jumping as a training method for jumping ability. *Sports Medicine, 9*(1), 7-22.

Bobbert, M. F., Huijing, P. A., & van Ingen Schenau, G. J. (1987a). Drop jumping. I. The influence of jumping technique on the biomechanics of jumping. *Medicine & Science in Sports & Exercise, 19*(4), 332-338.

Bobbert, M. F., Huijing, P. A., & van Ingen Schenau, G. J. (1987b). Drop jumping. II. The influence of dropping height on the biomechanics of drop jumping. *Medicine & Science in Sports & Exercise, 19*(4), 339-346.

Bosco, C. (1999). *Strength assessment with Bosco's Test.* Rome: Italian Society of Sport Science.

Bosco, C., Komi, P. V., & Ito, A. (1981). Prestretch potentiation of human skeletal muscle during ballistic movement. *Acta physiologica Scandinavica, 111*(2), 135-140.

Bottinelli, R., Schiaffino, S., & Reggiani, C. (1991). Force-velocity relations and myosin heavy chain isoform compositions of skinned fibres from rat skeletal muscle. *The Journal of Physiology, 437*, 655-672.

Brown, A. C., Wells, T. J., Schade, M. L., Smith, D. L., & P.C., F. (2007). Effects of Plyometric Training Versus Traditional Weight Training on Strength, Power, and Aesthetic Jumping Ability in Female Collegiate Dancers. *Journal of Dance Medicine & Science, 11*(2), 38-44.

Bruhn, S., Kullmann, N., & Gollhofer, A. (2004). The effects of a sensorimotor training and a strength training on postural stabilisation, maximum isometric contraction and jump performance. *International Journal of Sports Medicine, 25*(1), 56-60.

Buchanan, C. I., & Marsh, R. L. (2001). Effects of long-term exercise on the biomechanical properties of the Achilles tendon of guinea fowl. *Journal of applied physiology, 90*(1), 164-171.

Buchanan , T. S., Almdale, D. P., Lewis, J. L., & Rymer, W. Z. (1986). Characteristics of synergistic relations during isometric contractions of human elbow muscles. *Journal of Neurophysiology, 56*(5), 1225-1241.

Cohen, J. (1988). *Statistical power analysis for the behavioral sciences* (2. ed.). Hillsdale, NJ u.a.: Lawrence Erlbaum Associates.

Duchateau, J., & Baudry, S. (2011). Training adaptation of the neuromuscular system. In P. V. Komi (Ed.), *Neuromuscular aspects of sport performance* (Vol. 17, pp. 216-253). Oxford: Wiley-Blackwell.

Duclay, J., Robbe, A., Pousson, M., & Martin, A. (2009). Effect of angular velocity on soleus and medial gastrocnemius H-reflex during maximal concentric and eccentric muscle contraction. *Journal of Electromyography and Kinesiology, 19*(5), 948-956.

Flanagan, E. P., Ebben, W. P., & Jensen, R. L. (2008). Reliability of the reactive strength index and time to stabilization during depth jumps. *Journal of Strength & Conditioning Research, 22*(5), 1677-1682.

Fleck, S. J., & Kraemer, W. J. (2004). *Designing resistance training programs* (3rd ed.). Champaign, IL: Human Kinetics.

Gamble, P. (2010). *Strength and conditioning for team sports : sport-specific physical preparation for high performance*. London u.a.: Routledge.

Gollhofer, A., & Kyrolainen, H. (1991). Neuromuscular control of the human leg extensor muscles in jump exercises under various stretch-load conditions. *International Journal of Sports Medicine, 12*(1), 34-40.

Hakkinen, K., Pakarinen, A., Kyrolainen, H., Cheng, S., Kim, D. H., & Komi, P. V. (1990). Neuromuscular adaptations and serum hormones in females during prolonged power training. *International Journal of Sports Medicine, 11*(2), 91-98.

Hortobagyi, T., Hill, J. P., Houmard, J. A., Fraser, D. D., Lambert, N. J., & Israel, R. G. (1996). Adaptive responses to muscle lengthening and shortening in humans. *Journal of Applied Physiology, 80*(3), 765-772.

Kirch, S. (1995). *Handbuch für Rock'n'Roll*. Aachen: Meyer & Meyer.

Komi, P. V. (1984). Physiological and biomechanical correlates of muscle function: effects of muscle structure and stretch-shortening cycle on force and speed. *Exercise and Sport Sciences Reviews, 12*, 81-121.

Komi, P. V. (2000). Stretch-shortening cycle: a powerful model to study normal and fatigued muscle. *Journal of Biomechanics, 33*(10), 1197-1206.

Komi, P. V. (2003). Stretch-Shortening Cycle. In P. V. Komi (Ed.), *Strength and Power in Sport* (Vol. 2nd ed, pp. 184-202). Oxford: Blackwell Science.

Kubo, K., Kanehisa, H., Kawakami, Y., & Fukunaga, T. (2001). Effects of repeated muscle contractions on the tendon structures in humans. *European Journal of Applied Physiology, 84*(1-2), 162-166.

Kubo, K., Morimoto, M., Komuro, T., Yata, H., Tsunoda, N., Kanehisa, H., & Fukunaga, T. (2007). Effects of plyometric and weight training on muscle-tendon complex and jump performance. *Medicine & Science in Sports & Exercise, 39*(10), 1801-1810.

Kyrolainen, H., Avela, J., McBride, J. M., Koskinen, S., Andersen, J. L., Sipila, S., . . . Komi, P. V. (2005). Effects of power training on muscle structure and neuromuscular performance. *Scandinavian Journal of Medicine & Science in Sports, 15*(1), 58-64.

Kyrolainen, H., Komi, P. V., Hakkinen, K., & D., H. K. (1998). Effects of Power Training With Stretch-Shortening Cycle (SSC) Exercises of Upper Limbs in Untrained Women. *Journal of Strength & Conditioning Research, 12*(4), 248-252.

LaStayo, P. C., Pierotti, D. J., Pifer, J., Hoppeler, H., & Lindstedt, S. L. (2000). Eccentric ergometry: increases in locomotor muscle size and strength at low training intensities. *American Journal of Physiology - Regulatory, Integrative and Comparative Physiology, 278*(5), R1282-1288.

Lindstedt, S. L., LaStayo, P. C., & Reich, T. E. (2001). When active muscles lengthen: properties and consequences of eccentric contractions. *Physiology, 16*(6), 256-261.

Lindstedt, S. L., Reich, T. E., Keim, P., & LaStayo, P. C. (2002). Do muscles function as adaptable locomotor springs? *Journal of Experimental Biology, 205*(Pt 15), 2211-2216.

Linke, W. A., Ivemeyer, M., Mundel, P., Stockmeier, M. R., & Kolmerer, B. (1998). Nature of PEVK-titin elasticity in skeletal muscle. *Proceedings of the National Academy of Sciences USA, 95*(14), 8052-8057.

Lloyd, R. S., Oliver, J. L., Hughes, M. G., & Williams, C. A. (2012). The effects of 4-weeks of plyometric training on reactive strength index and leg stiffness in male youths. *Journal of Strength and Conditioning Research, 26*(10), 2812-2819.

Malisoux, L., Francaux, M., Nielens, H., & Theisen, D. (2006). Stretch-shortening cycle exercises: an effective training paradigm to enhance power output of human single muscle fibers. *Journal of Applied Physiology, 100*(3), 771-779.

Malisoux, L., Francaux, M., & Theisen, D. (2007). What do single-fiber studies tell us about exercise training? *Medicine & Science in Sports & Exercise, 39*(7), 1051-1060.

Markovic, G. (2007). Does plyometric training improve vertical jump height? A meta-analytical review. *British Journal of Sports Medicine, 41*(6), 349-355.

Markovic, G., Jukic, I., Milanovic, D., & Metikos, D. (2007). Effects of sprint and plyometric training on muscle function and athletic performance. *Journal of Strength and Conditioning Research, 21*(2), 543-549.

Matavulj, D., Kukolj, M., Ugarkovic, D., Tihanyi, J., & Jaric, S. (2001). Effects of plyometric training on jumping performance in junior basketball players. *The Journal of Sports Medicine and Physical Fitness, 41*(2), 159-164.

Matveev, L. P. (1981). *Grundlagen des sportlichen Trainings* (1. Aufl. ed.). Berlin: Sportverl.

McBride, J. M., Triplett-McBride, T., Davie, A. J., Abernethy, P. J., & Newton, R. U. (2003). Characteristics of titin in strength and power athletes. *European journal of applied physiology, 88*(6), 553-557.

Moritani, T., & deVries, H. A. (1979). Neural factors versus hypertrophy in the time course of muscle strength gain. *American Journal of Physical Medicine & Rehabilitation, 58*(3), 115-130.

Pousson, M., Van Hoecke, J., & Goubel, F. (1990). Changes in elastic characteristics of human muscle induced by eccentric exercise. *Journal of Biomechanics, 23*(4), 343-348.

Prado, L. G., Makarenko, I., Andresen, C., Kruger, M., Opitz, C. A., & Linke, W. A. (2005). Isoform diversity of giant proteins in relation to passive and active contractile properties of rabbit skeletal muscles. *The Journal of General Physiology, 126*(5), 461-480.

Prilutsky, B. (2005). Eccentric muscle action in sport and exercise. *Biomechanics in sport: performance enhancement and injury prevention*, 56-86.

Ratamess, N. A., Alvar, B. A., Housh, T. J., Kibler, W. B., Kraemer, W. J., & Triplett, N. T. (2009). American College of Sports Medicine position stand. Progression models in resistance training for healthy adults. *Medicine & Science in Sports & Exercise, 41*(3), 687-708.

Reich, T., Lindstedt, S., LaStayo, P., & Pierotti, D. (2000). Is the spring quality of muscle plastic? *American Journal of Physiology-Regulatory, Integrative and Comparative Physiology, 278*(6), R1661-R1666.

Rode, C., Siebert, T., & Blickhan, R. (2009). Titin-induced force enhancement and force depression: a 'sticky-spring' mechanism in muscle contractions? *Journal of Experimental Biology, 259*(2), 350-360.

Ronnestad, B. R., Kvamme, N. H., Sunde, A., & Raastad, T. (2008). Short-term effects of strength and plyometric training on sprint and jump performance in professional soccer players. *Journal of Strength & Conditioning Research, 22*(3), 773-780.

Sale, D. G. (1988). Neural adaptation to resistance training. *Medicine & Science in Sports & Exercise, 20*(5 Suppl), S135-145.

Stutzig, N., & Siebert, T. (2015). Influence of joint position on synergistic muscle activity after fatigue of a single muscle head. *Muscle & Nerve, 51*(2), 259-267. doi: 10.1002/mus.24305

Taube, W., Leukel, C., Lauber, B., & Gollhofer, A. (2011). The drop height determines neuromuscular adaptations and changes in jump performance in stretch-shortening cycle training. *Scandinavian Journal of Medicine & Science in Sports.*

Toumi, H., Best, T. M., Martin, A., F'Guyer, S., & Poumarat, G. (2004). Effects of eccentric phase velocity of plyometric training on the vertical jump. *International Journal of Sports Medicine, 25*(5), 391-398.

Voigt, M., Chelli, F., & Frigo, C. (1998). Changes in the excitability of soleus muscle short latency stretch reflexes during human hopping after 4 weeks of hopping training. *European Journal of Applied Physiological and Occupational Physiology, 78*(6), 522-532.

Wilkerson, G. B., Colston, M. A., Short, N. I., Neal, K. L., Hoewischer, P. E., & Pixley, J. J. (2004). Neuromuscular Changes in Female Collegiate Athletes Resulting From a Plyometric Jump-Training Program. *Journal of Athletic Training, 39*(1), 17-23.

WRRC. (2012). Rock'n'roll rules RR/1/0112. Retrieved from http://www.wrrc.org/data/wrrc.org/doc/Rules_Competition_RnR/30_RR_RULES_0112.pdf (January, 2012)

Young, W. B., & Farrow, D. (2006). A Review of Agility: Practical Applications for Strength and Conditioning. *Strength and conditioning journal, 28*(5), 38-39.

Zemková, E., Dzurenková, D., & Pelikán, H. (2001). Assessment of jump abilities in rock'n'roll performers. *Homeostasis, 41*(6), 265-267.

Zemková, E., & Hamar, D. (2005). Jump ergometer in sport performance testing. *Acta Universitatis Palackianae Olomucensis, Gymnica, 35*(1), 7-16.

12

The Effects of a Self-Adapted, Jaw Repositioning Mouthpiece and Jaw Clenching on Muscle Activity during Vertical Jump and Isometric Clean Pull Performance

Charles Allen (Corresponding author)

Exercise Science Program, Florida Southern College, 111 Lake Hollingsworth Drive, Lakeland, FL 33801, USA

E-mail: callen@flsouthern.edu

Yang-Chieh Fu

Department of Health, Exercise Science and Recreation Management, University of Mississippi, P.O. Box 1848, University, Mississippi 38677, USA

E-mail: ycfu@olemiss.edu

John C. Garner

Department of Kinesiology and Health Promotion, Troy University, 600 University Avenue, Troy, Alabama 36082, USA

E-mail: jcgarner@troy.edu

Abstract

Purpose: The purpose of this study was to investigate the effects of a self-adapted, jaw repositioning mouthpiece and jaw clenching on muscle activity during the countermovement vertical jump (CMVJ) and isometric mid-thigh clean pull (MTCP). **Methods:** Thirty-six healthy, recreationally trained males (n=36; age, 23 ± 2.8 years; height, 178.54 ± 9.0 cm; body mass, 83.09 ± 7.8 kg) completed maximal CMVJ and MTCP assessments under six experimental conditions: jaw repositioning mouthpiece plus clenching (MP+C), jaw repositioning mouthpiece with jaw relaxed (MP), traditional mouthguard plus clenching (MG+C), traditional mouthguard with jaw relaxed (MG), no mouthpiece plus clenching (NoMP+C) and no mouthpiece with jaw relaxed (NoMP) while muscle activity of the dominant leg medial gastrocnemius (G), medial hamstring (H), vastus medialis (VMO), and erector spinae (ES) was recorded. **Results:** Repeated measures ANOVA revealed no changes in MTCP muscle activation for any mouthpiece or clench condition. Jaw clenching, regardless of mouthpiece condition, significantly improved prime mover muscle activation during CMVJ ($p < .001$). Prime mover muscle activation was significantly greater during CMVJ assessment for jaw repositioning mouthpiece and no mouthpiece conditions over the use of a traditional mouthguard ($p < .001$), but the repositioning mouthpiece did not lead to improved muscle activation compared to no mouthpiece ($p > .05$). **Conclusion:** These findings support jaw clenching as a viable technique to elicit concurrent activation potentiation (CAP) of prime mover muscle activity during dynamic but not isometric physical activity.

Keywords: jaw repositioning mouthpiece, jaw clenching, concurrent activation potentiation, muscle activation

1. Introduction

The use of jaw-aligning mouthpieces to alleviate the symptoms associated with temporomandibular joint disorder (TMD) is quite common and has been purported to improve various aspects of performance (Smith, 1978; Kaufman, 1980; Kaufman and Kaufman, 1984). Recently, the popularity of jaw-aligning devices for the purposes of performance enhancement has grown. These mouthguards, which in addition to the jaw repositioning properties, provide protection to the orofacial structures similar to traditional protective mouthguards. They also come in mouthpiece form, which changes the mandibular-maxillary relationship without the protective properties. Dental impressions taken by a dental practitioner are used to custom fit the jaw repositioning devices to the individual, which leads to an expensive end product; however, there are self-adaptable boil-and-bite versions available. These products can be designed to fit the upper or lower jaw, depending on the specific oral appliance model and individual preference, and have small acrylic bite plates that inhibit direct contact of the upper and lower molar teeth when the mouth is closed. This changes the temporomandibular joint relationship, pulling the mandible down and slightly forward, which mimics the jaw position achieved with the TMD treatment devices.

Several studies have examined these devices and their effects on a variety of physiological variables with mixed results (Garner & McDivitt, 2009; Garner & Miskimin, 2009; Garner et al, 2011a; Garner et al, 2011b). A positive relationship between a customized, jaw repositioning mouthpiece and aerobic endurance exercise performance has been reported with changes in airway openings (Garner & McDivitt, 2009) and several parameters of respiratory exchange including VO_2, VO_2/kg, and VCO_2 (Garner et al, 2011a). Another investigation reported significant improvements in auditory reaction times when the same customized repositioning mouthpiece was worn compared to no mouthpiece use (Garner & Miskimin, 2009). Stress hormone response following a vigorous bout of resistance exercise was significantly attenuated when a customized, jaw repositioning mouthpiece was implemented in comparison to no mouthpiece conditions (Garner et al, 2011b). Researchers examined salivary cortisol levels at various time points during and post-resistance training exercise. While cortisol levels were similar for the duration of the exercise bout for both the mouthpiece and no mouthpiece conditions, cortisol levels at 10 minutes post exercise was significantly lower when the mouthpiece was used, suggesting a direct relationship between jaw repositioning mouthpiece use and post-exercise attenuation of cortisol.

Studies examining the effects of jaw repositioning devices on various measures of force production have also been conducted (Arent et al, 2010; Dunn-Lewis et al, 2012; Allen et al, 2014). No improvement in vertical jump performance variables or one-repetition maximum bench press performance was reported with the use of a self-adapted, jaw repositioning mouthpiece compared to no mouthpiece (Allen et al, 2014). Similarly, the effects of two jaw repositioning mouthguards on strength, power and a myriad of other assessments were investigated with no improvements in any performance measure compared to placebo mouthguard and no mouthguard (Golem & Arent, 2015). Conversely, significant improvements in vertical jump height and peak power during the 30 second Wingate Anaerobic Power Test were reported when a neuromuscular dentistry-based, customized mouthguard was used by professional and collegiate athletes compared to tests without a mouthguard in the same participant group (Arent et al, 2010). Dunn-Lewis et al, (2012) examined a self-adapted, jaw repositioning mouthguard's effects on a myriad of performance variables in highly trained males and females. Power and force production during the bench throw test were significantly greater in both sexes under the mouthpiece condition. Additionally, significant improvements were reported for the mouthpiece condition in males only for force production and power during the plyo-press power quotient assessment and rate of power production during the vertical jump assessment. The use of a customized, jaw repositioning mouthguard was also reported to enhance the concurrent activation potentiation (CAP) effects of jaw clenching by promoting a more aligned and forceful contraction of the masticatory muscles (Busca et al, 2016). Grip strength performance, which was greater when the jaw was clenched than when the jaw was relaxed, improved to a greater extent when participants clenched the jaw while wearing the customized jaw repositioning mouthguard.

Proposed mechanisms underlying jaw repositioning mouthguard and mouthpiece use are varied depending upon the performance outcome of interest. Early practitioners of neuromuscular dentistry proposed improved proprioceptive function (Jakush, 1982). Another proposed mechanism of interest involves improved neuromuscular response due to proper jaw alignment (Garner et al, 2011b). Increased genioglossus muscle contraction, demonstrated to lead to a relaxation of the pharyngeal airway, was proposed as one explanation for improved gas exchange parameters during treadmill running when a performance mouthpiece was worn compared to no mouthpiece condition (Garner et al, 2011b). These authors also reported increased electromyography activity of the genioglossus muscle when the jaw repositioning mouthpiece was worn (Garner et al, 2011b). An increase in neuromuscular activity may explain, at least in part, the previously reported improvements in muscle force production. However, the effects of jaw repositioning mouthpiece use on prime mover muscle activation during physical activity have not yet been reported in the literature. Consequently, this investigation sought to examine the effects of a self-adapted, jaw-repositioning mouthpiece on muscle activation during power and force production activities. Additionally, the effects of maximal jaw clenching while wearing the jaw-repositioning mouthpiece were also examined as jaw clenching has been shown to impact force production and muscle activation during physical activity (Ebben et al, 2010b). It was hypothesized that jaw clenching during the selected assessments would lead to improvements in muscle activation over non-clenched conditions and the addition of the jaw repositioning mouthpiece might further improve muscle activation.

2. Methods

This study examined how jaw clenching and jaw alignment via a self-adapted, jaw repositioning mouthpiece impacted muscle activation during maximum countermovement vertical jump (CMVJ) and maximum isometric mid-thigh clean pull (MTCP) assessments. A within-subjects design was used in which participants repeated the assessments under each experimental condition.

2.1 Subjects

Thirty six (n = 36) physically active and recreationally resistance trained males, aged 18-30 years, completed the research protocol. Participants were considered physically active if they engaged in routine resistance training exercise for a minimum of three days per week for the previous month. None of the participants (n=36; age, 23 ± 2.8 years; height, 178.54 ± 9.0 cm; body mass, 83.09 ± 7.8 kg) reported current or past history of TMD, and all were free of physical injury and illness at the time of testing. All participants signed the University approved Institutional Review Board consent documents.

2.2 Experimental Controls

To ensure no dietary abnormalities throughout testing, a dietary journal documenting all food and beverage intake for the 72 hours prior to the initial testing session was required. Additionally, 24-hour dietary recalls were also reported for both remaining testing days. Participants were also asked to refrain from any non-prescription supplementation/drug use throughout the study with caffeine being the only exception. Participants were asked to maintain normal use or nonuse of caffeine for the duration of the study. To ensure adequate hydration status for assessment, consumption of 5-7 milliliters of water per kilogram of body weight four hours prior to each testing session was prescribed (American

Dietetic Association, 2009). A urine sample was provided by all participants on each testing day which was analyzed for specific gravity via dipstick (BTNX Inc; Markham, Ontario, Canada) to ensure euhydration status prior to testing. Participants maintained their normal exercise routines, however, they were asked to refrain from exercise 24 hours prior to a testing session. Finally, participants were asked to maintain their normal sleeping patterns as best as possible throughout their study participation. Dietary records were analyzed by a registered dietitian to ensure individual consistency throughout study participation, and questioning by the primary investigator was conducted each testing day prior to the onset of assessment to determine participant adherence to exercise, nutritional, and sleep requests.

2.3 Procedures

Experimental testing consisted of four laboratory visits. The initial visit involved participant prescreening, obtaining informed consent, basic anthropometric measurements, provision of mouthpieces, and familiarization with all testing procedures. The three remaining laboratory visits were data collection sessions lasting approximately one hour and were separated by approximately one week. All testing times were scheduled within one hour of the time of day of the previous testing session to account for diurnal variation. There were three oral appliance conditions which consisted of a self-adapted, jaw repositioning mouthpiece (ArmourBite Mouthpiece; Under Armour, Baltimore, MD, USA), a traditional mouthguard (Cramer Mouth Guard; Cramer Products Inc, Gardner, KS, USA), and no mouthpiece. To account for jaw clenching during assessment, two jaw musculature conditions, jaw clenched and jaw relaxed, were included for a total of six experimental conditions which were as follows: jaw repositioning mouthpiece plus clenching (MP+C), jaw repositioning mouthpiece with jaw relaxed (MP), traditional mouthguard plus clenching (MG+C), traditional mouthguard with jaw relaxed (MG), no mouthpiece plus clenching (NoMP+C) and no mouthpiece with jaw relaxed (NoMP). The experimental conditions were randomized for all participants. Both jaw clenched and jaw relaxed trials for each respective mouthpiece condition were performed within a testing session separated by a twenty minute washout period to allow for recovery. To control for clenching during the jaw relaxed trials, the participants were instructed to breathe through pursed lips which is consistent with previously published research (Ebben et al, 2008b; Ebben et al, 2010a).

2.3.1 Maximum Voluntary Contraction Assessment

During each testing visit, the maximum CMVJ and isometric MTCP trials were preceded by maximum voluntary contraction (MVC) assessment. Following dynamic warm up and prior to each assessment of CMVJ and MTCP, participants were asked to perform three MVCs for each of the selected musculature. Participants maximally contracted the selected muscles for three seconds, and EMG activity was collected for five seconds including one second prior to and immediately following those contractions. These MVC were analyzed for peak signals, and were used to determine percent activation of the selected musculature during performance of the assessments.

2.3.2 Countermovement Jump Assessment

CMVJ assessment procedures via a Vertec® device (Sports Imports, Columbus, OH, USA) were consistent with previously described methods (McGuigan, 2016). The participants were instructed to determine their maximum reach height by standing flat-footed, directly underneath the Vertec device, reaching up with the dominant hand to push forward the highest vane that could be reached. The height of the device was then increased to accommodate a maximal effort CMVJ. The participant was then instructed to perform each CMVJ trial without moving the feet prior to take off, to jump maximally, and to tap the highest vane possible at the apex of the jump. Trials were recorded as the vertical distance, to the nearest one-half inch between the reach height and height of vane tapped during the jump. Each participant was permitted three trials separated by 30 seconds for each testing condition. The trial producing the highest jump was used for analysis.

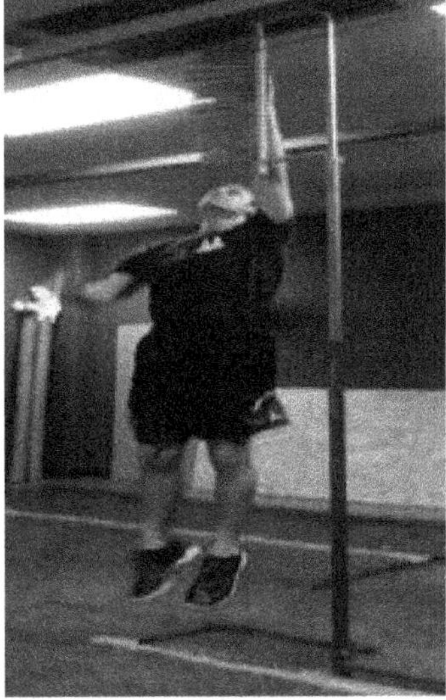

Image 1. Countermovement Vertical Jump Assessment

Description: Participant reaches up with the dominant hand at the apex of the jump to tap the highest vane possible.

2.3.3 Isometric Mid-Thigh Clean Pull Assessment

Procedures for MTCP assessment were consistent with those previously reported (Kawamori, 2006). A Jones machine (BodyCraft, Inc., Sunbury, OH, USA) was used to facilitate MTCP assessment. The machine was modified so that the bar was fixed and unmovable. A goniometer was used to standardize hip and knee angles to flexed positions of 125° and 140° respectively, with as little variance between participants as the Jones machine adjustments would allow. The participants used a double overhand, closed grip in which the thumb was wrapped around the bar. Additionally, nylon weightlifting straps were used to remove hand size and grip strength as potentially limiting factors. When instructed, the participant exerted maximal force onto the floor while pulling against the fixed barbell for three seconds. Thirty seconds rest was provided between trials to ensure recovery. Three trials were afforded to each participant. The trials yielding the best performance were utilized for further analysis.

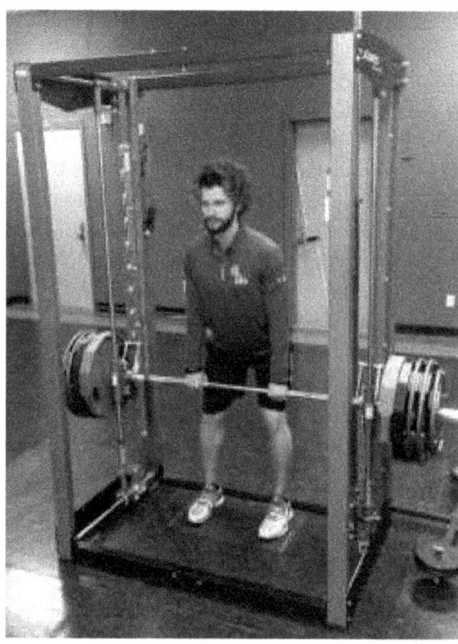

Image 2. Mid-Thigh Clean Pull Assessment

Description: The barbell is affixed by nylon straps and weight added to the barbell to prevent movement of the Jones machine.

2.4 Electromyography

Bipolar surface electromyography (EMG) was recorded at 1000Hz during CMVJ and MTCP assessment on the participants' dominant side during all three laboratory testing visits. Electrodes (EME Company, Baton Rouge, LA, USA) 5cm in length and 3cm in width were placed 3cm apart, as measured from the electrode center, at each location with a ground electrode on the tibial head. Skin preparation for all electrodes included shaving of the hair and abrasion of the skin around electrode site followed by cleansing with an alcohol swab. Data was recorded from the medial head of the gastrocnemius (G), medial hamstring (H), oblique fibers of the vastus medialis (VMO), and erector spinae (ES). Specific electrode placement followed the recommendations found on the Surface Electromyography for the Non-Invasive Assessment of Muscles website (The SENAM Project). EMG data collection was facilitated using an 8-channel electromyography system (Noraxon USA Inc., Scottsdale, AZ, USA) and raw EMG data were processed with a 4th order Butterworth bandpass filter (10-300Hz) via MatLab software (The MathWorks, Inc., Natick, MA, USA).

2.5 Statistical Analyses

A 3 x 2 (mouthpiece x clench condition) repeated measures ANOVA was conducted to analyze each of the dependent variables for interaction and main effect significance. In cases where conditions of sphericity were not met, the Greenhouse-Geisser correction estimate was used if $\varepsilon < .75$, and the Huynh-Feldt correction estimate was used if $\varepsilon > .75$. Pair-wise comparisons utilized a Bonferroni confidence interval adjustment. Paired sample t-tests were utilized to determine specific differences when interactions between mouthpiece and clench condition were observed. All analyses were performed with an a priori alpha level of $p \leq 0.05$. Sample size was also determined a priori using G*Power 3.1 software (Faul et al, 2009). Data were analyzed using IBM Statistics package software, version 22.0 (IBM SPSS Statistics, Armonk, NY, USA).

3. Results

For all CMVJ and MTCP EMG measures, data are expressed as a percentage of activation relative to MVC EMG signal. For MVC EMG, data represents the peak EMG signal recorded during the trial with greatest muscle activity.

3.1 MVC Data

Peak EMG signal for all four muscles assessed are presented in Table 1 below. There was main effect significance for jaw clenching (p = 0.019) for gastrocnemius muscle activity only. There was mouthpiece*clench interaction significance for both the gastrocnemius and erector spinae peak EMG signal. Further analysis revealed that the peak gastrocnemius EMG signal was significantly greater for the MG+C compared to MG condition, and peak erector EMG signal was significantly greater for the NoMP compared to the NoMP+C condition.

Table 1. Peak EMG signal during MVC trials (mV)

	MP	MP+C	MG	MG+C	NoMP	NoMP+C
G	.570 ± .22	.562 ± .24	.498 ± .21	*.604 ± .25	.544 ± .24	.589 ± .27
H	.514 ± .30	.518 ± .25	.525 ± .29	.546 ± .30	.515 ± .31	.497 ± .29
VMO	.349 ± .19	.347 ± .19	.307 ± .16	.334 ± .18	.304 ± .17	.328 ± .18
ES	.239 ± .08	.241 ± .08	.260 ± .12	.262 ± .12	*.290 ± .15	.244 ± .11

Description: Data are expressed as mean ± standard deviation. An asterisk (*) indicates a significant difference ($p < 0.05$) between clench conditions. G= medial gastrocnemius; H=medial hamstring; VMO=vastus medialis obliquus; ES=erector spinae; MP=jaw repositioning mouthpiece; MP+C=jaw repositioning mouthpiece and jaw clenching; MG=protective mouthguard; MG+C=protective mouthguard and jaw clenching; NoMP=no mouthpiece; NoMP+C=no mouthpiece, clenching only.

3.2 *CMVJ EMG Data*

There was significant main effects for mouthpiece and clench conditions for the G, H, and VMO but not ES muscle activity. Data illustrating these findings are found in Tables 2 and 3 respectively. A significant mouthpiece*clench interaction was also observed for muscle activity of all four muscles of interest. Post-hoc analysis of this interaction revealed that the MG+C condition elicited significantly greater percentages of muscle activation than the MG condition for all four muscles.

Table 2. Percentage of muscle activation during CMVJ relative to MVC

	MP	MG	NoMP
G	76.88 ± 3.18	*48.44 ± 3.55	74.55 ± 3.83
H	90.82 ± 7.13	*76.32 ± 6.48	96.21 ± 9.01
VMO	246.99 ± 19.34	*153.54 ± 12.11	233.19 ± 21.46
ES	146.61 ± 13.07	150.297 ± 13.22	155.86 ± 23.50

Description: Data are expressed as mean ± standard error. An asterisk (*) indicates a significant difference ($p < 0.05$) relative to the other mouthpiece conditions. G= medial gastrocnemius; H=medial hamstring; VMO=vastus medialis obliquus; ES=erector spinae; MP=jaw repositioning mouthpiece; MG=protective mouthguard; NoMP=no mouthpiece.

Table 3. Percentage of muscle activation during CMVJ relative to MVC

	Jaw Clenched	Jaw Relaxed	p Value
G	76.36 ± 3.09*	56.89 ± 2.64	$p < 0.001$
H	97.27 ± 6.42*	78.29 ± 6.61	$p = 0.001$
VMO	236.48 ± 16.31*	186.00 ± 14.29	$p < 0.001$
ES	156.20 ± 13.34	145.65 ± 13.73	$p = 0.327$

Description: Data are expressed as mean ± standard error. An asterisk (*) indicates a significant difference ($p < 0.05$) between clench conditions. G= medial gastrocnemius; H=medial hamstring; VMO=vastus medialis obliquus; ES=erector spinae.

3.3 MTCP EMG Data

MTCP EMG data are represented in Tables 4 and 5. There were no significant interaction or main effects for percent activation of any muscle for any treatment condition.

Table 4. Percentage of muscle activation during MTCP relative to MVC

	MP	MG	NoMP
G	20.14 ± 2.09	20.67 ± 2.08	19.57 ± 1.96
H	42.20 ± 4.11	47.55 ± 6.51	49.48 ± 5.17
VMO	73.39 ± 6.83	73.46 ± 7.05	76.32 ± 8.18
ES	125.54 ± 7.66	126.81 ± 7.86	124.27 ± 8.86

Description: Data are expressed as mean ± standard error. G= medial gastrocnemius; H=medial hamstring; VMO=vastus medialis obliquus; ES=erector spinae; MP=jaw repositioning mouthpiece; MG=protective mouthguard; NoMP=no mouthpiece.

Table 5. Percentage of muscle activation during MTCP relative to MVC

	Jaw Clenched	Jaw Relaxed	*p* Value
G	20.45 ± 1.77	19.80 ± 2.01	$p = 0.574$
H	48.97 ± 5.47	43.84 ± 3.93	$p = 0.217$
VMO	74.23 ± 6.17	74.55 ± 7.27	$p = 0.927$
ES	126.20 ± 6.74	124.88 ± 7.75	$p = 0.764$

Description: Data are expressed as mean ± standard error. G= medial gastrocnemius; H=medial hamstring; VMO=vastus medialis obliquus; ES=erector spinae.

4. Discussion

The aim of this investigation was to determine changes in muscle activity due to wearing a self-adapted, jaw repositioning mouthpiece during maximum CMVJ and isometric MTCP assessment. Additionally, due to jaw clenching potentially impacting the results, the authors sought to determine whether the observed changes could be attributed exclusively to jaw clenching, jaw alignment by the use of a repositioning mouthpiece, or if the presence of both conditions led to synergistic results.

4.1 Mouthpiece Conditions

There was no difference in percent activation between MP and NoMP conditions during CMVJ and MTCP performance for any of the four muscles examined. While performance enhancements such as improved respiratory exchange parameters (Garner et al, 2011a), increased vertical jump height and anaerobic power (Arent et al, 2010), and improved force production variables (Dunn-Lewis et al, 2012) have been attributed to the use of jaw repositioning appliances, increased relative muscle activation does not appear to be among them. One possible explanation for this may be related to the jaw repositioning mouthpiece design. Many of the previous investigations demonstrating performance improvements as the result of jaw repositioning appliance use employed customized versions fabricated by dental practitioners specifically for the individual user (Arent et al, 2010; Garner & McDivitt, 2009; Garner & Miskimin, 2009; Garner et al, 2011a; Garner et al, 2011b) . The current study utilized a self-adapted, jaw repositioning mouthpiece which utilizes a typical boil-and-bite fitting procedure. It is possible that a customized jaw repositioning appliance may prove beneficial in augmenting muscle activation during forceful exertion.

Interestingly, percent activation for the G, H, and VMO was significantly lower during the MG condition compared to the MP and NoMP conditions during the CMVJ assessment. This is an important finding considering the recommended and requisite usage of similar mouthguards during sports such as lacrosse and American football (ADA, 2006; NCAA, 2011). Although important in providing safety and protection of the teeth and mouth from potential injury during competition, many athletes have negative perceptions of mouthguards due to breathing and verbal communication difficulties (Ferrari et al, 2002). Additionally, some athletes suspect that mouthguards have detrimental effects on performance (Bourdin et al, 2006; Gardiner et al, 2000). Upon the completion of the current investigation, participants were polled regarding their preference of the oral appliance conditions in the study. The responses reflect similar discontent with the MG used compared to the MP and NoMP conditions. Thirty one of 36 participants indicated a preference for either MP or NoMP conditions over the MG condition, with the most common reason given being discomfort in the MG condition. Of the five participants who indicated a preference for the MG condition, all cited familiarity from previous participation in sports requiring such mouthguards as the reason for their preference. It is possible that the MG condition, being unfamiliar and uncomfortable to the majority of the participants, created an awkward and distracting performance environment, leading to the observed detriment in muscle activation.

4.2 Jaw Clenching Conditions

Clenching the jaw elicited significantly greater percent activation of the G, H, and VMO but not the ES, compared to the non-clench condition and regardless of mouthpiece condition during CMVJ performance. Erector spinae activity was not different between clench conditions. Ebben (2006) introduced and defined concurrent activation potentiation (CAP) as the ergogenic advantage of increased prime mover performance as the result of simultaneous remote voluntary contraction (RVC) such as clenching the jaw, and touted CAP as the reason for improved force production variables during various physical activities (Ebben et al, 2008a; Ebben et al, 2008b; Ebben et al, 2010a; Ebben et al, 2010b). Considering this definition, the current findings are logical. For the CMVJ, the G, H, and VMO would be considered prime movers. The ES, although active during the CMVJ, would not be considered a prime mover for this activity, and as such, would not be potentiated during CMVJ performance. A previous study investigating muscle activity during isokinetic knee extension and flexion revealed significantly higher muscle activity for prime mover musculature when RVC including jaw clenching were utilized (Ebben et al, 2010b). Muscle activity of the movement antagonist as well as homologous contralateral musculature was not changed. These findings, as well as the findings of the current investigation, support the specificity of CAP to the prime movers involved in the activity of interest.

In contrast, jaw clenching failed to lead to a significant change in muscle activity in comparison to the non-clench condition for any muscle examined during performance of the isometric MTCP. These findings are consistent with previous research as well (Garceau et al, 2012). Muscle activity during isometric knee extension with the incorporation of jaw clenching as well as other RVC was no different than isometric knee extension without RVC (Garceau et al, 2012). Although muscle activity was not significantly different between RVC and no RVC conditions, PF and RFD were significantly improved under RVC conditions (Garceau et al, 2012). Increased neural drive as a result of functional cortical connections and motor overflow has been proposed as the primary mechanism underlying CAP (Ebben, 2006; Ebben et al, 2008a; Ebben et al, 2008b; Ebben et al, 2010a; Ebben et al, 2010b). The findings of the current study, coupled with those reported by Garceau et al, (2012), suggest that any observed CAP performance improvement during isometric activity would not be due to increased neural drive but other mechanisms not yet known. As stated previously, this investigation sought to discern whether jaw clenching or jaw repositioning mouthpiece use was exclusively responsible for any observed changes in muscle activity and was not designed to determine specific mechanisms leading to those changes. Future research should attempt to reveal those mechanisms. It is important to note that while the current results do not support motor overflow as the underlying mechanism of CAP during isometric activity, it does not negate it either.

Previous research has demonstrated that aggregate RVC elicited CAP to a greater extent than isolated RVC (Ebben et al, 2008b). During isometric knee extension, mean and peak torque values were significantly improved when a single RVC was utilized, however, conditions that combined multiple RVC led to knee extensor torque values greater than the single RVC condition (Ebben et al, 2008b). The current study was concerned specifically with jaw clenching as a variable impacting muscle activity and not with maximizing CAP via the incorporation of multiple RVC. As such, other examples of RVC, such as the Valsalva maneuver, were not incorporated. All participants in the current investigation were given instructions to breathe as normally as possible during the performance assessments, in an attempt to control for the potential CAP effects of holding the breath. It is possible that, with the incorporation of additional RVC, CAP may have been stimulated to a greater degree, and increased muscle activity to the level of statistical significance.

5. Conclusions

This is the first study to determine whether observed improvements in muscle activation can be attributed exclusively to jaw repositioning mouthpiece use, jaw clenching, or if both conditions are necessary to achieve ergogenic effects. Jaw clenching, regardless of mouthpiece condition, improved muscle activation during countermovement vertical jump (CMVJ) compared to non-clench conditions. Although muscle activation was greater during CMVJ assessment for jaw repositioning mouthpiece and no mouthpiece conditions over the use of a traditional mouthguard, the repositioning mouthpiece did not lead to improved muscle activation compared to no mouthpiece. No changes were observed in isometric mid-thigh clean pull (MTCP) muscle activation for any mouthpiece or clench condition. These findings support jaw clenching as a viable technique to elicit concurrent activation potentiation (CAP) of prime mover muscle activity during dynamic but not isometric physical activity. Future studies should examine customized jaw repositioning mouthguards or mouthpieces and their effects on muscle activation.

References

ADA council on access, prevention and inter-professional relations; ADA council on scientific affairs. (2006). Using mouthguards to reduce the incidence and severity of sports-related oral injuries. *The Journal of the American Dental Association, 137*, 1712-1720.

Allen, CR, Dabbs, NC, Zachary, CS, Garner, JC. (2014). The acute effect of a commercial bite-aligning mouthpiece on strength and power in recreationally trained men. *Journal of Strength and Conditioning Research, 28(2)*, 499-503.

American Dietetic Association. (2009). Position of the American Dietetic Association, Dietitians of Canada, and the American College of Sports Medicine: Nutrition and Athletic Performance. *The Journal of the American Dental Association, 109*, 509-527.

Arent, SM, McKenna, J, Golem, DL. (2010). Effects of a neuromuscular dentistry-designed mouthguard on muscular endurance and anaerobic power. *Comparative Exercise Physiology, 7*, 73-79.

Bourdin, M, Brunet-Patru, I, Hager, PE, Allard, Y, Hager, JP, Lacour, JR, Moyen, B. (2006). Influence of maxillary mouthguards on physiological parameters. *Medicine & Science in Sports & Exercise, 38*(8), 1500-1504.

Busca, B, Morales, J, Solana-Tramunt, M, Miro, A, and Garcia, M. (2016). Effects of jaw clenching while wearing a customized bite-aligning mouthpiece on strength in healthy young men. *Journal of Strength and Conditioning Research, 30(4)*, 1102-1110.

Dunn-Lewis, C, Luk, H, Comstock, BA, Szivak, TK, Hooper, DR, Kupchak, BR, Watts, AM, Putney, BJ, Hydren, JR, Volek, JS, Denegar, CR, Kraemer, WJ. (2012). The effects of a customized over-the-counter mouth guard on neuromuscular force and power production in trained men and women. *Journal of Strength and Conditioning Research, 26*, 1085-1093.

Ebben, WP. (2006). A brief review of concurrent activation potentiation: theoretical and practical constructs. *Journal of Strength and Conditioning Research, 20*, 985-991.

Ebben, WP, Flanagan, EP, Jensen, RL. (2008). Jaw clenching results in concurrent activation potentiation during the countermovement jump. *Journal of Strength and Conditioning Research, 22*, 1850-1854.

Ebben, WP, Kaufmann, CE, Fauth, ML, Petushek EJ. (2010). Kinetic analysis of concurrent activation potentiation during back squats and jump squats. *Journal of Strength and Conditioning Research, 24*(6), 1515-1519.

Ebben, WP, Leigh, DH, Geiser, CF. (2008). The effect of remote voluntary contractions on knee extensor torque. *Medicine & Science in Sports & Exercise, 40*(10), 1805-1809.

Ebben, WP, Petushek, EJ, Fauth, ML, Garceau, LR. (2010). EMG analysis of concurrent activation potentiation. *Medicine & Science in Sports & Exercise, 42*(3), 556-562.

Faul, F, Erdfelder, E, Buchner, A, Lang, AG. (2009). Statistical power analyses using G*Power 3.1: Tests for correlation and regression analyses. *Behavior Research Methods, 40*(4), 1149-1160.

Ferrari, CH, Ferreria de Mederios, JM. (2002). Dental trauma and level of information: mouthguard use in different contact sports. *Dental Traumatology, 18*, 144-147.

Garceau, LR, Petushek, EJ, Fauth, ML, Ebben, WP. (2012). Effect of remote voluntary contractions on isometric prime mover torque and electromyography. *Journal of Exercise Physiology Online, 15*(4), 40-46.

Gardiner, DM, Ranalli, DN. (2000). Attitudinal factors influencing mouthguard utilization. *Dental Clinics of North America, 44*, 53-65.

Garner, DP, Dudgeon, WD, McDivitt, EJ. (2011). The effects of mouthpiece use on cortisol levels during an intense bout of resistance exercise. *Journal of Strength and Conditioning Research, 25*, 2866-2871.

Garner, DP, Dudgeon, WD, Scheett, TP, McDivitt, EJ. (2011). The effects of mouthpiece use on gas exchange parameters during steady-state exercise in college-aged men and women. *The Journal of the American Dental Association,* 142, 1041-1047.

Garner, DP, McDivitt, EJ. (2009). Effects of mouthpiece use on airway openings and lactate levels in healthy college males. *Compendium of Continuing Education in Dentistry, 30*, 9-13.

Garner, DP, Miskimin, J. (2009). Effects of mouthpiece use on auditory and visual reaction time in college males and females. *Compendium of Continuing Education in Dentistry, 30*, 14-17.

Golem, DL, Arent, SM. (2016). Effects of over-the-counter jaw-repositioning mouth guards on dynamic balance, flexibility, agility, strength, and power in college-aged male athletes. *Journal of Strength and Conditioning Research, 29*, 500-512.

Jakush J. (1982). Divergent views: Can dental therapy enhance athletic performance? *The Journal of the American Dental Association, 104*, 292-298.

Kaufman, RS. (1980). Case reports of TMJ repositioning to improve scoliosis and the performance by athletes. *New York State Dental Journal, 46*, 206-209.

Kawamori, N, Rossi, SJ, Justice, BD, Haff, EE, Pistilli, EE, O'Bryant, HS, Stone, MH, Haff, GG. (2006). Peak force and rate of force development during isometric and dynamic mid-thigh clean pulls performed at various intensities. *Journal of Strength and Conditioning Research, 20*(3), 483-491.

McGuigan, M. (2016). Administration, scoring, and interpretation of selected tests. In G. G. Haff & N. T. Triplett (Eds.), *Essentials of Strength Training and Conditioning* (pp 259-316). Champaign, IL: Human Kinetics.

NCAA. (2011). *2011-12 NCAA Sports Medicine Handbook.* Indianapolis, IN: The National Collegiate Athletic Association.

Smith, SD. (1978). Muscular strength correlated to jaw posture and the temporomandibular joint. *New York State Dental Journal, 48*, 278-285.

The SENIAM Project. [Online] Available: http://www.seniam.org (October 28, 2014).

13

Differences in Lower Body Kinematics during Forward Treadmill Skating Between Two Different Hockey Skate Designs

Mike R. Hellyer
TESTify Performance, Winnipeg, Canada
91 Lowson Crescent, Winnipeg, R3P 0T3, Canada
E-mail: mikerhellyer@gmail.com

Marion J.L. Alexander (Corresponding author)
Faculty of Kinesiology and Recreation Management,
University of Manitoba, Winnipeg, Canada
306 Max Bell Center, Winnipeg, R3T 2N2, Canada
E-mail: marion.alexander@umanitoba.ca

Cheryl M. Glazebrook
Faculty of Kinesiology and Recreation Management,
University of Manitoba, Winnipeg, Canada
319 Max Bell Center, Winnipeg, R3T 2N2, Canada
E-mail: cheryl.glazebrook@umanitoba.ca

Jeff Leiter
Pan Am Clinic, Winnipeg, Canada
75 Poseidon Bay, Winnipeg, R3M 3E4, Canada
E-mail: jleiter@panamclinic.com

Abstract

Purpose: The purpose of this study was to investigate the differences in ankle flexibility and skating technique between a traditional hockey skate boot and a hockey skate boot with a flexible rear tendon guard. Skating technique was further investigated at different speeds to give insight on how skating technique alters as skating speed is increased. **Methods:** Eight elite hockey players were selected for the present study, which was conducted while skating on an Endless Ice Skating Treadmill. Variables were recorded using a three-camera setup and measured from video records at five selected treadmill speeds using the Dartfish Team Pro v6 software. Kinematic variables were then compared between the two skate designs with a doubly multivariate repeated measures design. Statistical significance was set at $p<0.05$. **Results:** Post hoc univariate tests comparing skate designs displayed significant increases in plantar flexion, plantar flexion angular velocity, hip extension, hip extension angular velocity, stride length, and stride velocity while participants were wearing the skates that had a flexible rear tendon guard. Significant increases were also displayed in plantar flexion, plantar flexion angular velocity, knee extension, knee extension angular velocity, hip extension, hip extension angular velocity, hip abduction range of motion, hip abduction angular velocity, stride width, stride length, and stride velocity as the treadmill speed increased. There was also a significant decrease in the time the skate was in contact with the treadmill as treadmill speed increased. **Conclusion:** The results suggested that while skating forward, hockey players could improve their hockey skating technique by using hockey skates that have a flexible rear tendon guard. This flexible tendon guard improved skating technique by increasing the time of force application to the ice by increasing the range of ankle plantar flexion during propulsion of the forward skating stride.

Keywords: skate design, plantar flexion, tendon guard

1. Introduction

Hockey is a sport that requires a high level of strength, power, and skill. To be successful at the professional level athletes need to be proficient in all the skills required to play the game. Among them, skating is one of the most important (McPherson, Wrigley, & Montelpare, 2004). Players must be able to skate forwards and backwards, as well as to crossover, pivot, start, and stop during a hockey game. A player that is able to skate fast and change direction rapidly has an advantage in puck possession and puck handling. The skilled skater is more often in a position to score a goal or help to stop a goal.

1.1 Hockey Skate Design

Past literature has primarily focused on the analysis of the kinematic variables determining skating performance while neglecting the impact of biomechanical changes in skate design (Chang, Turcotte, & Pearsall, 2009; Lafontaine, 2007; Marino & Weese, 1979; Upjohn, Turcotte, Pearsall, & Loh, 2008). There has been minimal research conducted on how the biomechanical design of equipment can affect skating performance (Robert-Lachaine, Turcotte, Dixon, & Pearsall, 2012). Nevertheless, the performance of a hockey player depends on several factors, including strength, agility, shooting ability, and skating skill, which includes the equipment used during play. A study conducted by Hoshizaki et al. (Hoshizaki, Kirchner, & Hall, 1989) compared ankle range of motion while skating using different ice hockey skates and concluded that conventional hockey skates restrict the range of motion at the ankle joint for the average hockey player due to the stiff ankle guard. These authors suggested that skate manufacturers should consider altering skate flexibility when designing skates in the future.

The sport of speed skating went through a change in skate design that saw athletes improve skating performance dramatically (Houdijk, Heijnsdijk, de Koning, de Groot, & Bobbert, 2000). The introduction of the klapskate in 1997-98 allowed speed skaters to keep their blade in contact with the ice longer as they pushed off down the ice. This was done with a hinge placed under the ball of the foot between the skate boot and the blade (Houdijk, Heijnsdijk, et al., 2000). This new hinge allowed the skater to increase the amount of plantar flexion at the end of push off which is correlated to the amount of time the blade is in contact with the ice surface during force production of the forward skating stride. The increase in time the blade is in contact with the ice during force production increases the impulse a forward skater can create against the ice as impulse is the product of force and time (Behm, Wahl, Button, Power, & Anderson, 2005). This increase in impulse allows the skater to travel faster down the ice.

Although a hinge under the ball of the foot is impractical in the sport of ice hockey due to the variety of skills a hockey player must complete during a game, other design modifications can be made to the traditional hockey skate in order to take advantage of the klapskate design without compromising performance in other skills in which a player must be proficient. Easton hockey has developed a new skate that houses a flexible rear tendon guard (Figure 2). This tendon guard is said to allow added plantar flexion as a hockey skater pushes off the ice surface just as the klapskate does for a speed skater. This added plantar flexion is said to occur without reducing the player's ability to complete other skills that are needed to be an elite ice hockey skater. This skate also has an asymmetrical skate boot with the lateral side constructed five millimeters lower than the medial portion of the boot. This characteristic was designed to promote a larger angle of eversion, which could potentially lead to a longer hockey stride while skating forward (Easton Hockey, 2014).

The results of this study will provide insight into the biomechanical changes a hockey skater can experience while wearing a new skate design that includes a flexible rear tendon guard.

1.2 Skating and Skate Development

This study has been designed due to the recent trend in the hockey community to pursue biomechanical advancements in the design of the hockey skate (Hancock, Lamontagne, Stothart, & Sveistrup, 1999; Pearsall, Paquette, Baig, Albrecht, & Turcotte, 2012; Pitkin, Smirnova, Scherbina, & Zvonareva, 2002; Robert-Lachaine et al., 2012; Turcotte, Pearsall, & Montgomery, 2001). Skate researchers have started to focus on new ways to increase the range of motion at the ankle joint in the traditional hockey skate design. The attempt to develop innovative hockey skate designs, shares the same revolutionary concept of increasing ankle range of motion that the klapskate brought to the sport of speed skating (Hoshizaki, Hall, & Bourque, 1989; Madore, 2003). This new type of hockey skate design allowing greater ankle plantar flexion should be thoroughly investigated as it has the potential to provide ice hockey players with added joint range of motion, potentially increasing forward skating speed as well as enhancing mobility on skates.

Hockey skate manufacturers have improved skating performance by making skates more stable, reducing their weight, and adding protection for the foot (Robert-Lachaine et al., 2012). The modern hockey skate consists of a skate boot with upper and lower portions, blade holder, and skate blade (Bourque, 1985). Skate boots are now more rigid, possess higher ankle collars and have stiff Achilles tendon guards providing players with stability to help balance over the small skate blade. These characteristics also protect the skater's ankle from the opponent's sharp skate blades and sticks along with hard rubber pucks travelling at excessive speeds.

Although these characteristics provide the athlete with stability and protection they also limit the skater from producing a full range of motion at the ankle (Robert-Lachaine et al., 2012). This reduction in ankle range of motion could possibly lead to limiting the range of motion not only at the ankle but also at the knee and hip, ultimately reducing a player's maximum skating speed.

1.3 The Klapskate

The ice skates used in speed skating went through a revolutionary transformation in 1997-98. This time period saw the introduction of the klapskate which enabled athletes to instantly improve skating performance as they shattered all of the current world speed skating records (Houdijk, Wijker, De-Koning, Bobbert, & De-Groot, 2001). The speed at which speed skaters could skate increased by 0.3m/s in the first year alone (Kuper & Sterken, 2003). It was presented by

Houdijk et al. (Houdijk, De Koning, De Groot, Bobbert, & Van Ingen Schenau, 2000) that klapskates not only enabled skaters to skate at a higher velocity, 10m/s compared to 9.6m/s, but also maintained an equal velocity at a lower metabolic level compared to the conventional skate. The difference between the conventional speed skate and the klapskate was that the klapskate was equipped with a hinge between the boot and blade under the ball of the foot. This hinge allowed the skater to plantarflex the foot at the end of push-off while the entire blade of the skate remained in contact with the ice (Houdijk, De Koning, et al., 2000).

It has been established that the range of motion occurring at the ankle joint influences the range of motion at the knee joint during sport performance (Haguenauer, Legreneur, & Monteil, 2006). When comparing push-offs in speed skating between conventional speed skates and klapskates, experts (Houdijk, Heijnsdijk, et al., 2000) concluded that klapskates, which enabled the skater to increase the range of motion at the ankle, also increased the work output at the knee joint. In the final 50 ms of force production during the skating stride the center of pressure of the propulsion force reaches the ball of the skaters foot. The center of pressure will stay under the ball of the foot for speed skaters wearing the klapskate, as the hinge placed under the ball of the foot allows the entire skate blade to stay in contact with the ice as the skater plantarflexes the ankle. A skater wearing a conventional skate design will see the center of pressure pass from the ball of the foot and move forward to the end of the blade. This occurs because the entire skate blade is fixed to the boot of the conventional skate design (Houdijk, De Koning, et al., 2000).

The skate blade must also be rotated laterally and positioned perpendicular to the direction of force applied by the skater. This is necessary to grip the ice with the inside edge of the blade producing enough friction to develop a propulsive force. If this perpendicular position of the skate blade is not met the skate will slip forwards or backwards due to the lack of frictional force applied to the ice by the skate blade. The klapskate design allows the skater to direct the propulsive force perpendicular to the blade of the skate as the ankle is plantar flexed and the knee is fully extended.

This transpires as the klapskate keeps the blade in a perpendicular position until the knee reaches full extension. As a skater reaches the maximum amount of plantar flexion while wearing the restrictive conventional skate, fully extending the knee will now create a forward directed force relative to the skate blade. Therefore, it is a position of knee flexion during the latter stages of propulsion that is required to direct the propulsive force perpendicular to the skate blade while wearing the conventional skate. This prevents the knee from fully extending and contributing in the later stages of force production during forward skating (Houdijk, De Koning, et al., 2000).

1.4 Ankle Range of Motion

Haguenauer et al. (Haguenauer et al., 2006) also compared the effects ankle range of motion has on the knee joint. Elite figure skaters performed vertical jumps on a force plate for three separate conditions: barefoot, wearing a 1.5 kg ankle mass on both legs simulating the weight of the skates, and while wearing figure skates. These authors found that the stiff design of the figure skate boot decreased the athlete's ability to jump by limiting plantar flexion at the ankle joint. This decrease in ankle joint range of motion had significant implications on the knee joint during leg extension. Haguenauer et al. (Haguenauer et al., 2006) concluded that participants displayed significant decreases in knee extension at the instant of toe-off when wearing the restrictive skate boot. This finding is in agreement with that of Houdijk et al. (Houdijk, De Koning, et al., 2000) that reducing the amount of ankle plantar flexion an athlete has will reduce the amount of knee extension during extension of the lower limbs which is crucial in force production during forward skating in ice hockey.

The purpose of this study was to investigate the differences in ankle flexibility and skating technique between a traditional hockey skate boot and a hockey skate boot with a flexible rear tendon guard. Skating technique was further investigated at different speeds to give insight on how skating technique alters as skating speed is increased.

2. Methods

2.1 Participants

The participants for this study consisted of highly skilled male hockey players with Canadian Interuniversity Sport or professional hockey experience. A power analysis based on data from the pilot study was conducted to determine the sample size required for this study. A significance level (alpha) of 0.05 and type two-error beta of 0.2 was set to produce a desired power of at least 0.80. Using G*Power version 3 software it was determined that a minimum of eight participants were required to ensure adequate power (Faul, Erdfelder, Lang, & Buchner, 2007). There was no compensation offered to participants for taking part in this study. The Easton Mako skates (Easton Hockey, 2014) were obtained for the duration of the study from an Easton sales representative located in Winnipeg, Manitoba.

Prior to the study, participants were required to provide written consent by signing an informed consent form approved by the ENREB research group from the University of Manitoba. Participants then signed a Physical Activity Readiness Questionnaire for Everyone from the Canadian Society for Exercise Physiology (CSEP) (Quinn, 2015) and answered a short questionnaire to collect information including: height (cm), mass (kg), age, hockey experience, and brand of the current skate.

Table 1. Descriptive characteristics of participants

	Mean ± SD	Range
Age	25.50 ± 3.42	20.0 - 30.0
Height (m)	1.80 ± 0.08	1.68 - 1.90
Mass (kg)	82.55 ± 11.29	68.04 - 102.06
Hockey Experience (Years)	18.5 ± 2.14	16.00 - 22.00

All skates were sharpened with a 0.5 inch hollow and similar rocker radius by Custom Edge Skate Service to help eliminate differences between the two pairs of skates.

2.2 Skates Used

Each participant's personal skates were considered the traditional skate design for this study. The materials the participant's personal skates were made from may have differed slightly from other skates on the current market but the biomechanical properties of a high ankle collar, and stiff Achilles tendon guard are consistent with other modern skates on store shelves.

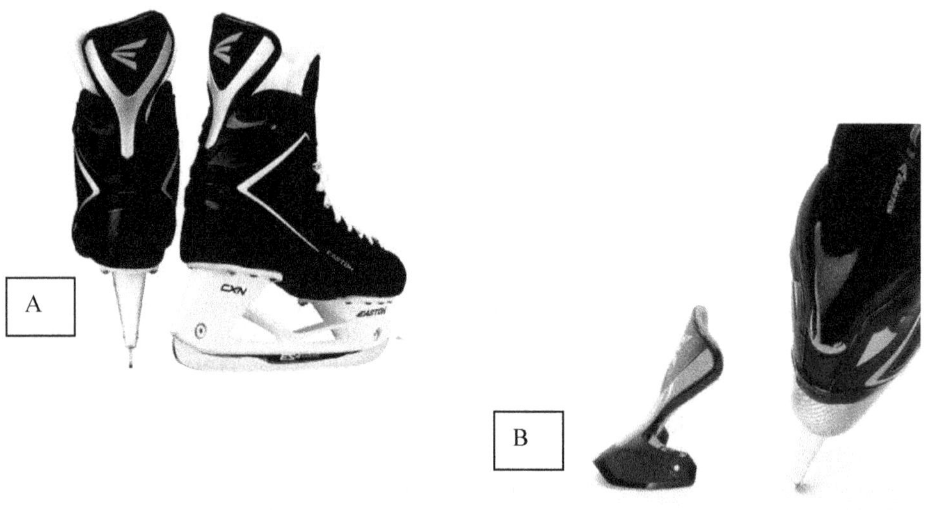

Figure 1. Easton Mako skate (retrieved from: http://hockeysupremacy.com) (A); Flexible rear tendon guard on Easton Mako (retreived from: http://purehockey.com) (B)

The Easton Mako hockey skate (Figure 1) served as the experimental skate design during this study. This skate was chosen due to the unique biomechanical characteristics it possesses. This new skate design includes a raised heel, an asymmetrical skate boot with the medial side sitting five millimeters taller than the lateral side of the boot and an active extendon guard on the rear of the skate boot (Figure 1)(Easton Hockey, 2014).

2.3 Ankle Flexibility Measurements

Ankle flexibility measurements were taken with a Canon GL2 video camera. Ankle movements were clearly seen in the video footage, which were then determined using Dartfish Team Pro v6 (Dartfish, 2014). This included both passive and active range of motion testing for the ankle in three different conditions: wearing no skate, wearing the current skate they were using (traditional design), and wearing the Easton Mako skate (Easton Hockey, 2014). Ankle dorsiflexion and plantar flexion were measured with participants lying supine on a table (Clarkson, 2000) (Figure 3). To simulate the position of the lower limb during hockey skating, a rolled towel was placed under the knee to maintain 20° to 30 ° of knee flexion.

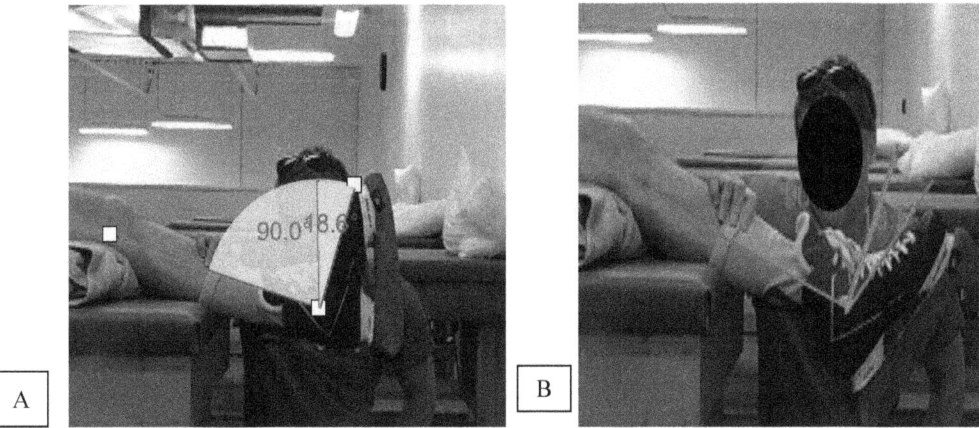

Figure 2. Measurement of ankle dorsiflexion (18.6 °) and plantarflexion (18.5 °) while wearing the Easton Mako skate.

The tibia and fibula were stabilized with the axis of rotation marked just inferior to the lateral malleolus. The stationary arm of the joint was placed parallel to the longitudinal axis of the fibula with the movable arm of the joint marked parallel to the inferior aspect of the heel eliminating forefoot movement from the measurement. Ankle dorsiflexion and plantar flexion were measured while wearing the hockey skate with the same procedure. This was accomplished by measuring the distance between points on the lower limb and the lateral malleolus to help estimate it's position within the hockey skate boot (Figure 2).

Inversion and eversion of the subtalar joint were measured with the participant lying prone and the feet positioned beyond the end of the table (Clarkson, 2000) (Figure 3). The ankle was set in a neutral position with two markings on the skin being placed over the midline of the superior aspect of the calcaneus. The stationary arm of the joint was placed parallel to the longitudinal axis of the lower leg with the movable arm of the joint being placed along the midline of the posterior aspect of the calcaneus in line with the mark on the heel pad posteriorly (Clarkson, 2000). Inversion and eversion with the hockey skate was measured with the same procedure however the movable arm was modified to align with the center of the skate blade, as the mark on the heel pad was not visible.

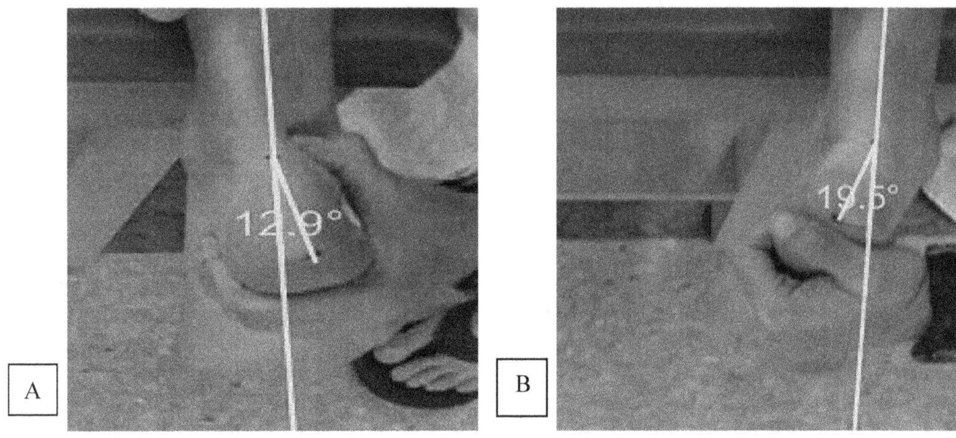

Figure 3. Measurement of subtalar inversion (19.5°) and eversion(12.9°) with no skate.

2.4 Skating Data Collection

Filming of the participants while skating took place on an Endless Ice skating treadmill (Figure 4). A three-camera set-up was used to capture video for the right side of the body. A Canon GL2 camera was used to film the sagittal view from the right. This camera was placed on a tripod approximately 2.30 m from the skating zone. A Fujifilm EXR camera was attached to a tripod and fixed to the wall in front of the skating treadmill at an approximate distance of 2.4 m from the skating zone capturing data in the frontal plane. A third camera (Canon GL2) was placed in the direction of the stride of the right leg. The position of this camera varied according to the participant to remain in line with his/her right leg.

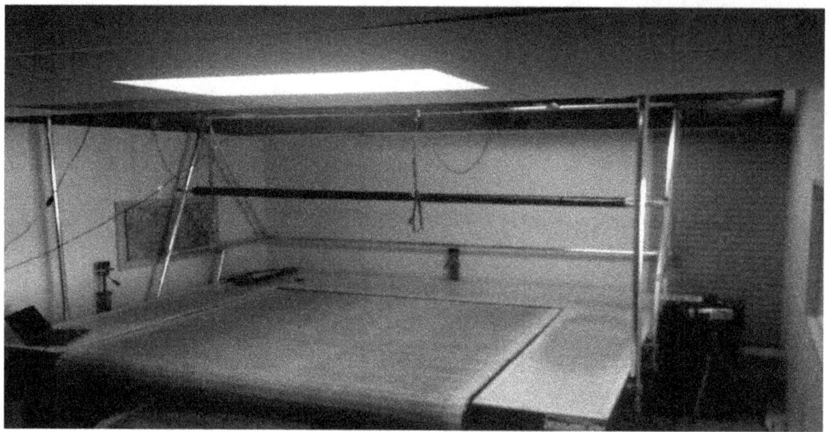

Figure 4. Endless ice skating treadmill.

Participants were instructed by the researcher to perform a dynamic warm-up consisting of approximately five minutes of aerobic activity and five minutes of total body calisthenics. Following the warm up participants were randomly selected to the traditional group (nr = 4; wearing the traditional skates) or the Easton Mako group (nr = 4; wearing the Easton Mako skates). Each participant was then outfitted with body markers at the right hip (RHIP) and right knee (RKNE). RHIP was located at the superior aspect of the right greater trochanter while RKNE was located at the lateral femoral epicondyle of the right knee. These marker locations are consistent with the protocol normally used in the University of Ottawa's gait laboratory and proved to be robust for consistently estimating joint angles (Robertson, 2012).

Participants were then attached to a safety harness that was connected to an overhead tracking system by a weighted kill switch. This weighted switch was wired to the control panel and served as an emergency shut off. In addition to the weighted switch a padded bar was positioned across the front of the treadmill for participants to grasp helping prevent injury in the case of a fall. A fifteen-minute familiarization period was then given to the participants so they could become accustomed to skating on the treadmill. This familiarization period was instructed by a WinnPro Hockey (Winnpro Hockey, 2015) instructor and included forward skating, both bilateral and unilateral edge control drills, and one legged squats. Participants then skated at three different velocities 3.33 m/s (8 mph), 5.00 m/s (11 mph), and 6.66m/s (14 mph) for 20 s each with a two-minute rest between trials. These speeds were based on self-selected treadmill skating speeds of elite hockey players, while the time-interval gives sufficient time for the video cameras to gather at least 20 consecutive strides at each speed (Chang et al., 2009).

Participants then skated at two additional speeds. This portion of the test consisted of skating at speeds of 6.71 m/s (15 mph) and 8.05 m/s (18 mph) for 20 s with a 30 s rest period between intervals. Participants then changed into the second pair of skates depending on their initial skate selection group. Another familiarization period was completed, then participants performed the same task while wearing the second pair of skates.

2.5 Skating data processing

The measurement of joint angles was conducted using the angle tool in analyzer mode of Dartfish v6 (Dartfish, 2014). All variables were expressed with respect to reference anatomical position, i.e. upright posture, arms down at the sides, and the palms face forward (Baechle, Earle, & National Strength, 2008). There were two positions of interest when calculating variables related to the position of the push off leg while skating: weight acceptance and propulsion. Weight acceptance was considered the position when the heel of the skate blade came in contact with the treadmill just after recovery of the right leg. Propulsion was considered the position when the toe of the right skate blade was last seen in contact with the treadmill prior to takeoff.

Ankle dorsiflexion, knee flexion, hip flexion, hip adduction, hip abduction, and hip adduction were measured at weight acceptance. Ankle plantar-flexion, knee flexion, hip flexion, and hip abduction were measured at propulsion. Each variable was measured for each subject during ten consecutive strides at each of the five speeds while wearing both skate designs. For the purposes of this study a stride was defined as the time from weight acceptance to propulsion. To ensure the most accurate angle possible the display video full screen mode was used. Ankle plantar-flexion range of motion was obtained from the positions of ankle dorsiflexion at weight acceptance and ankle plantar-flexion at propulsion.

Knee extension range of motion was calculated by subtracting the amount of knee flexion the participant had at propulsion from the amount of knee flexion obtained at weight acceptance (Figure 5). Hip extension range of motion was measured by subtracting the amount of hip flexion at propulsion from the amount of hip extension at weight acceptance (Figure 6). In the case where a participant did not show a recovery past a neutral position, hip abduction range of motion was calculated by subtracting the amount of hip abduction at weight acceptance from the amount of hip abduction at propulsion (Figure 7). If the participant showed hip adduction at weight acceptance, it was added to the amount of hip abduction at propulsion to calculate the range of hip abduction.

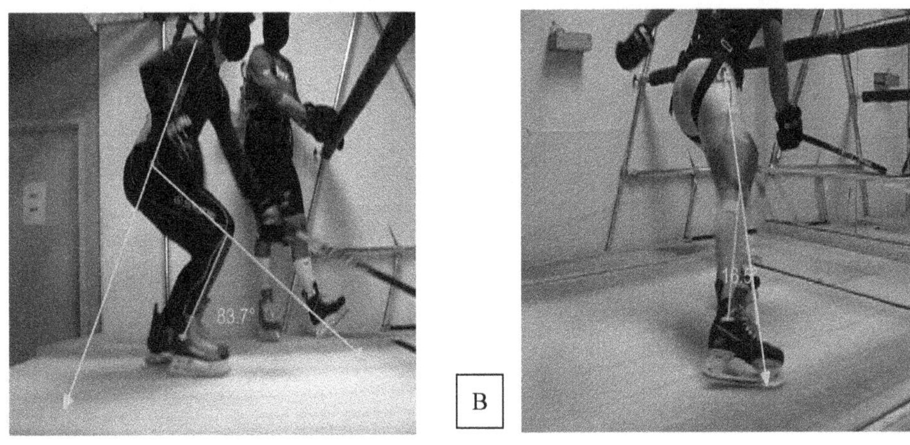

Figure 5. Knee flexion at weight acceptance (A); Knee flexion at propulsion (B)

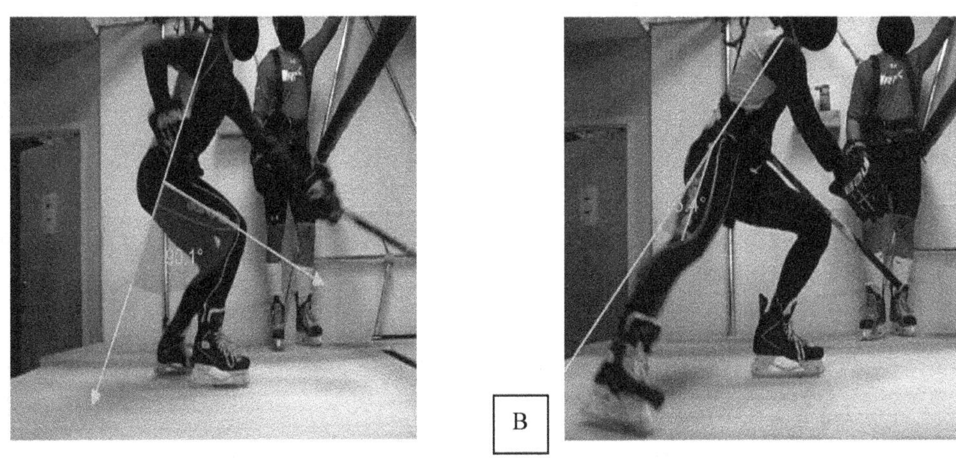

Figure 6. Hip flexion at weight acceptance (A); Hip flexion at propulsion (B)

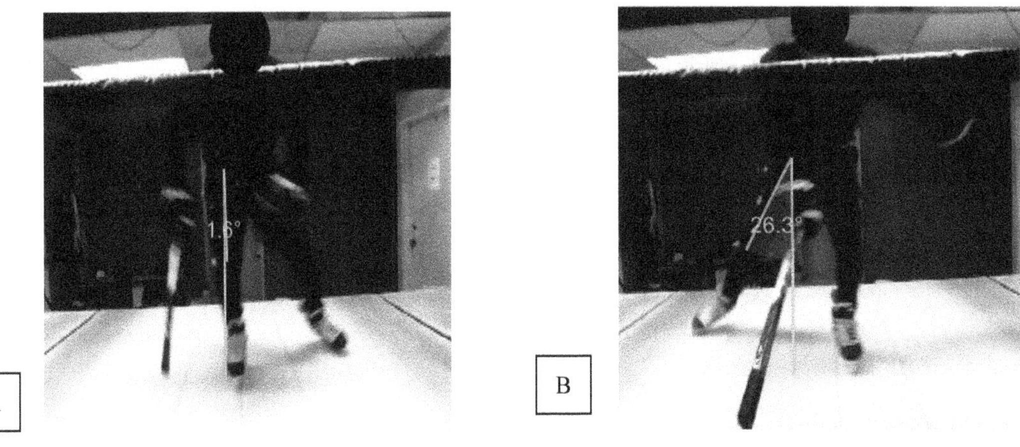

Figure 7. Hip adduction at weight acceptance (A); Hip abduction at propulsion (B)

Stride length was calculated by using the distance tool in the analyzer mode of Dartfish (Dartfish, 2014). Stride length in the sagittal plane was then measured as the distance the skate blade travelled from weight acceptance to propulsion. The distance the skate blade traveled in the frontal plane from weight acceptance to propulsion was then calculated to be stride width (Figure 8). Total stride length was then calculated by using Pythagorean theorem.

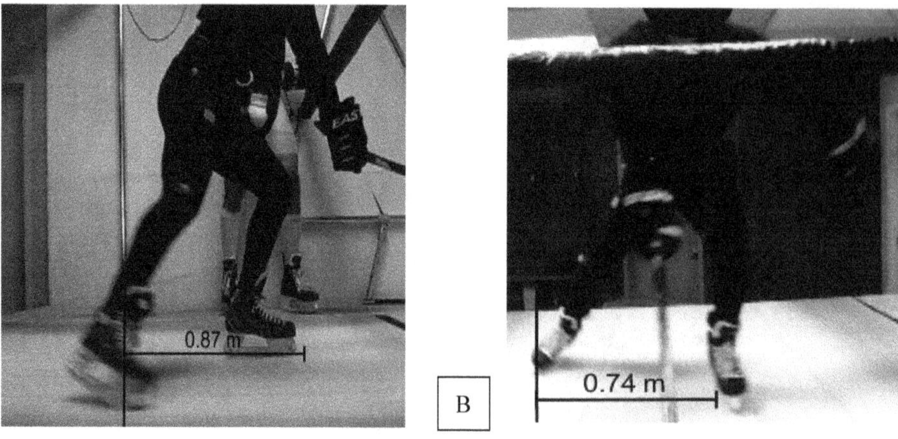

Figure 8. Stride length in the sagittal plane (A); Stride width in the frontal plane (B)

Blade time on the treadmill was calculated as the time from weight acceptance to propulsion by using the time tool in analyzer mode (Dartfish, 2014). Ankle plantar-flexion angular velocity, knee extension angular velocity, hip extension angular velocity, hip abduction angular velocity, and stride velocity were then calculated by dividing their prospective range of motions by blade time on ice. All variables were measured for ten consecutive strides of the right leg while wearing both the traditional skate and Easton Mako skate at 3.33 m/s (8 mph), 5.00 m/s (11 mph), 6.66 m/s (14 mph), 6.71 m/s (15 mph), and 8.05 m/s (18 mph).

2.6 Statistical Analyses

Statistical analyses were undertaken to compare the skating technique between two skate types and were performed using the SPSS 20 statistical software ("IBM SPSS software," 2013). Means and standard deviations of all the variables estimated during the testing were calculated when participants were wearing no skate, the traditional skate, and the Easton Mako skate. Differences in passive and active ranges of motion along with the type of skate were examined using a doubly multivariate repeated-measures test. *Post hoc* univariate tests and planned pairwise comparisons were then completed to determine where the differences in range of motion occurred between the three conditions of no skate, traditional skate, and Easton Mako skate. A Bonferroni correction was used as it is recommended when the univariate tests produce values that are not exactly equal to alpha, but are less than alpha in most situations (Lix & Sajobi, 2010).

Means and standard deviations of all the variables measured while participants were skating on a treadmill were calculated for 10 consecutive strides per condition. A total of 10 conditions were analyzed in the present study, the traditional skate at five speeds and the Easton Mako skate at five speeds. Differences between skate design and treadmill speed were then calculated with a doubly multivariate repeated-measures design. In the present study there were two independent variables (skate type/treadmill speed) and 13 dependent variables. There were two levels of skate type (Traditional/Easton Mako), and 5 levels of treadmill speed (3.33 m/s, 5.00 m/s, 6.66 m/s, 6.71 m/s, 8.05m/s). *Post hoc* univariate tests and planned pairwise comparisons were also completed to determine where the differences in skating kinematics occurred. A Bonferroni adjustment was once again used to help control for a Type 1 error (Lix & Sajobi, 2010). Statistical significance was set at $p<0.05$ for all tests. A correlation analysis was also completed to determine which variables were associated with increased skating speed.

3. Results

3.1 Participants

3.2 Ankle Flexibility Measurements

The doubly multivariate repeated-measures test displayed significant differences between passive and active range of motion yielding a significance value of p=.025 (Table 2).

Table 2. Multivariate results for pre-procedure range of motion

Within Subjects Effect	F	Hypothesis df	Error df	Significance
Passive ROM vs Active ROM	9.526	4.000	4.000	.025
Skate Type	7.104	8.000	22.000	.000

Post hoc univariate tests (Table 3) displayed significant differences between eversion (p=.001) and inversion (p=.003) along with non-significant differences in dorsiflexion (p=.919) and plantar flexion (p=.655). Further complex contrast comparisons revealed that passive eversion range of motion displayed a mean increase of 3.1° (p=.001) when compared to active eversion range of motion. Passive inversion range of motion displayed a mean increase of 6.3° p=.003) greater than active inversion range of motion.

Table 3. Univariate tests comparing passive and active range of motion (*p<.05).

Measure	Range of Motion	Mean	Std.Error	F	Significance
Dorsiflexion	Passive	20.2	0.78	0.011	.919
	Active	20.1	0.90		
Plantar flexion	Passive	21.2	.0.88	0.218	.655
	Active	20.9	0.73		
Eversion	Passive	11.4	0.79	27.419	.001*
	Active	8.3	0.75		
Inversion	Passive	20.2	1.77	20.311	.003*
	Active	13.9	0.93		

Table 4. Unvariate tests comparing no skate, traditional skate, and Easton Mako skate (*p<.05).

Measure	Skate Type	Mean	Std.Error	F	Significance
Dorsiflexion	No skate	21.1	1.84		
	Traditional	20.7	1.06	.950	.410
	Easton Mako	18.8	0.62		
Plantar flexion	No skate	31.3	2.23		
	Traditional	13.0	1.49	28.555	.000*
	Easton Mako	18.9	0.66		
Eversion	No skate	10.8	1.16		
	Traditional	8.7	0.67	1.006	.376
	Easton Mako	10.0	1.40		
Inversion	No skate	20.4	2.24		
	Traditional	16.3	0.60	7.237	.007*
	Easton Mako	14.4	1.33		

The doubly multivariate repeated-measures test also produced a significant difference (p=.000) when comparing the three conditions: wearing no skate, wearing their own skate, and wearing the Easton Mako skate (Table 2). *Post hoc* univariate tests (Table 4) indicated differences in plantar flexion range of motion (p=.000) and inversion range of motion (p=.007) with non-significant differences in dorsiflexion (p=.410) and eversion (p=.376). Complex contrast comparisons further determined that plantar flexion while wearing no skate was shown to have an increase of 18.4° (p=.001) when compared to the participant's own skate. As well, plantar flexion was greater by 12.5° (p=.003) when compared to the Easton Mako skate. There was a mean increase in plantar flexion of 5.9° (p=.003) when participants were wearing the Easton Mako skate compared to their own skate. Participants wearing no skate displayed a mean increase of 6.0° (p=.012) of inversion range of motion when compared to wearing the Easton Mako skate.

3.3 Skating Experimental Acquisitions

The means and standard errors of the 13 variables were calculated for all eight participants while wearing their own traditional hockey skate and the Easton Mako skate. The results of the doubly multivariate repeated measures test suggested significant differences in skating technique within both skate design (p=.022) and treadmill speed (p=.000) (Table 5).

Table 5. Multivariate results for the skating treadmill test

Within Subjects Effect	F	Hypothesis df	Error df	Significance
Skate	1248.638	7.000	1.000	.022
Speed	3.512	52.000	64.079	.000

Post hoc univariate tests were then completed on each variable to determine differences in skating kinematics while participants skated using the two different skate designs. Significant differences were observed between ankle plantar flexion range of motion (p=.000), ankle plantar flexion angular velocity (p=.003), hip extension range of motion (p=.039), hip extension angular velocity (p=.020), stride length (p=.041), and stride velocity (p=.011). In all cases the variables related to range of motion and angular velocity increased when using the Easton Mako skate. There were no significant differences shown in knee extension range of motion (p=.133), knee extension angular velocity (p=.098), hip abduction range of motion (p=.299), hip abduction angular velocity (p=.553), sagittal stride length (p=.065), stride width (p=.520), and skate time on the treadmill (p=.087) when comparing skate designs.

The planned contrast comparisons, Table 6 and Table 7 display the differences between skate design in both range of motion and angular/linear velocity respectively. Ankle plantar flexion range of motion was 6.2° larger while participants were wearing the Easton Mako skate. Ankle plantar flexion angular velocity was also significantly larger while participants were wearing the Easton Mako skate showing an increase of 9.8 °/s. Participants also displayed significant increases in hip extension range of motion (1.7 °) and hip extension angular velocity (5.4 °/s) while wearing the Easton Mako skate. Significant increases in stride length (0.1 m) and stride velocity (0.2 m/s) were also evident with participants sporting the Easton Mako skate.

Table 6. Mean range of motion measured comparisons between skate designs while skating on a treadmill (*=p<.05).

Measure	Skate	Mean	Absolute Mean Difference	Standard Error
Plantar flexion (degrees)	Traditional	13.5	6.2*	1.94
	Mako	19.7		1.97
Knee extension (degrees)	Traditional	45.4	2.8	2.56
	Mako	48.2		3.61
Hip extension (degrees)	Traditional	50.3	1.7*	1.81
	Mako	52.0		1.81
Hip abduction (degrees)	Traditional	34.1	0.8	3.16
	Mako	33.3		2.84
Sagittal stride length (meter)	Traditional	0.9	0.1	0.04
	Mako	1.0		0.03
Stride width (meter)	Traditional	0.7	0.0	0.03
	Mako	0.7		0.04
Stride length (meter)	Traditional	1.2	0.1*	0.03
	Mako	1.3		0.02

3.4 Treadmill Speed and Skating Technique

Significant differences were displayed in ankle plantar flexion range of motion (p=.000), ankle plantar flexion angular velocity (p=.000), knee extension range of motion (p=.000), knee extension angular velocity (p=.000), hip extension range of motion (p=.000), hip extension angular velocity (p=.000), hip abduction range of motion (p=.000), hip abduction angular velocity (p=.000), stride width (p=.000), stride length (p=.006), stride velocity (p=.000), and skate time on the treadmill (p=.000) as treadmill speed increased from 3.33 m/s to 8.05 m/s. No significant difference was found between speed and sagittal stride length (p=.101).

Table 7. Mean angular and linear velocity measured comparisons between skate designs while skating on a treadmill (*=p<.05).

Measure	Skate	Mean	Absolute Mean Difference	Standard Error
Plantar flexion angular velocity (degrees/s)	Traditional	19.4	9.8*	2.47
	Mako	29.3		3.00
Knee extension angular velocity (degrees/s)	Traditional	66.0	5.9	3.52
	Mako	71.9		5.16
Hip extension angular velocity (degrees/s)	Traditional	73.2	5.4*	4.42
	Mako	78.6		5.04
Hip abduction angular velocity (degrees/s)	Traditional	48.3	0.8	2.18
	Mako	49.1		1.53
Stride velocity (meter/s)	Traditional	1.7	0.1*	0.08
	Mako	1.8		0.09
Skate time on treadmill (seconds)	Traditional	.70	0.0	0.03
	Mako	.70		0.04

Table 8 and 9 display planned pairwise comparisons between 3.33 m/s and 8.05 m/s. Participants exhibited an increase in ankle plantar flexion range of motion of 5.1° (p=.000) as speed went from 3.33 m/s to 8.05 m/s. A significant increase in ankle plantar flexion angular velocity of 13.1 °/s (p=.000) was also shown as speed increased. Knee extension range of motion (12.2°, p=.000) and angular velocity (34.6 °/sec, p=.036) also increased with skating speed.

Significant increases in hip extension range of motion (8.3°, p=.001) and hip extension angular velocity (30.9 °/s, p=.000) were also observed as speed increased from 3.33 m/s to 8.05 m/s. Increases of 6.4° in hip abduction range of motion (p=.001) and 20.8 °/sec of hip abduction angular velocity (p=.000) were also observed as speed increased. As participants skating speed increased sagittal stride length (0.1 m, p=.016), stride width (0.1 m, p=.001), stride length (0.2 m, p=.001), and stride velocity (0.6 m/s, p=.000) all increased significantly. Finally as skating speed increased from 3.33 m/s to 8.05 m/s there was a significant decrease in the amount of time participants skates were in contact with the treadmill of 0.2 seconds (p=.000).

Table 8. Mean range of motion measured comparisons between 3.33 m/s and 8.05 m/s (*=p<.05).

Measure	Speed (m/s)	Mean	Absolute Mean Difference	Standard Error
Plantar flexion (degrees)	3.33	13.4	5.1*	1.78
	8.05	18.5		1.81
Knee extension (degrees)	3.33	39.6	12.2*	3.37
	8.05	51.8		3.26
Hip extension (degrees)	3.33	47.2	8.3*	2.05
	8.05	55.5		1.91
Hip abduction (degrees)	3.33	30.1	6.4*	2.86
	8.05	36.5		3.17
Sagittal stride length (meter)	3.33	0.9	0.1	0.03
	8.05	1.0		0.04
Stride width (meter)	3.33	0.6	0.1*	0.03
	8.05	0.7		0.04
Stride length (meter)	3.33	1.1	0.2*	0.03
	8.05	1.3		0.04

Table 9. Mean angular and linear velocity measured comparisons between treadmill speeds 3.33 m/s and 8.05 m/s (*=p<.05).

Measure	Speed (m/s)	Mean	Absolute Mean Difference	Standard Error
Plantar flexion angular velocity (degrees/s)	3.33	16.7	13.1*	1.83
	8.05	29.8		2.76
Knee extension angular velocity (degrees/s)	3.33	49.6	34.6*	2.93
	8.05	84.2		5.88
Hip extension angular velocity (degrees/s)	3.33	60.1	30.9*	2.92
	8.05	91.0		5.79
Hip abduction angular velocity (degrees/s)	3.33	37.2	20.8*	1.69
	8.05	58.0		2.10
Stride velocity (meter/s)	3.33	1.4	0.6*	0.07
	8.05	2.0		0.09
Skate time on treadmill (seconds)	3.33	0.8	0.2*	0.04
	8.05	0.6		0.03

3.5Variables associated with Skating Speed

The correlations between the treadmill speed and the variables measured during the skating treadmill test are reported in Table 10. Through examination of the correlation analysis it was evident that the angular velocity occurring at each joint displayed a higher correlation with treadmill speed than did the range of motion occurring about the joint. Hip abduction angular velocity had the highest correlation with treadmill speed. This variable had a high positive correlation (0.778) with treadmill speed, indicating that as the treadmill speed was increased the skaters increased their angular velocity of hip abduction. Knee extension angular velocity also had a high positive correlation (0.658) with increasing treadmill speed, which suggests that increases in the skater's angular velocity at the knee was associated with the increase in treadmill speed. Stride velocity was the variable to produce the next highest positive correlation (0.605) followed by hip extension angular velocity (0.587) and plantar flexion angular velocity (0.442). Positive correlations between treadmill speed and the range of motion occurring about each joint displayed moderate r values for hip extension (0.435) and knee extension (0.427), with small r- values being observed in ankle plantar flexion (0.267) and hip abduction (0.263).

Sagittal stride length had a small r value of 0.250, suggesting a weak positive association. Moderate r values were calculated for both stride width (0.377) and stride length (0.381), indicating that stride width and stride length increased as the treadmill speed increased. An r-value of -0.466 representing skate blade contact time suggested that there was a moderate negative correlation between the time the skate blade was on the treadmill and treadmill speed. This means that as treadmill speed increased the time the skate blade was on the treadmill decreased.

Table 10. Correlation between treadmill speed and variables measured. (*p<.05,**p<.01)

	Correlation n=80	
Variable	r-value	Significance
Ankle Plantar Flexion	0.267	0.017*
Ankle Plantar Flexion Angular Velocity	0.442	0.000**
Knee Extension	0.427	0.000**
Knee Extension Angular Velocity	0.658	0.000**
Hip Extension	0.435	0.000**
Hip Extension Angular Velocity	0.587	0.000**
Hip Abduction	0.263	0.018*
Hip Abduction Angular Velocity	0.778	0.000**
Sagittal Stride Length	0.250	0.025*
Stride Width	0.377	0.001**
Stride Length	0.381	0.000**
Stride Velocity	0.605	0.000**
Skate Blade Time on Ice	-0.466	0.000**

4. Discussion

4.1 Ankle Flexibility Measurements

The purpose of the present study was to investigate the effect skate design has on ankle flexibility and lower body kinematics during the propulsive phase of forward hockey skating. Changing the biomechanical design of the hockey skate, which is a piece of equipment that plays a huge role in determining whether an athlete is successful, may lead to significantly improving a player's ability to excel over their opponents. The present study analyzed differences in passive and active dorsiflexion, plantar flexion, eversion, and inversion while participants were wearing no skate, their own skate, and the Easton Mako skate.

Significant differences were found between both plantar flexion (p=.000) and inversion (p=.007). Plantar flexion was greatest when players were wearing no skate (31.3°) followed by the Easton Mako skate (18.9°) and finally the traditional skate design (13.0°). Although the Easton Mako skate increased ankle plantar flexion range of motion when compared to the traditional skate design it was evident that the player was still restricted from using their entire range of motion. New skate designs that allow participants to use more of this available range of motion at the ankle joint should be investigated in future studies. This may have a positive effect on increasing forward skating performance. The Easton Mako skate did not show any significant difference in eversion range of motion when compared to the traditional skate design (p=0.376). The design of the new skate boot with the medial side sitting five millimeters higher than the lateral side was designed to promote eversion and increase a player's ability to turn on the ice. Future studies should investigate differences in eversion while skating to understand the implications an asymmetrical skate boot such as the Easton Mako has on performance.

4.2 Skating Experimental Acquisitions

Lower body kinematic comparisons while skating on a treadmill were the primary focus of this study. Thirteen variables were measured during the propulsive phase of the hockey stride, for eight participants, while skating forwards on a skating treadmill. Through the statistical analysis there were significant differences found in lower body kinematics between the two skate designs (p=.022). These findings are consistent with two authors (Robert-Lachaine et al., 2012; Tidman, 2014) who also reported that a change in the biomechanical design of the hockey skate can alter skating kinematics. There was also an observed significant difference in lower body kinematics as the speed of the treadmill increased (p=.000). These findings are consistent with several authors (Haguenauer et al., 2006; Houdijk, De Koning, et al., 2000; Page, 1975; Upjohn et al., 2008) that found lower body kinematics change as skating speed is increased.

The results of this study supported the primary research hypothesis, i.e. that lower limb kinematics are influenced by skate design. In fact both plantar flexion range of motion and plantar flexion angular velocity significantly differed as athletes utilized the two different skate designs. Plantar flexion range of motion was found to be 6.2° larger while participants were wearing the Easton Mako skate (19.7°) when compared to the traditional skate design (13.5°). These findings are similar to those of Robert-Lachaine et al. (Robert-Lachaine et al., 2012) who found plantar flexion values of 16° in participants using a skate with a flexible rear tendon guard and Upjohn et al. (Upjohn et al., 2008) who found plantar flexion values of 13.5° for participants using a traditional skate design. This increased range of motion will increase the propulsive output aiding players to skate faster down the ice. Plantar flexion angular velocity was also significantly increased by 9.8°/s with the use of the Easton Mako skate (29.2°/s) when compared to the traditional design (19.4°/s). This difference together with the increased range of motion exhibited by the use of this new skate design indicates that not only was the range of motion larger while wearing the Easton Mako, but also the movement was occurring at a faster rate. Assuming the recovery phase of the stride does not change while using this new skate design, the increase in angular velocity will increase the stride rate, which is a characteristic of faster skaters (Page, 1975; Upjohn et al., 2008).

While investigating a hockey skate with a flexible back tendon Robert-Lachaine et al. (Robert-Lachaine et al., 2012) discovered that the "total peak force occurred later during plantar flexion which suggested the increased range of motion resulted in a more prolonged effective force generation during a given skating stride" (pg. 205). The increased range of motion displayed in the current study by the implementation of the Easton Mako skate therefore suggests that players will generate greater force from the plantar flexors during the hockey stride when compared to the traditional skate design. This increase in force generation, along with the increase in angular displacement of the ankle, increases the total work produced by the skater. Due to this increase in total work (W) and the increase in angular velocity (ω) seen while participants were wearing the Easton Mako skate we know that the power output ($P = T \times \omega$), which is a characteristic of faster skaters, was higher when participants were using the Easton Mako skate compared to the traditional design. Increasing both work and power during a given time period enables a skater to travel faster down the ice (Vaughan, 1988).

Luhtanen and Komi (Luhtanen & Komi, 1978) found the plantar flexors of the ankle to be important contributors in vertical jumping. They found the plantar flexors to contribute 22% of the total vertical jump height. This suggests that, as the ankles are concentrically plantar flexed during the forward hockey stride the plantar flexors play an important role in producing force into the ice. Given the evidence provided by these studies hockey players should be using skates that enable them to use the plantar flexors to their maximal capability.

As the treadmill speed increased from 3.33 m/s to 8.05 m/s there were again significant differences in both plantar flexion range of motion (5.1°) and plantar flexion angular velocity (13.1°/s). While skating at 3.33 m/s plantar flexion range of motion was shown to be 13.4° and increased to 18.5° at a speed of 8.05 m/s. Participants exhibited 16.7°/s of plantar flexion angular velocity while skating at 3.33 m/s and 29.83 °/s of plantar flexion angular velocity at 8.05 m/s. This again agrees with authors Robert-Lachaine et al. and Vaughn (Robert-Lachaine et al., 2012; Vaughan, 1988) that increased plantar flexion range of motion and increased plantar flexion angular velocity lead to faster skating. Taking into account that plantar flexion range of motion and angular velocity increased as speed increased we can conclude the Easton Mako improves performance at the ankle joint allowing participants to skate faster as it led to an increase in both plantar flexion range of motion and plantar flexion angular velocity.

4.3 Skate Design implications on Knee Extension

In the present study there was no significant difference in knee extension range of motion or knee extension angular velocity as skate design was altered. Recent literature has concluded that the range of motion occurring at the ankle joint during athletic movements affects the kinematics of the knee joint. When comparing push-offs in speed skating between conventional speed skates and klapskates, Houdijk et al. (Houdijk, De Koning, et al., 2000) concluded that klapskates, which increased the range of motion at the ankle, increased the work output at the knee joint. Another study investigating the effects ankle range of motion has on the vertical jump during figure skating Haguenauer (Haguenauer et al., 2006) concluded that the stiff design of the figure skating boot decreased performance by limiting plantar flexion, decreasing work at the ankle joint, and decreasing knee angular velocity. According to Upjohn et al. (Haguenauer et al., 2006), this was done by restricting movement at the ankle joint causing a "redistribution of the energy produced by the knee extensors to the hip and ankle joints" (p. 706). The findings of the current study do not agree with these previous studies, as there was no increase in knee extension range of motion or knee extension angular velocity as plantar flexion range of motion and angular velocity increased.

Although not significant the present study calculated a mean increase of 2.8° in knee extension range of motion while participants were wearing the Easton Mako skate (48.2°) when compared to the traditional skate design (45.4°). These values are similar to those reported by Lafontaine (Lafontaine, 2007) that knee extension values of 55.6° and Upjohn et al. (Upjohn et al., 2008) who reported knee extension values of 34.8°. The slight increase in knee extension during the present study when compared to those of Upjohn et al. (Upjohn et al., 2008) may be attributed to the use of faster treadmill speeds. An increase of 5.9° in knee extension angular velocity was also a non-significant observation when comparing the Easton Mako skate (71.9 °/s) to the traditional skate design (66.0°/s). Contrary to previous studies by Haguenauer et al. and Houdijk et al. (Haguenauer et al., 2006; Houdijk, De Koning, et al., 2000) the present study does not substantiate that producing significant increases in joint range of motion at the ankle leads to significantly increasing the knee extension range of motion during propulsion in forward ice skating. However the Easton Mako skate did not limit range of motion or angular velocity at the knee joint which is important to hockey players as faster skaters exhibit increases in both of these characteristics when compared to slower skaters (Upjohn et al., 2008). As the treadmill speed increased from 3.33 m/s to 8.05 m/s knee extension range of motion significantly increased from 39.6° to 51.8°, while knee extension angular velocity significantly increased from 49.6 °/s to 84.2 °/s. The results of the current study agree with authors Upjohn et al. (Upjohn et al., 2008) and Page (Page, 1975) that faster skaters exhibit greater knee extension and knee angular velocity. It is therefore important to further investigate the effects that increasing ankle range of motion may have on the knee during forward skating in hockey as it could lead to an increase in skating speed.

Hip extension range of motion and hip extension angular velocity were significantly different as participants changed skate designs. The Easton Mako skate outperformed the traditional skate design once again when it came to hip extension kinematics. Hip extension range of motion was increased by 1.7° while participants were wearing the Easton Mako skate (52.0°) when compared to the traditional skate design (50.3°). These values are similar to those of Upjohn et al. (Upjohn et al., 2008) who reported hip extension range of motion to be 40.3°. The slight increase in hip extension between the two studies could once again be attributed to the different treadmill speeds. This increase in hip extension allows skaters to increase the force production by the hip extensors during the propulsion phase. This increase in range of motion also places the hip flexor muscles in a position of greater tension as they reach toe off. The greater tension induces the hip flexors to be pre-stretched which stores energy in both of its elastic and contractile components. This ultimately induces a stronger force as the hip flexors contract at the beginning of recovery (Nordin & Frankel, 2012). This stronger contraction will make for a faster recovery during the swing phase of the hockey stride increasing stride rate, which is a characteristic of faster skaters (Page, 1975; Upjohn et al., 2008).

The Easton Mako skate (78.6 °/s) also improved angular velocity of the hip extensors during propulsion when compared to the traditional skate design (73.2 °/s). This increase in angular velocity, which is a characteristic of elite skaters, increases the power they have in the lower legs to propel them down the ice at faster speeds. Hip extension and hip extension angular velocity were also significantly affected by the speed in which participants were skating. Hip extension range of motion increased 8.3° from 47.2° to 55.5°. These values are slightly larger than the 40.3° of hip extension range of motion reported by Upjohn et al. (Upjohn et al., 2008) due to the variance in treadmill speeds. Hip extension angular velocity was increased by 30.9 °/s from 60.1 °/s to 91.0 °/s as the treadmill speed increased from 3.33 m/s to 8.05 m/s. These increases are in agreement with de Koning et al. (de Koning, de Groot, & van-Ingen-Schenau, 1989) who concluded as skating speed is increased, hip extension range of motion and hip extension angular velocity also increase. Due to this increased activity at the hip joint players wearing this skate design rather than a traditional skate design will potentially skate faster.

4.5 Correlation Analysis

The correlation analysis completed from the skating treadmill test variables produced significant associations between all 13 variables and treadmill speed (Table 10). The highest r-values were present in the angular velocities occurring at each joint. These results indicated that as skating speed increased the angular velocities in the hip, knee and ankle also increased. The higher correlations observed in angular velocities when compared to the correlations present in the range of motion of the lower limbs suggest that increases in angular velocity may be more important than increases in joint range of motion when it comes to increasing skating speed. This high correlation of angular velocity agrees with several authors (Bracko, 2009; de Koning, Thomas, Berger, De Groot, & van Ingen Schenau, 1995; Upjohn et al., 2008) who found increases in angular velocities of the joints of the lower limbs to be a characteristic of faster skaters.

The stride characteristics presented similar results. Although a moderate correlation existed between treadmill speed and both stride width (0.377) and stride length (0.381), the r-value was higher for stride velocity (0.605). These results suggest that stride velocity or the rate in which it takes a player to go from weight bearing to propulsion, may be the most important stride characteristic a player should focus on when trying to increase skating speed.

5. Conclusion and Practical Applications

The purpose of this study was to investigate the differences in ankle flexibility and skating technique between a traditional hockey skate boot and a hockey skate boot with a flexible rear tendon guard. Skating technique was further investigated at different speeds to give insight on how skating technique alters as skating speed is increased.

It was hypothesized that the skate design with a flexible rear tendon guard would increase both range of motion and angular velocity occurring at the ankle , knee, and hip during propulsion of the forward skating stride. It was also hypothesized that this new skate design would increase stride length, stride width, and stride velocity during propulsion.

Based on the findings of this study the following conclusions appear justified:

- Ankle plantar flexion range of motion and ankle plantar flexion angular velocity during propulsion of the forward skating stride are increased when using a skate with flexible rear tendon guard.
- Hip extension range of motion and hip extension angular velocity during propulsion of the forward skating stride are increased when using a skate with flexible rear tendon guard.
- Hockey players increased stride length and stride velocity of propulsion when using a skate that has a flexible rear tendon guard.
- The time the skate was in contact with the treadmill during propulsion was decreased with the implementation of a flexible rear tendon guard.

Improvements in hockey skate design have important implications for the skating skill of elite hockey players. Success in ice hockey is closely related to skating skill and is partially dependent on push off forces and joint ranges of motion allowed by a particular skate design. A skate design that allows for increased range of motion at the ankle joint during push off has the potential to increase skating speed and agility by increasing the contribution from the ankle plantarflexors such as gastrocnemius and soleus as well as the knee extensors. A slight tilt of the skate sole in the direction of eversion may also improve the angle of the skate blade with regard to utilizing the inside edge for a longer period during push off. More study is required examining other unique skate designs that increase the range of motion at key skating joints to determine which designs have the greatest potential for improving hockey skating speed and agility.

References

Baechle, T. R., Earle, R. W., & National Strength, C. A. (2008). *Essentials of Strength Training and Conditioning*. Champaign, IL: Human Kinetics.

Behm, D. G., Wahl, M. J., Button, D. C., Power, K. E., & Anderson, K. G. (2005). Relationship between hockey skating speed and selected performance measures. *The Journal of Strength & Conditioning Research, 19*(2), 326-331.

Bourque, R. (1985). Canada Patent No.: US Patent No. 4, 276. .

Bracko, M. R. (2009). Enhancing Performance in ice hockey. In M. Duncan & M. Lyons (Eds.), *Advances in Strength and Conditioning Research* (pp. 243-254). Hauppauge, NY: Nova Publishers.

Chang, R., Turcotte, R., & Pearsall, D. (2009). Hip adductor muscle function in forward skating. *Sports Biomechanics, 8*(3), 212-222.

Clarkson, H. M. (2000). *Musculoskeletal assessment: joint range of motion and manual muscle strength.* Philadelphia: Lippincott Williams & Wilkins.

Dartfish, I. (2014). Dartfish Digital Video Analysis System. Retrieved from http://www.dartfish.com/en/sports-enhancements/sport_performance_software/index.htm

de Koning, J. J., de Groot, G., & van-Ingen-Schenau, G. J. (1989). Mechanical aspects of the sprint start in Olympic speed skating. *Int J Sport Biom, 5*(2), 151-168.

de Koning, J. J., Thomas, R., Berger, M., De Groot, G., & van Ingen Schenau, G. J. (1995). The start in speed skating: from running to gliding. *Medicine and Science in Sports and Exercise, 27*(12), 1703-1708.

Easton Hockey. (2014). Easton Hockey. Retrieved from http://eastonhockey.com/gear/products/skates/mako-skate

Faul, F., Erdfelder, E., Lang, A. G., & Buchner, A. (2007). G* Power 3: A flexible statistical power analysis program for the social, behavioral, and biomedical sciences. *Behavior Research Methods, 39*(2), 175-191.

Haguenauer, M., Legreneur, P., & Monteil, K. M. (2006). Influence of figure skating skates on vertical jumping performance. *Journal of Biomechanics, 39*(4), 699-707.

Hancock, S., Lamontagne, M., Stothart, J. P., & Sveistrup, H. (1999). *The influence of three hockey skate boots on the range of motion, elastic moment and stiffness of the human ankle joint complex.* Paper presented at the Proceedings from XVIth Conference of the International Society of Biomechanics, Calgary, Canada.

Hoshizaki, T. B., Hall, K., & Bourque, R. (1989). Montreal, Canada Patent No.: US. Patent No. 4, 885.

Hoshizaki, T. B., Kirchner, G., & Hall, K. (1989). Safety in Ice Hockey: Kinematic analysis of the talocrural and subtalar joints during the hockey skating stride. *American Society for Testing and Materials, 1*, 141.

Houdijk, H., De Koning, J. J., De Groot, G., Bobbert, M. F., & Van Ingen Schenau, G. J. (2000). Push-off mechanics in speed skating with conventional skates and klapskates. *Medicine and Science in Sports and Exercise, 32*(3), 635-641.

Houdijk, H., Heijnsdijk, E. A., de Koning, J. J., de Groot, G., & Bobbert, M. F. (2000). Physiological responses that account for the increased power output in speed skating using klapskates. *European Journal of Applied Physiology and Occupational Physiology, 83*(4-5), 283-288.

Houdijk, H., Wijker, A. J., De-Koning, J. J., Bobbert, M. F., & De-Groot, G. (2001). Ice friction in speed skating: can klapskates reduce ice frictional loss? *Medicine-and-science-in-sports-and-exercise-, 33*(3), 499-504.

Kuper, G. H., & Sterken, E. (2003). Endurance in speed skating: The development of world records. *European Journal of Operational Research, 148*(2), 293-301.

Lafontaine, D. (2007). Three-dimensional kinematics of the knee and ankle joints for three consecutive push-offs during ice hockey skating starts. *Sports Biomechanics, 6*(3), 391-406

Lix, L. M., & Sajobi, T. (2010). Testing multiple outcomes in repeated measures designs. *Psychological Methods, 15*(3), 268.

Luhtanen, P., & Komi, P. V. (1978). Segmental contribution to forces in vertical jump. *European Journal of Applied Physiology and Occupational Physiology, 38*(3), 181-188.

Madore, C. (2003). Montreal, Canada Patent No.: U. Patent.

Maor, E. (2007). *The Pythagorean Theorem: A 4,000-year History*. Princeton: Princeton University Press.

Marino, G. W., & Weese, R. G. (1979). A kinematic analysis of the ice skating stride. In J. Terauds (Ed.), *Science in Skiing, Skating and Hockey*. Del Mar, CA: Academic Publishers.

McPherson, M. N., Wrigley, A., & Montelpare, W. J. (2004). The biomechanical characteristics of development-age hockey players: Determining the effects of body size on the assessment of skating technique. *American Society for Testing and Materials (ASTM), Special Technical Publication* (pp. 272-287).

Nordin, M., & Frankel, V. H. (2012). *Basic biomechanics of the musculoskeletal system*

(4th ed.). Philadelphia, PA: Lippincott Williams & WIlkins.

Page, P. (1975). *Biomechanics of forward skating in ice hockey.* (MSc), Dalhousie University, Halifax.

Pearsall, D. J., Paquette, Y. M., Baig, Z., Albrecht, J., & Turcotte, R. A. (2012). Ice hockey skate boot mechanics: Direct torque and contact pressure measures. *Procedia Engineering, 34*, 295-300.

Pitkin, M., Smirnova, L., Scherbina, K., & Zvonareva, E. (2002). *Biomechanics of ice hockey skating in amputees with foot and ankle prostheses.* Paper presented at the Proceedings of the 7th Annual Russian National Congress, St. Petersburg, Russia.

Quinn, E. (2015). PAR-Q- The physical activity readiness questionnaire. *About Health.* Retrieved from http://sportsmedicine.about.com/od/fitnessevalandassessment/qt/PAR-Q.htm

Robert-Lachaine, X., Turcotte, R. A., Dixon, P. C., & Pearsall, D. J. (2012). Impact of hockey skate design on ankle motion and force production. *Sports Engineering, 15*(4), 197-206.

Robertson, D. G. E. (2012). *Vicon Workstation Quick Reference Guide* (PDF). Retrieved from http://www.health.uottawa.ca/biomech/courses/apa4311/Vicon%20Workstation%20Quick%20Reference%20Guide.pdf

Robertson, D. G. E. (2004). *Research Methods in Biomechanics*. Champaign, IL: Human Kinetics.

Tidman, R., Lambert, L., Cruikshank, D., & Silver-Thorn, M. . (2014). *Hockey Skating Kinematics.* Paper presented at the Proceedings of the Marquette University Biomedical Engineering Symposium, Milwaukee, WI.

Turcotte, R. A., Pearsall, D. J., & Montgomery, D. L. (2001). An apparatus to measure stiffness properties of ice hockey skate boots. *Sports Engineering, 4*(1), 43-48.

Upjohn, T., Turcotte, R., Pearsall, D. J., & Loh, J. (2008). Three-dimensional kinematics of the lower limbs during forward ice hockey skating. *Sports Biomechanics, 7*(2), 206-221.

Vaughan, C. L. (1988). Biomechanics of Speed Skating *Biomechanics of Sport (1st edition)*. Boca Raton: CRC Press.

Winnpro Hockey. (2015). Winnpro Hockey. Retrieved from http://www.winnprohockey.com/About.html

14

Influence of Whole Body Vibration and Specific Warm-ups on Force during an Isometric Mid-Thigh Pull

Vanessa L. Cazás-Moreno (Corresponding author)
School of Applied Sciences, University of Mississippi, 215 Turner Center, P.O. Box 1848 University, MS 38677-1848
E-mail: vlcazas@olemiss.edu

Jacob R. Gdovin
School of Applied Sciences, University of Mississippi, 215 Turner Center, P.O. Box 1848 University, MS 38677-1848
E-mail: jrgdovin@olemiss.edu

Charles C. Williams
School of Applied Sciences, University of Mississippi, 215 Turner Center, P.O. Box 1848 University, MS 38677-1848
E-mail: ccwilli1@olemiss.edu

Charles R. Allen
School of Applied Sciences, University of Mississippi, 215 Turner Center, P.O. Box 1848 University, MS 38677-1848
E-mail: crallen@olemiss.edu

Yang-Chieh Fu
School of Applied Sciences, University of Mississippi, 215 Turner Center, P.O. Box 1848 University, MS 38677-1848
E-mail: ycfu@olemiss.edu

Lee E. Brown
College of Health and Human Development, California State University, Fullerton, 800 North State College Blvd., Fullerton, CA 92834
E-mail: leebrown@fullerton.edu

John C. Garner III
School of Applied Sciences, University of Mississippi, 215 Turner Center, P.O. Box 1848 University, MS 38677-1848
E-mail: jcgarner@olemiss.edu

5

Abstract

Purpose: The purpose of this study was to investigate the effects of general and specific warm-up protocols on rate of force development (RFD), relative RFD (rRFD), ground reaction force (GRF) and relative ground reaction force (rGRF) during an isometric mid-thigh pull (IMTP), after WBV exposure. **Methods:** Fifteen healthy recreationally trained males (age: 24.1 ± 2.3 yrs, height: 72.9 ± 7.8 cm; mass: 86.9 ± 8.3) completed five protocols: baseline, isometric vibration (iVib), isometric no vibration (iNV), dynamic vibration (dVib) and dynamic no vibration (dNV). The baseline was completed without any warm-up prior to the IMTP. The intervention protocols had the same prescription of 4 sets of 30-second bouts of quarter squats (dynamic [DQS] and isometric [IQS]) on the WBV platform with or without vibration. Following a one-minute rest period after each protocol, participants completed three maximal IMTPs. **Results:** Repeated measures ANOVA with a Bonferroni post hoc demonstrated that RFD in dNV (7657.8 ± 2292.5 N/s) was significantly greater than iVib (7156.4 ± 2170.0 N/s). However, the other experimental trials for RFD demonstrated no significant differences ($p>0.05$). There were also no significant differences for rRFD, GRF or rGRF between protocols. **Conclusion:** These results demonstrate that a dynamic warm-up without WBV elicits greater RFD than an isometric warm-up with WBV prior to a maximal isometric exercise. Further research needs to be investigated utilizing dynamic and isometric warm-ups in conjunction with WBV and power output.

Keywords: males, recreationally trained, power

1. Introduction

Improvements in power, developed from multiple training sessions, have been shown to enhance sport performance (Adams et al., 2009; Gerakaki et al., 2013; Haff et al., 2005; Kurt et al., 2014; Lamont et al., 2010). There are a number of traditional methods such as anaerobic and aerobic protocols that are utilized which lead to an increase in power production; however, athletes and coaches alike are continually looking for novel methods that are more efficient at improving performance (Cardinale & Bosco, 2003; Chmielewska et al., 2014; Dabbs et al., 2010; Dabbs et al., 2011; Dabbs et al., 2012; Dallas et al., 2014; Kurt et al., 2014; Lamont et al., 2010; Marin et al., 2013; Rittweger et al., 2000; Ritzmann et al., 2013; Ronnestad et al.,2012). Traditionally, a warm-up is recommended prior to performing an exercise (Thompson et al., 2013). Warm-ups typically consist of both general and specific activities. The general warm-up consists of full body movements that are used to increase the body's temperature, blood flow, functional mobility, and muscle activation (i.e. jogging or jumping jacks) (Thompson et al., 2013). The specific warm-up consists of movements directly related to the performance related tasks (i.e. mimicking movements utilized during performance) (Thompson et al., 2013).

Participating in a specific warm-up prior to a vigorous activity has been shown to enhance lower body strength and power (Alikhajeh et al.,2011; Hamada et al., 2000; Ribeiro et al., 2014). However, if the intensity of the specific warm-up is too low, it may not augment performance (Anderson, et al., 2014; Ribeiro et al., 2014). Incorporating a supplementary, specific warm-up, may lead to increased motor unit recruitment and synchronization (Gerakaki et al., 2013; Lamont et al., 2010). It has been demonstrated that an increase in performance may occur as a result of applying a specific warm-up that utilizes dynamic and isometric exercises that are aimed at eliciting an increase in force production (Lamont et al., 2010). In addition to dynamic and isometric exercises, whole body vibration (WBV) may be an alternative warm-up method prior to an explosive bout of exercise. In an acute study conducted by Holt et al. (2008), they demonstrated the use of a dynamic specific warm-up resulted in an increased vertical jump performance in comparison to a general warm-up and stretching protocol. Similarly, a study by Thompsen et al. demonstrated that both horizontal and vertical jumps were enhanced in female collegiate athletes after utilizing a body weight dynamic warm-up in comparison to a static or weighted warm-up. Frantz et al. (2011), demonstrated that collegiate baseball players had significant enhancements in lower body power after utilizing body weight exercise dynamic warm-up in comparison to a static stretching warm-up. Anderson et al. (Anderson et al., 2014) found that high intensity warm-ups elevated trained individuals' heart rate to near maximal intensity, and this significantly increased high intensity sprint intervals. These results indicate that the use of a dynamic specific warm-up may be beneficial for trained individuals prior to an acute bout of power exercises.

The purpose of warm-ups are to prepare an athlete for competition (Thompson et al., 2013). However, some warm-ups have failed to increase lower body performance (Anderson et al., 2014; Cardinale & Bosco, 2003; Reiman et al., 2010; Ribeiro et al., 2014). Ribeiro et al. (2014) reported that the effects of three different warm-ups did not enhance the number of repetitions to failure during a submaximal squat exercise in recreationally trained individuals'. Aerobic, anaerobic, and stretching exercises did not influence vertical jump performance according to Christensen et al. (2008) Furthermore, Reiman et al. (2010) revealed that teenage athletes did not demonstrate significant differences in lower body power when warming-up with a weighted vest that was 5% of their body weight in comparison to a body weight dynamic protocol. These results indicate that the intensity of the warm-up activities may have been too fatiguing or there was not an adequate amount of rest in between the warm-up and the explosive activity.

Whole-body vibration has been implemented as a specific warm-up alone and in conjunction with dynamic exercises (i.e. squats) prior to explosive activity (Cardinale & Bosco, 2003; Chmielewska et al., 2014; Dabbs et al., 2010; Dabbs et al., 2011; Dabbs et al., 2012; Dallas et al., 2014; Kurt et al., 2014; Lamont et al., 2010; Marin et al., 2013; Rittweger et al., 2000; Ritzmann et al., 2013; Ronnestad et al., 2012; Turner, 2011). Dallas et al. (2014) utilized a low vibration frequency of 30 Hz prior to vertical jump performance and found that jump height significantly increased. Similarly, Dabbs et al. (2010) demonstrated that maximum jump height also significantly improved after WBV exposure at 30 Hz. In another study, jump height significantly increased at a higher frequency of 40 Hz (Turner et al., 2011). This demonstrates that utilizing WBV as a specific warm-up, may lead to acute increased neuromuscular performance (force and power) prior to an explosive bout of exercise (Cardinale & Bosco, 2003; Dabbs et al., 2010; Dabbs et al., 2011; Dabbs et al., 2012; Dallas et al., 2014; Marin et al., 2013; Rittweger et al., 2000; Ritzmann et al., 2013; Ronnestad et al., 2012).

Conversely, the literature has also shown that WBV has failed to demonstrate significant increases in performance (Chmielewska et al., 2014; Rittweger et al., 2000; Ritzmann et al., 2013). Chmielewska (2014) demonstrated that WBV did not alter motor unit recruitment of the rectus femoris after exposure to either low- or high- frequency vibration during repeated squats. Similarly, in an applied setting, Rittweger et al. (2000) indicated that acute explosive power decreased after WBV exposure. Furthermore, Ritzmann (2013) reported that the H-reflex was negatively altered following WBV which led to a lack of performance enhancement. As debates continues in the literature regarding WBV, it is important to note that its effects may be highly individualized (Chmielewska et al., 2014) indicating the time to enhancement may be individualized.

An isometric mid-thigh pull (IMTP) is an explosive and complimentary exercise to the Olympic lifts. The IMTP manipulates the start of the second pull of the clean exercise and attempts to reach triple extension of the ankles, knees and hips (Comfort et al., 2011; Jones et al., 2015; Haff et al., 2005). An IMTP requires maximal effort, yet the exercise is isometric and joint angles do not change from the starting hang position. The IMTP has been used in research settings to measure applied forces and has also been used as a training tool to possibly eliminate poor technique (Haff et al., 2005). There have been a number of studies that have investigated RFD and GRF during an IMTP (Comfort et al., 2011; Haff et al., 2005; Haff et al., 2015; Khamoui et al., 2011) with Haff et al., (2015) demonstrating that the IMTP is an acceptable and reliable exercise.

To date, there are no standardized warm-up protocols prior to a maximal isometric power output. The literature reflects multiple combinations of time and exercise methods utilizing static, dynamic and WBV (Adams et al., 2009; Chmielewska et al., 2014; Dabbs et al., 2010; Dabbs et al., 2011; Dabbs et al., 2012; Dallas et al., 2014; García-López et al., 2012; Gerakaki et al., 2013; Kurt et al., 2014; Lamont et al., 2010; Marin et al., 2013; Rittweger et al., 2000; Ronnestad et al., 2012; Turner et al., 2011) making it important to further examine its applicability to improvements in the rate of force development (RFD), relative RFD (rRFD), ground reaction force (GRF) and relative ground reaction force (rGRF) during sport performance after warm-up exposure (Alikhajeh et al., 2011; Chmielewska et al., 2014; Cilli et al., 2014; Dabbs et al., 2010; Dabbs et al., 2011; Dallas et al., 2014; García-López et al., 2012; Marin et al., 2013; Rittweger et al., 2000; Ritzmann et al., 2013; Ronnestad et al., 2012; Thompson et al., 2013; Turner et al., 2011). As previously mentioned, utilizing a specific warm-up is highly recommended prior to any maximal effort lower body power activity. It has been shown (Lamont et al., 2010) that the use of WBV as a specific warm-up resulted in an acute increase in power and force production during a maximal isometric muscle action. Further investigation is needed to determine the effects of a dynamic, isometric and combination mode of warm-up prior to a maximal isometric muscle action. It is plausible that WBV in conjunction with a specific warm-up may lead to an increase in acute power and force production during an IMTP. Furthermore, research has demonstrated that there is a significant correlation between IMTP and dynamic and explosive exercises (Haff et al., 2005; Khamoui et al., 2011; Marin et al., 2013). The IMTP exercise was selected for this study to minimize the variance between participants, isolate the dependent variables of interest (Comfort et al., 2011) and test the applicability of the findings (Haff et al., 2015; Lamont et al., 2010). Therefore, the purpose of this study was to determine the influence of isometric and dynamic exercises in conjunction of WBV versus no WBV on the RFD, rRFD, GRF and rGRF during an IMTP.

2. Methods

Each participant completed one-familiarization, a baseline and four intervention sessions separated by a minimum of one hour. Three maximal IMTP's were performed one minute after each intervention session (specific warm-up) was completed. Therefore, a within subject repeated measures study design was used to examine RFD, rRFD, GRF and rGRF.

2.1 Participants

Fifteen healthy, recreationally trained males who were free of any lower body orthopedic and/or musculoskeletal injuries completed the study (age: 24.1 ± 2.3 yrs, height: 72.9 ± 7.8 cm; mass: 86.9 ± 8.3). Recreationally trained was defined as completing a minimum of three hours per week of resistance training over the last year prior to the initiation of the study. All participants read and signed a University Institutional Review Board (IRB) approved informed consent.

2.2 Procedures

Each participant was asked to avoid any lower body aerobic or anaerobic training 24 hours prior to the start and for the duration of the study. During the familiarization session, participants had their anthropometrics recorded, followed by verbal instructions and visual demonstration of the general warm-up and the IMTP. Three non-recorded, self-selected effort pulls of the IMTP were completed at this time. Participants were instructed to pull at minimal to moderate effort. Following this, each participant was given verbal instructions and a demonstration of how to perform the isometric quarter squat (IQS) and the dynamic quarter squats (DQS) during vibration and no vibration exposure while standing on the WBV platform. As participants stood on the vibration platform, IQS were completed simultaneously until they felt comfortable with the task; DQS were completed after the isometric condition. For the familiarization without vibration, participants simply stood on the platform while performing both quarter squat conditions. Participants were instructed to wear the same footwear throughout the remainder of the study.

During the first testing session, baseline testing of the IMTP was conducted prior to any warm-up. The baseline test consisted of three maximal IMTP on the modified Jones Machine (BODYCRAFT, Lewis Center, OH) (Figure 1). Participants were given the following instructions prior to each maximal IMTP: "pull as hard as you can, as fast as you can, while driving your feet down into the ground". Encouragement was given during each pull. The IMTP was held for 3-seconds and a 15-second rest period was given between each maximal pull. Lifting straps were worn for all pulls.

After baseline testing, each participant performed a general warm-up and completed the following protocols based on a counterbalanced design: IQS with vibration (iVib), IQS with no vibration (iNV), DQS with vibration (dVib), and DQS with no vibration (dNV). After completing the specific warm-up, one-minute of rest was given prior to the post-test (Cazas et al., 2013). Post-testing utilized the same protocol as baseline testing. This procedure was repeated until each participant completed each specific warm-up protocol. Each condition was separated by a minimum of one hour.

2.3 Warm Up Descriptions

The general warm-up was completed prior to each specific warm-up protocol and consisted of 10 bodyweight squats, 10 m of walking knee hugs and 10 m Frankenstein marches. During the walking knee hugs participants stepped forward with one foot and went into full range of motion of plantar-flexion, as the opposite leg flexed at the knee and the hip while the participant pulled their knee into their chest simultaneously. Frankenstein marches consisted of stepping forward with one foot and kicking the opposite leg into the air at maximal range of motion, while maintaining straight legs. After their perceived maximum range of motion had been achieved, the kicking leg returned to starting position and then switched legs.

The specific warm-up consisted of 4 sets of 30-second bouts in conjunction with the following: IQS with vibration. (iVib), IQS with no vibration (iNV), DQS with vibration (dVib), DQS with no vibration (dNV) while standing on the vibration plate. Thirty-seconds of rest was given between each bout. All vibration conditions were completed at 30 Hz and the no vibration protocols were completed at 0 Hz while standing on the vibration platform. During the 30-second bouts, participants completed one of the intervention conditions at a time. The IQS was defined as a muscle action that did not alter any changes in the joint angles, thus maintaining a constant musculotendinous length for the duration of the 30-second bout (Garner, 2008). The DQS was defined as repetitive eccentric to concentric muscle actions at a 1 to 1 ratio. The researcher monitored the IQS and the 1-second to 1-second ratio for each participant.

2.4 Isometric Mid-thigh Pull

A standard Olympic barbell and a modified Jones Machine were used to perform the IMTP. The Jones Machine hooks had been reversed, so the barbell could not move when an external load was placed on it. The barbell was held directly under the hooks by straps (Figure 1). To mimic a power stance, participants started in a hang position between 120- and 130-degree knee flexion (West et al., 2011). Hip flexion was maintained in a comfortable position in response to the knee flexion throughout the exercise. By placing the participant in an optimal force-generating angle, the power stance may potentially result in the greatest amount of power production (Comfort et al., 2011; Haff et al., 2015; Kawamori et al., 2006). The barbell placement was adjusted with respect to the height of each participant; a goniometer was used to measure the knee joint angle. Hip flexion was in a fixed angle relative to the comfort of the participant. Foot placement was slightly greater than shoulder width while an overhand grip placement was used on the barbell; this grip position was directly on the lateral sides of the participant's quadriceps. Prior to initiation of the exercise, participants set up in the power position with their weight distributed evenly on both feet. A certified strength and conditioning specialist (CSCS) monitored all participants to ensure safety and proper technique was performed. Proper technique consisted of maintaining a flat back, head placement in a neutral position, and shoulders positioned slightly over the bar. To initiate the action, participants were instructed to explosively drive through their feet, in an attempt to extend at the ankles, knees and hips. For this study, the IMTP was defined as a maximal concentric loading exercise, yet there were no changes in joint angle (Garner et al., 2008). This resulted in a concentrically loaded, maximal isometric muscle action, where no mechanical movement occurred.

2.5 Equipment

The force plate was a 0.6 m x 0.4 m force platform (Bertec Corporation, Columbus, OH, Inc.) embedded in floor and was used to measure IMTP RFD and GRF with a sampling rate of 1000 Hz.

The Power Plate pro5 (Northbrook, IL), which had a 86 cm x 94 cm (W x D) vibration platform was used. It administered a pivotal vibration frequency at 30 Hz with a vertical amplitude of 2-4 mm.

2.4 Data Analysis

Data analysis was conducted by a self-developed code written in Matlab (Mathworks, Inc., Natick, MA, USA). The interval of movement during the analysis was from the time point of when the vertical ground reaction force (VGRF) returned back to the participant's body mass to the end of the pull (see figure 1). RFD was defined by the amount of force produced over the change in time (200 Nm/s) initiated at the beginning of the movement interval (Haff et al., 2015; Lamont et al., 2010). Relative RFD was defined as the absolute RFD divided by the participant's bodyweight in kilograms (Nm/s/kg). GRF was defined as the maximum VGRF throughout the entire movement interval. GRF was analyzed at the time point at which the participants force peaked throughout the pull. Relative GRF was defined as the absolute GRF divided by the participant's bodyweight in kilograms (N/kg). Multiple 1 x 5 repeated measures analysis of variance (ANOVA) were used to determine differences between conditions. All statistical procedures were conducted using SPSS (version 22, Chicago, IL, USA). An a priori alpha level was set at 0.05. A Bonferroni post hoc was used to highlight any between condition differences.

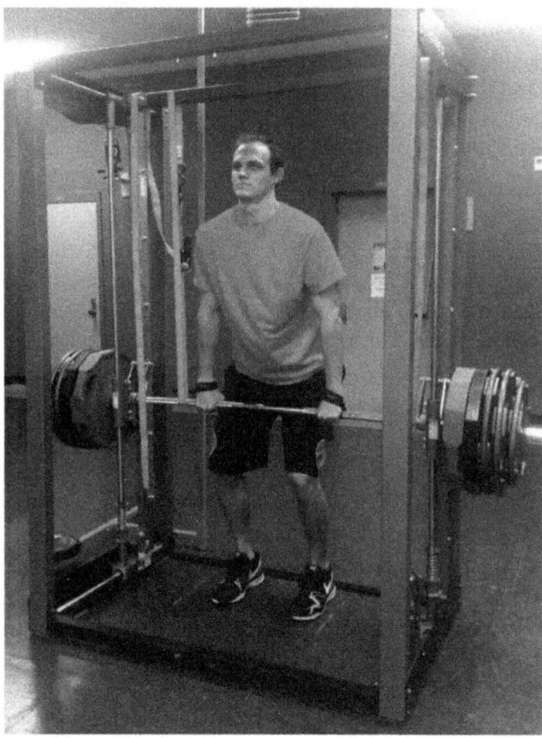

Figure 1. Isometric Mid-Thigh Pull
Description: the barbell was securely fixed with straps, while the weight added to the barbell was added to ensure the Jones Machine would not move.

3. Results

There was a significant main effect for RFD. Post hoc testing revealed dNV was significantly greater than iVIB with an overall effect size of .84. No other conditions were different (figure 2). There were no significant ($p>0.05$) differences between conditions for rRFD, GRF or rGRF (table 1). Individual percent change from baseline for GRF, rGRF, RFD and rRFD are illustrated for each condition in figure 3, 4, 5 and 6, respectively.

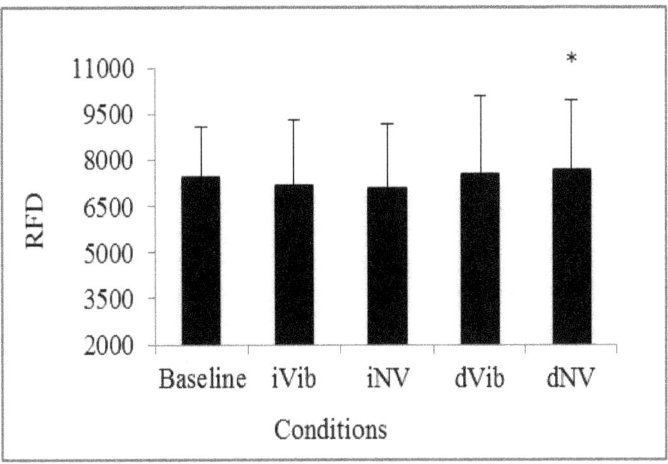

Figure 2. Rate of Force Development
Description: Maximum RFD values for all five conditions: isometric vibration (iVib); isometric no vibration (iNV); dynamic vibration (dVib); and dynamic no vibration (dNV); Group means: mean ± SD; (Nm/s); * significantly greater than iVib.

Table 1. Mean ± SD for relative RFD (Nm/s/kg), GRF (N) and relative GRF (N/kg) for all five conditions: isometric vibration (iVib); isometric no vibration (iNV); dynamic vibration (dVib); and dynamic no vibration (dNV).

Variable	Baseline	iVib	iNV	dVib
rRFD	85.31 ± 17.38	82.77 ± 24.72	81.53 ± 22.87	87.14 ± 29.08
GRF	3132.6 ± 509.5	3124.4 ± 598.6	3083.9 ± 496.7	3134.7 ± 509
rGRF	36.09 ± 5.64	36.11 ± 6.77	35.62 ± 5.32	36.31 ± 6.25

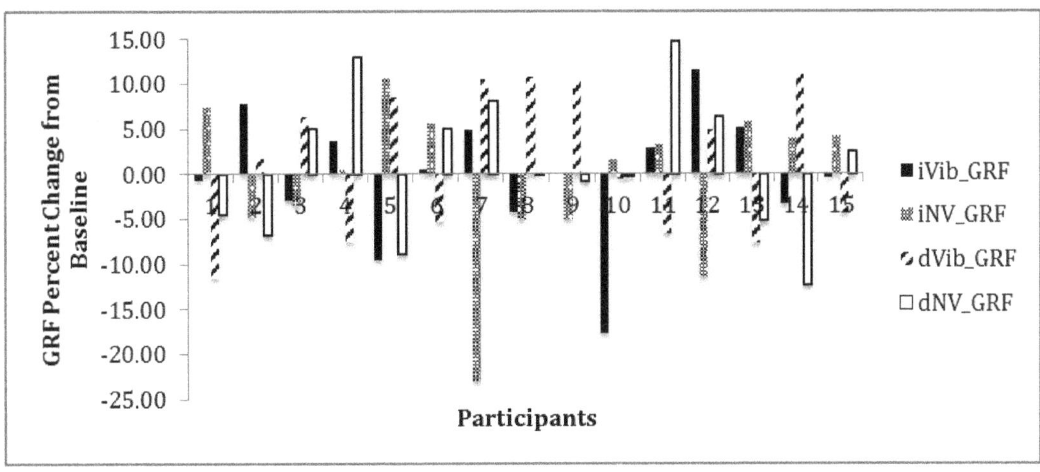

Figure 3. Ground Reaction Force Percent Change from Baseline.
Description: GRF percent change from baseline for each participant and condition.

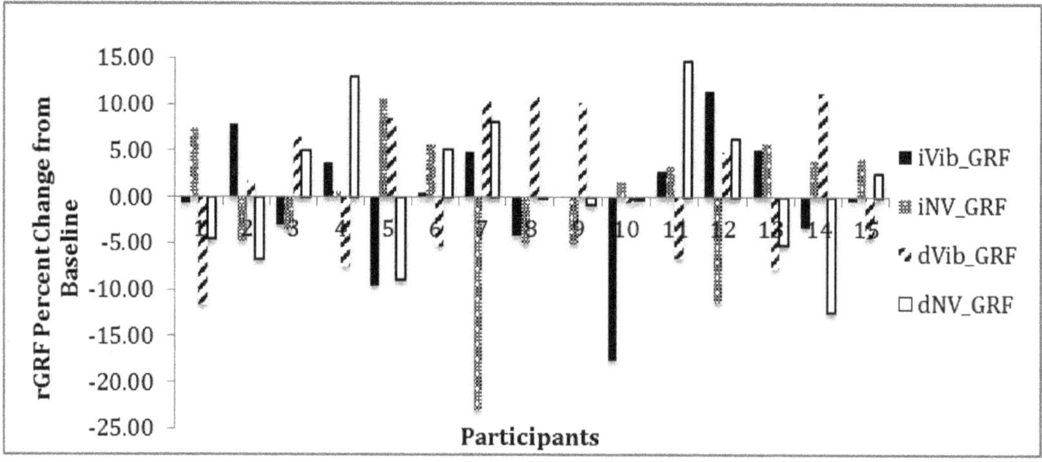

Figure 4. Relative Ground Reaction Force Percent Change from Baseline.
Description: rGRF percent change from baseline for each participant and condition.

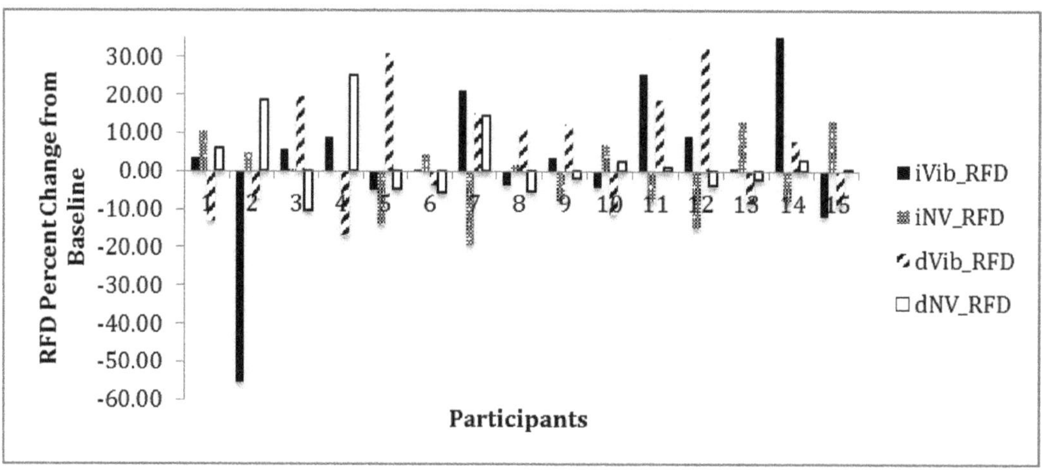

Figure 5. Rate of Force Development Percent Change from Baseline.
Description: RFD percent change from baseline for each participant and condition.

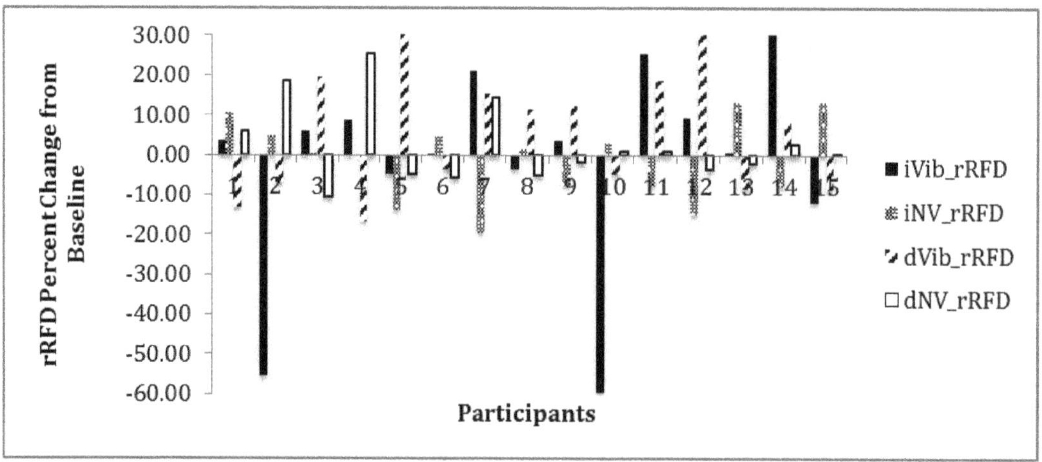

Figure 6. Relative Rate of Force Development Percent Change from Baseline.
Description: rRFD percent change for each participant and condition.

4. Discussion

The purpose of this study was to investigate the influence of dynamic and isometric specific warm-ups in conjunction with WBV on acute GRF and RFD during an IMTP. The main finding of this study was that no warm-up condition demonstrated any significant differences from baseline. A secondary finding was that the dynamic, specific warm-up without WBV elicited greater absolute RFD in comparison to the isometric, specific warm-up with WBV, but was not different from any other condition. To our knowledge, this is the first study to investigate the effect of WBV in conjunction with different specific warm-ups on RFD, and GRF during an IMTP.

Currently, there is a lack of research investigating WBV in conjunction with dynamic and isometric specific warm-ups on an isometric exercise. Therefore, it is difficult to directly compare current literature to the present study. However, the design of this study was based off WBV, resistance training and resistance exercise protocols (Adams et al., 2009; Chmielewska et al., 2014; Dabbs et al., 2010; Dabbs et al., 2011; Dabbs et al., 2012; Dallas et al., 2014; Gerakaki et al., 2013; Kurt et al., 2014; Lamont et al., 2010; Marin et al., 2013; Rittweger et al., 2000). As WBV has been shown to prime the higher order motor units prior to an explosive exercise.

There are a number of variables that influence the ability of a warm-up to enhance performance, such as intensity, load, training age, biological age, and fiber type (Alikhajeh et al., 2011). The present study used recreationally trained individuals to investigate lower body isometric strength after various warm-up protocols. Berning et al. (2010), reported that a general warm-up (5-minutes of cycling) in conjunction with one, 3-second heavy isometric squat (150% of the participants 1RM) elicited greater vertical jump height in recreationally trained individuals indicating that a supramaximal isometric muscle action enhances performance. This suggests the isometric intensity utilized in the present study may not have been great enough to elicit increased strength. Thompsen et al. (2007) investigated the influence of a weighted specific warm-up in comparison to a body weight specific warm-up in division III athletes. They reported that vertical and horizontal jump distance was enhanced following a dynamic warm-up in comparison to a static warm-up protocol. Similarly, Lowery et al. (2012) investigating the effects of low (56%), moderate (70%) and high intensity (93%) warm-ups on vertical jump performance, and showed that low intensity did not enhance performance. However, with an adequate amount of recovery (~4 minutes), moderate and high intensity increased performance. Similarly, Frantz et al. (2011) demonstrated that a dynamic warm-up consisting of body weight exercises stimulated an increase in vertical jump height and horizontal jump distance, but horizontal jump distance decreased after an isometric warm-up compared to no warm-up. This suggests that a low intensity isometric warm-up prior to an explosive power exercise may not enhance or even reduce performance. In contrast, the present study demonstrated no significant negative effects on performance following an isometric warm-up.

Lamont et al. (2010) compared isometric quarter squat training with a combination of WBV and resistance training versus resistance training alone and demonstrated that neither post-training GRF or RFD at 250 ms were significantly different from baseline measures. Their results are similar to the present study in that there were no significant differences between groups for GRF. This suggests that WBV in conjunction with isometric exercises could be utilized as a general or specific warm-up. An acute investigation by Bush et al. (2015) analyzed dynamic and isometric warm-ups with and without WBV in untrained individuals on knee extension strength. They demonstrated that there were significant increases in force production after the dynamic vibration protocol, but a significant decrease for all other conditions (dynamic and isometric without vibration and isometric with vibration). Furthermore, it was indicated that the decline in force production occurred during post-testing and was a result of fatigue (Bush et al., 2015). In the present study, none of the conditions elicited a significant difference in force production. This suggests that untrained individuals may demonstrate acute force increases following dynamic squats with WBV, while resistance trained individuals may require increased volume or intensity. Additionally, as the dynamic protocol used by Bush et al. (2015) had a longer eccentric to concentric ratio for dynamic squats, this and the 1- to 1-second ratio used in the present study may support why a decrease in the applied force output was not seen presently.

WBV has demonstrated that it may elicit improvements in acute force and power performance in resistance trained individuals (Adams et al., 2009; Cormie et al., 2006; Dabbs et al., 2010; Dabbs et al., 2011; Dabbs et al., 2012; Ronnestad et al., 2012). It has been hypothesized to activate the alpha-motor neurons, which may improve performance measures in an acute bout of explosive performance during an isometric muscle action (Lamont et al., 2010). In theory, the combination of WBV with dynamic or isometric resistance exercises may alter the neuromuscular contractile activity, leading to an increase in applied force production by recruiting higher order motor units. An acute study conducted by Cormie et al. (2006) found that jump height was significantly increased following WBV at 30 Hz when performing an isometric squat. This may infer that the combination of WBV and an isometric warm-up may increase applied force prior to a dynamic movement questioning the rule of specificity. Ronnestad et al. (2012) reported an increase in acute peak power in an explosive dynamic exercise after a bout of WBV at 50 Hz with no significant differences in dynamic strength in comparison to no WBV . In contrast to the present study, explosive exercise elicited a significant increase RFD after a dynamic protocol without vibration in comparison to the isometric warm-up with vibration. This may indicate that the total volume or intensity of WBV may have been too low in the present study to see an increase in IMTP performance.

5. Conclusion

These results suggest that WBV consisting of 4 bouts of 30-seconds, while performing DQS or IQS with 30s rest, does not influence RFD or GRF in an IMTP. However, DQS without vibration for 4 bouts of 30s demonstrated an increase in RFD compared to iVib, but no other conditions. This suggests that athletes and coaches who are in search of various methods of eliciting an acute increase in power should consider implementing this protocol. In addition, utilizing WBV does not negatively effect force or power production. Thus, this specific methodology could be conducted as a general warm-up. These results may also suggest that a stimulus similar to a dynamic movement should be used prior to a maximal isometric action. Further research is needed to determine an optimal protocol for explosive isometric exercise subsequent to a specific warm-up in conjunction with WBV.

References

Adams, J. B., Edwards, D., Serravite, D. H., Bedient, A. M., Huntsman, E., Jacobs, K. A., . . . Signorile, J. F. (2009). Optimal frequency, displacement, duration, and recovery patterns to maximize power output following acute whole-body vibration. *J Strength Cond Res, 23*(1), 237-245.

Alikhajeh, Y., Ramezanpour, M. R., & Moghaddam, A. (2011). The Effect of Different Warm-up Protocols on young Soccer Players' sprint. *Procedia-Social and Behavioral Sciences, 30*, 1588-1592.

Anderson, P., Landers, G., & Wallman, K. (2014). Effect of warm-up on intermittent sprint performance. *Res Sports Med, 22*(1), 88-99.

Berning, J. M., Adams, K. J., DeBeliso, M., Sevene-Adams, P. G., Harris, C., & Stamford, B. A. (2010). Effect of functional isometric squats on vertical jump in trained and untrained men. *J Strength Cond Res, 24*(9), 2285-2289.

Bush, J. A., Blog, G. L., Kang, J., Faigenbaum, A. D., & Ratamess, N. A. (2015). Effects of quadriceps strength after static and dynamic whole-body vibration exercise. *J Strength Cond Res, 29*(5), 1367-1377.

Cardinale, M., & Bosco, C. (2003). The use of vibration as an exercise intervention. *Exercise and sport sciences reviews, 31*(1), 3-7.

Cazas, V. L., Brown, L. E., Coburn, J. W., Galpin, A. J., Tufano, J. J., Laporta, J. W., & Du Bois, A. M. (2013). Influence of rest intervals after assisted jumping on bodyweight vertical jump performance. *J Strength Cond Res, 27*(1), 64-68.

Chmielewska, D., Piecha, M., Blaszczak, E., Krol, P., Smykla, A., & Juras, G. (2014). The effect of a single session of whole-body vibration training in recreationally active men on the excitability of the central and peripheral nervous system. *J Hum Kinet, 41*, 89-98.

Christensen, B. K., & Nordstrom, B. J. (2008). The effects of proprioceptive neuromuscular facilitation and dynamic stretching techniques on vertical jump performance. *J Strength Cond Res, 22*(6), 1826-1831.

Cilli, M., Gelen, E., Yildiz, S., Saglam, T., & Camur, M. (2014). Acute effects of a resisted dynamic warm-up protocol on jumping performance. *Biol Sport, 31*(4), 277-282.

Comfort, P., Allen, M., & Graham-Smith, P. (2011). Comparisons of peak ground reaction force and rate of force development during variations of the power clean. *The Journal of Strength & Conditioning Research, 25*(5), 1235-1239.

Comfort, P., Jones, P. A., McMahon, J. J., & Newton, R. (2015). Effect of knee and trunk angle on kinetic variables during the isometric midthigh pull: test-retest reliability. *Int J Sports Physiol Perform, 10*(1), 58-63.

Cormie, P., Deane, R. S., Triplett, N. T., & McBride, J. M. (2006). Acute effects of whole-body vibration on muscle activity, strength, and power. *J Strength Cond Res, 20*(2), 257-261.

Dabbs, N.C., Brown, L. E., Coburn, J. W., Lynn, S. K., Biagini, M. S., & Tran, T. T. (2010). Effect of whole-body vibration warm-up on bat speed in women softball players. *J Strength Cond Res, 24*(9), 2296-2299.

Dabbs, N.C., Munoz, C. X., Tran, T. T., Brown, L. E., & Bottaro, M. (2011). Effect of different rest intervals after whole-body vibration on vertical jump performance. *J Strength Cond Res, 25*(3), 662-667.

Dabbs, N.C., Tran, T. T., Garner, J. C., & Brown, L. E. (2012). A brief review: Using whole-body vibration to increase acute power and vertical jump performance. *Strength & Conditioning Journal, 34*(5), 78-84.

Dallas, G., Kirialanis, P., & Mellos, V. (2014). The acute effect of whole body vibration training on flexibility and explosive strength of young gymnasts. *Biol Sport, 31*(3), 233-237.

Frantz, T.L., & Ruiz, M. D. (2011). Effects of dynamic warm-up on lower body explosiveness among collegiate baseball players. *J Strength Cond Res, 25*(11), 2985-2990.

García-López, D., Garatachea, N., Marín, P. J., Martín, T., & Herrero, A. J. (2012). Acute effects of whole-body vibrations on balance, maximal force and perceived exertion: Vertical platform versus oscillating platform. *European Journal of Sport Science, 12*(5), 425-430.

Garner, J. C., Blackburn, T., Weimar, W., & Campbell, B. (2008). Comparison of electromyographic activity during eccentrically versus concentrically loaded isometric contractions. *J Electromyogr Kinesiol, 18*(3), 466-471.

Gerakaki, M. E., Evangelidis, P. E., Tziortzis, S., & Paradisis, G. P. (2013). Acute effects of dynamic whole body vibration in well trained track & field sprinters. *J Phys Ed Sport, 13*(3), 270-277.

Haff, G. G., Carlock, J. M., Hartman, M. J., Kilgore, J. L., Kawamori, N., Jackson, J. R., Stone, M. H. (2005). Force-time curve characteristics of dynamic and isometric muscle actions of elite women olympic weightlifters. *J Strength Cond Res, 19*(4), 741-748.

Haff, G. G., Ruben, R. P., Lider, J., Twine, C., & Cormie, P. (2015). A comparison of methods for determining the rate of force development during isometric midthigh clean pulls. *J Strength Cond Res, 29*(2), 386-395.

Hamada, T., Sale, D. G., MacDougall, J. D., & Tarnopolsky, M. A. (2000). Postactivation potentiation, fiber type, and twitch contraction time in human knee extensor muscles. *J Appl Physiol (1985), 88*(6), 2131-2137.

Holt, B. W., & Lambourne, K. (2008). The impact of different warm-up protocols on vertical jump performance in male collegiate athletes. *J Strength Cond Res, 22*(1), 226-229.

Kawamori, N., Rossi, S. J., Justice, B. D., Haff, E. E., Pistilli, E. E., O'BRYANT, H. S., Haff, G. G. (2006). Peak force and rate of force development during isometric and dynamic mid-thigh clean pulls performed at various intensities. *The Journal of Strength & Conditioning Research, 20*(3), 483-491.

Khamoui, A. V., Brown, L. E., Nguyen, D., Uribe, B. P., Coburn, J. W., Noffal, G. J., & Tran, T. (2011). Relationship between force-time and velocity-time characteristics of dynamic and isometric muscle actions. *J Strength Cond Res, 25*(1), 198-204.

Kurt, C., Toksoz, I., & Dindar, M. D. (2014). The effects of two different whole-body vibration frequencies on isometric strength, anaerobic performance, and rating of perceived exertion. *Journal of Physical Education and Sport, 14*(2), 306.

Lamont, H. S., Cramer, J. T., Bemben, D. A., Shehab, R. L., Anderson, M. A., & Bemben, M. G. (2010). Effects of adding whole body vibration to squat training on isometric force/time characteristics. *J Strength Cond Res, 24*(1), 171-183.

Lowery, R. P., Duncan, N. M., Loenneke, J. P., Sikorski, E. M., Naimo, M. A., Brown, L. E., Wilson, J. M. (2012). The effects of potentiating stimuli intensity under varying rest periods on vertical jump performance and power. *J Strength Cond Res, 26*(12), 3320-3325.

Marin, P. J., Ferrero, C. M., Menendez, H., Martin, J., & Herrero, A. J. (2013). Effects of whole-body vibration on muscle architecture, muscle strength, and balance in stroke patients: a randomized controlled trial. *Am J Phys Med Rehabil, 92*(10), 881-888.

Reiman, M. P., Peintner, A. M., Boehner, A. L., Cameron, C. N., Murphy, J. R., & Carter, J. W. (2010). Effects of dynamic warm-up with and without a weighted vest on lower extremity power performance of high school male athletes. *The Journal of Strength & Conditioning Research, 24*(12), 3387-3395.

Ribeiro, A. S., Romanzini, M., Schoenfeld, B. J., Souza, M. F., Avelar, A., & Cyrino, E. S. (2014). Effect of different warm-up procedures on the performance of resistance training exercises. *Percept Mot Skills, 119*(1), 133-145.

Rittweger, J., Beller, G., & Felsenberg, D. (2000). Acute physiological effects of exhaustive whole-body vibration exercise in man. *Clin Physiol, 20*(2), 134-142.

Ritzmann, R., Kramer, A., Gollhofer, A., & Taube, W. (2013). The effect of whole body vibration on the H-reflex, the stretch reflex, and the short-latency response during hopping. *Scand J Med Sci Sports, 23*(3), 331-339.

Ronnestad, B. R., Holden, G., Samnoy, L. E., & Paulsen, G. (2012). Acute effect of whole-body vibration on power, one-repetition maximum, and muscle activation in power lifters. *J Strength Cond Res, 26*(2), 531-539.

Thompsen, A. G., Kackley, T., Palumbo, M. A., & Faigenbaum, A. D. (2007). Acute effects of different warm-up protocols with and without a weighted vest on jumping performance in athletic women. *J Strength Cond Res, 21*(1), 52-56.

Thompson, P. D., Arena, R., Riebe, D., Pescatello, L. S., & American College of Sports, M. (2013). ACSM's new preparticipation health screening recommendations from ACSM's guidelines for exercise testing and prescription, ninth edition. *Curr Sports Med Rep, 12*(4), 215-217.

Turner, A. P., Sanderson, M. F., & Attwood, L. A. (2011). The acute effect of different frequencies of whole-body vibration on countermovement jump performance. *J Strength Cond Res, 25*(6), 1592-1597.

West, D. J., Owen, N. J., Jones, M. R., Bracken, R. M., Cook, C. J., Cunningham, D. J., Crewther, B. T. (2011). Relationships between force–time characteristics of the isometric midthigh pull and dynamic performance in professional rugby league players. *The Journal of Strength & Conditioning Research, 25*(11), 3070-3075.

15

Isometric Thumb Exertion Induces B Cell and T Cell Lymphocytosis in Trained and Untrained Males: Physical Aptitude Determines Response Profiles

Adam Michael Szlezak (Corresponding author)
Division of Sports Science, School of Allied Health Sciences,
Griffith University, Parklands Dr, Southport QLD 4215, Australia
E-mail: adam.szlezak@griffithuni.edu.au

Lotti Tajouri
Faculty of Health Science & Medicine, Bond University, Gold Coast QLD 4229, Australia
E-mail: ltajouri@bond.edu.au

James Keane
Faculty of Health Science & Medicine, Bond University, Gold Coast QLD 4229, Australia
E-mail: keanejames4@gmail.com

Siri Lauluten Szlezak
Faculty of Health Science & Medicine, Bond University,
Gold Coast QLD 4229, Australia
E-mail: siri.szlezak@gmail.com

Clare Minahan
Division of Sports Science, School of Allied Health Sciences,
Griffith University, Parklands Dr, Southport QLD 4215, Australia
E-mail: c.minahan@griffith.edu.au

Abstract

Purpose: The present study examined the effect of low-dose thumb exertion on lymphocyte subpopulation trafficking. The potential role of blood lactate in mediating lymphocyte redistribution was also investigated. **Methods:** 27 male participants (18 weightlifting-trained; 9 untrained) were separated into 3 groups of 9 (Weightlifting and Untrained Experimental: WL_{EXP}, UT_{EXP}; Weightlifting Placebo: WL_{PLA}). WL_{EXP} and UT_{EXP} performed 4x60 second isometric thumb intervals separated by 60 second rest intervals in a single-blinded placebo-controlled study. Participants were assessed over a 60 minute post-intervention recovery period for pain, blood lactate and lymphocyte subpopulation counts. **Results:** WL_{PLA} did not change for any measured variable ($p>0.05$). The two experimental groups increased significantly ($p<0.01$) in thumb pain post-intervention (WL_{EXP}:4.92/10; UT_{EXP}:2.92/10) however only WL_{EXP} remained elevated across all time-points. Blood lactate increased for both experimental groups post-intervention ($p<0.01$) whilst peak concentrations ($UT_{EXP:}$ 2.2mmol/L; $WL_{EXP:}$ 2.4mmol/L) and temporal profiles were not different between groups ($p>0.05$). No differences in cell count were seen for CD56+/CD16+ lymphocytes across time for any group ($p>0.05$). UT_{EXP} showed an early significant increase (20 min post-intervention) in CD4+CD3+ (20.78%, $p<0.01$), CD8+CD3+ (15.25%, $p<0.01$) and CD19+ (18.11%, $p=0.013$) cell count before returning to levels not different from baseline by the final time-point ($p>0.05$). Conversely, WL_{EXP} group showed no early increase followed by a delayed increase in cell count evident at the final time-point; CD4+CD3+ (19.06%, $p<0.01$), CD8+CD3+ (11.46%, $p=0.033$) and CD19+ (28.87%, $p<0.01$). Blood lactate was not correlated with lymphocyte counts. **Conclusions:** Physical aptitude and not cellular energy demand influences the lymphocyte response to resistance-exercise.

Keywords: B-Lymphocytes; Exercise; Lactic Acid; Lymphocytosis; Resistance Training; T-Lymphocytes

1. Introduction

Resistance-exercise is recognised as a key component of contemporary athletic training (Azeem & Kumar, 2011; Ranisavljev & Vladimir, 2010) and as such, the biological consequences of this exercise mode require thorough investigation. Considering the central role of the immune system in both host-defence and physiological adaptation (Luckheeram, Zhou, Verma, & Xia, 2012; Mosser & Edwards, 2008; Sonnet et al., 2006), a clinically relevant understanding of the interaction between the immune system and resistance-exercise is of great importance for exercise professionals. Before this can occur however, exercise-induced leukocyte responses and the mechanisms through which these responses transpire must be characterised.

Based on preliminary research, it is suggested that leukocyte responses to exercise are not random, but occur for specific functional purposes (Freidenreich & Volek, 2012; Walsh et al., 2011). Research is therefore warranted which investigates the relationship between resistance-exercise and those particular leukocytes involved in highly organised and regulated roles. Pleitrophic cells such as the lymphocytes are one important example, since they orchestrate fundamental biological tasks including cell-mediated and humoral immunity, coordination of innate immune responses and in regards to exercise, facilitate physiological adaption such as tissue remodelling (LeBien & Tedder, 2008; Luckheeram et al., 2012). Currently, the clinically relevant implications of exercise-induced changes to leukocyte homeostasis (distribution, proliferation and function) are unknown (Dohi et al., 2001; Mayhew, Thyfault, & Koch, 2005; Walsh et al., 2011). Additionally, there is a complete gap in the literature regarding potential immune responses to low-dose exercise (Walsh et al., 2011). Recent research has suggested that exercise intensity and duration are linked to leukocyte redistribution (Bush et al., 1999; Kraemer et al., 1999), however lymphocytes may respond through a different mechanism. Preliminary research in females has shown (Miles et al., 2003) that the greatest lymphocyte responses to resistance-exercise were associated with the highest post-exercise blood lactate levels; that is, high lactate responders ($\geq$11.92 mmol/L) showed significantly greater lymphocyte count elevations than lower lactate responders ($\leq$7.62 mmol/L). Furthermore, this response was not observed for monocytes and or granulocytes suggesting that cellular energy demand may selectively govern the lymphocytic response to resistance-exercise. Insight into the mechanisms through which resistance-exercise affects lymphocyte homeostasis is a key milestone in determining the functional consequences of this exercise mode, and thus warrants further investigation. Although blood lactate concentration cannot determine the exact rate or volume of energy produced anaerobically, it can be used to demonstrate a rise in cellular energy demand and anaerobic energy expenditure (Fernandez, Mendez-Villanueva, & Pluim, 2006; Spurway, 1992; Wirtz, Wahl, Kleinöder, & Mester, 2014). From a practical perspective, knowledge that blood lactate is associated with selective regulation of lymphocyte trafficking would influence the way in which anaerobic physical activity (e.g. resistance-training; Wirtz et al., 2014) is prescribed.

A significant challenge with investigating the relationship between lymphocytes and resistance-exercise is ensuring that the exercise intervention can be tightly controlled. A caveat with the existing literature is that it is dominated by large-dose exercise protocols encompassing multiple skeletal muscles and joints (Freidenreich & Volek, 2012). Due to potential inter-individual differences in biomechanics such as joint stability (Solomonow & Krogsgaard, 2001) and motor control (Frank, Kobesova, & Kolar, 2013), a researcher's ability to standardize performance of an exercise intervention is adversely affected when employing large dose, multiple-joint protocols. Since the link between blood lactate and lymphocyte redistribution was observed through a large exercise-dose (squat) protocol with previously untrained-female subjects (Miles et al., 2003), the present study aims to employ a more controllable exercise-intervention, i.e. an isometric thumb manoeuvre (Punsola-Izard, Salas-Gómez, Sirvent-Rivalda, & Esquirol-Caussà, 2012), and a male population. This approach will facilitate reliable examination of lymphocyte responses to resistance-exercise and associated blood lactate changes whilst producing findings relevant to males. Additionally, subjects of differing physical aptitude should be studied to identify if blood lactate or other variables influence lymphocyte-specific trafficking post-exercise. Finally, the study of lymphocyte responses to an isometric thumb exercise protocol will provide novel insight into the potential effect of low-dose exercise on the immune system. In the present study, the following hypotheses were made: i) Short duration isometric thumb exertion will mobilise lymphocyte subpopulations and increase blood lactate concentration; ii) An increase in circulating lymphocyte count is related to an increase in blood lactate concentration; iii) Lymphocyte responses will vary between experimental groups and this will be explained by variances in blood lactate responses.

2. Methods

2.1 Participants

Prior to recruitment of subjects, this study received full ethical approval from the Griffith University Human Research Ethics Committee. The study conformed to standards set out in the Declaration of Helsinki and its later amendments or comparable ethical standards. Before being admitted to the study, all participants were given a detailed explanation of the study procedures, experimental interventions and potential risks involved. Each participant then signed a written consent form. Twenty seven male subjects (18-40 yr) voluntarily participated in the present study and all twenty seven completed the study. Eighteen men were considered weightlifting athletes who ranged from local to state-level competitors and trained at a frequency of 2 or more weightlifting sessions per week (Table 1). The other nine men were untrained (not participating in any regular exercise and had not performed resistance-exercise for at least 12 months). The untrained subjects were grouped together into the Untrained experimental group (UT_{EXP}: n=9). Weightlifting athletes were randomly allocated into one of two groups (using the concealed, third party randomization method described by Schulz and associates (1995): i. Weightlifting experimental (WL_{EXP}: n = 9), or ii. Weightlifting placebo (WL_{PLA}: n = 9). All subjects were blinded to their group allocation. Subject characteristics are displayed in Table 1.

2.2 Experimental approach

The present study used a single-blinded, randomised, placebo-controlled study design. Every participant was given an appointment time and instructed to abstain from all forms of exercise for 48 h and fast for 2 h prior to attending their appointment. This controlled for prior physical stress and dietary intake affecting the study results (Carlson et al., 2008;

Freidenreich & Volek, 2012; Gleeson, 2007). Each participant attended the testing laboratory (temperature monitored at 23 °C) on one single occasion only. The session began with a pre-screening where a Doctor of Physical Therapy confirmed that subjects were apparently healthy. Subjects were excluded based on: past or present history of upper limb/hand musculoskeletal pathology, cardiovascular, metabolic, or respiratory illness; contraindications to resistance-exercise (Pollock et al., 2000). Subjects were then familiarised with the *B & L Pinch Gauge (PG-60) dynamometer* (B & L Engineering, CA, USA) and the MVC (maximum voluntary contraction) assessment using the familiarisation procedure described previously (Szlezak et al., 2015). Briefly, participants were seated in a standardised testing position as recommended by the American Society of Hand Therapists (Fess & Moran, 1981). Only the dominant hand was utilised for the purpose of achieving maximal efforts. Participants were instructed to perform 5 sub-maximal pinch efforts separated by 30 seconds rest before immediately completing a maximal-effort practice session identical to the testing session (see 2.3.1 MVC Assessment). This familiarisation procedure also ensured that any pre-fatiguing effect associated with this procedure was consistent across all research participants. Participants were also shown a copy of the Pain Visual Analogue Scale (VAS) and were instructed on how to complete it. Following familiarization, an Intravenous (IV) catheter was inserted into the median cubital vein of the participant's dominant hand and was left in-situ for serial blood sampling. This sampling method promoted precise timing of blood collection, and avoided repeat needle-trauma which could affect results. Blood for lymphocyte assessment was collected directly into an EDTA Vacutainer (Becton Dickinson, NJ, USA) and analysed within 60 minutes. Blood for lactate analysis was drawn with a syringe from the IV catheter and analysed immediately. At each collection point, 5ml of blood was drawn and discarded before collecting sample blood and catheter lines were maintained through saline flushing. After the catheter insertion, the participant rested for 10 minutes in the testing chair before baseline measures were collected to negate any potential affect the catheterisation could have on subsequent measures. Baseline measures were then recorded in the following order: i. Lateral pinch (see 2.3.1 MVC Assessment); ii. Pain perception (see 2.3.4 Pain Assessment); iii. Blood collection for lymphocyte assessment (see 2.3.5 Lymphocyte Assessment); iv. Blood collection for lactate analysis (see 2.3.6 Blood Lactate Analysis). Following baseline testing, participants undertook either an Exercise Intervention (WL_{EXP} and UT_{EXP} groups) or a Placebo Intervention (WL_{PLA} group). Once the interventions were completed, all participants immediately underwent the following rest and passive testing conditions in the order described: i. Pain Perception: immediately, 10 minutes, 20 minutes and 60 minutes post the interventions; ii. Blood collection for lymphocyte assessment: 20 minutes and 60 minutes post the interventions; iii. Blood collection for lactate analysis: 3 minutes, 10 minutes, 20 minutes and 60 minutes post the interventions. Of note, blood Lactate was first sampled at 3 minutes post-intervention to record peak concentrations (Goodwin, Harris, Hernández, & Gladden, 2007; Vucetic, Mozek, & Rakovac, 2015). Throughout the duration of the experiment, all subjects remained seated and were instructed against moving the tested limb to avoid any active recovery which could affect the results. IV catheters were removed after the final collection point. All blood samples and raw data were subsequently analysed and statistical analysis applied.

2.3 Procedures

2.3.1 MVC Assessment

Assessment occurred using a *B & L Engineering pinch gauge* (PG-60) with reported reliability and validity (Mathiowetz et al., 1985; Mathiowetz, Vizenor, & Melander, 2000; Mathiowetz, Weber, Volland, & Kashman,1984). All subjects undertook this assessment to determine their maximum lateral-pinch-strength of the dominant hand only. To eliminate testing bias, one researcher gave instructions and reset the dynamometer and a separate researcher viewed and recorded each test result. Subject encouragement during testing was standardised by using the verbal instructions described previously (Mathiowetz et al., 1984). Subjects were positioned in the standardised testing position (seated in a chair with arm rests and full back support, the shoulder adducted to neutral and neutrally rotated, elbow flexed at 90°, forearm in the neutral position, and wrist between 0° and 30° dorsiflexion and between 0° and 15° ulnar deviation [Fess & Moran, 1981; Mathiowetz et al., 1985]). This also controlled for contribution from accessory muscles. Subjects were tested using the protocol previously described (Mathiowetz et al., 1985). During testing, subjects were instructed to give a maximal effort. Immediately after the first effort was completed, the dynamometer was reset and a second (and final) effort was performed. Values were recorded and later averaged.

2.3.2 Exercise Intervention

A previously described low-dose exercise protocol (Szlezak et al., 2015) formed the exercise intervention. Briefly, this involved performing a lateral pinch-manoeuvre in a standardised testing position (Fess & Moran, 1981; Mathiowetz et al., 1985) and utilised a B & L Engineering pinch gauge (PG-60). A lateral-pinch manoeuvre was selected to minimise the potential effects of inter-individual biomechanical variation and accessory muscle exertion on study results (Punsola-Izard et al., 2012). A total of 4 minutes total-work (isometric thumb resistance-exercise) was performed, divided into four 60-s work-intervals each separated by one, 60-s rest interval. The total time for the exercise intervention was 7 minutes. The first two work intervals were performed at 50% MVC and the remaining two work intervals at 35% MVC (where MVC was determined during the MVC Assessment).

Participants continuously monitored the pinch gauge during the work-intervals to ensure they constantly applied the correct load (kg). The standardised command "keep the needle at your weight" was used by a researcher if the applied load changed from that specified (Szlezak et al., 2015).

2.3.3 Placebo Intervention

WL_{PLA} participants undertook the placebo intervention (previously described by Szlezak et al., 2015) which involved 4 work-intervals lasting 60-s separated by 60-s rest-intervals. In contrast to the exercise intervention, WL_{PLA} subjects held the pinch gauge without applying any downward pressure. This was considered a placebo since subjects could not know if they were performing a low-dose exercise intervention or not. Body positioning in the placebo intervention was identical to the exercise intervention. Participants rested during the rest-interval as described in the exercise intervention. A total-time of 7 minutes elapsed during the placebo intervention to maintain consistency with the exercise intervention.

2.3.4 Pain Assessment

A pain VAS was employed to validly and reliably assess each participant's perception of exercise-related muscle pain (Douris et al., 2006; Hawker, Mian, Kendzerska, & French, 2011; Sellwood, Brukner, Williams, Nicol, & Hinman, 2007). An unmarked horizontal 100 mm line with the terminal descriptors ''no pain'' (score of 0) and ''worst pain imaginable" (score of 10) was completed by the participants. Scoring occurred by measuring the distance (mm) on the 10-cm line between the "no pain" anchor and the respondent's mark thus providing a range of scores from 0–100 (Jensen, Karoly, & Braver, 1986).

2.3.5 Lymphocyte Assessment

Lymphocyte subpopulation analysis was performed using the *BD FACSVerse* flow cytometer and the Becton Dickinson Simultest™ IMK Lymphocyte kit for enumeration of B (CD19+) lymphocytes, helper/inducer T (CD3+CD4+) lymphocytes, suppressor/cytotoxic T (CD3+CD8+) lymphocytes and natural killer (CD16+and/or CD56+) lymphocytes (Becton Dickinson, Franklin Lakes, NJ, USA). Lymphocyte cell percentages and absolute counts were calculated and generated automatically on each blood sample using the Simultest IMK-Lymphocyte software once the operator entered the independent data (leukocyte count, leukocyte and lymphocyte percentages; HmX Hematology analyser, Beckman Coulter, Pasadena, CA, USA).

2.3.6 Blood Lactate Analysis

Analysis occurred using an automated blood lactate analyser (Lactate Pro, Arkray Inc., Tokyo, JPN) with reported reliability and accuracy (Pyne, Boston, Martin, & Logan, 2000). The device was calibrated prior to use as specified by the manufacturer. Venous blood was injected into a Lactate Pro test strip direct from the syringe. The analyser was left resting on a stationary table until the blood lactate calculation was finalised and recorded. Values were reported in millimoles per liter (mmol/L).

2.4 Statistical Analysis

Values presented are as means ± standard deviation. IBM SPSS Statistics 22 was used for all statistical testing. Fully-factorial ANOVA with repeated measures was used to determine any interaction among, or main effect of, the independent variables group and time. Least squares difference pairwise comparisons were used to detect the specific site of any significant effect identified. Pearson's correlation coefficients were calculated to determine any relationships among change in blood lactate concentration and change in lymphocyte subpopulation count for each of the participant groups (WL_{PLA}, UT_{EXP}, WL_{EXP}). Statistical significance was accepted at $p<0.05$.

3. Results

Subject characteristics are displayed in Table 1. The results of a one-way ANOVA revealed that no statistical differences were found for age ($F=0.114$, $p=0.892$), height ($F=0.561$, $p=0.578$) and body mass ($F=1.096$, $p=0.350$) variables among the three groups. Moreover, no differences among the three groups were found for any of the measured variables (reported pain, blood lactate, lymphocyte counts) at baseline ($p>0.05$).

Table 1. Subject characteristics

Group	UT_{EXP}	WL_{EXP}	WL_{PLA}
n	9	9	9
Age (yrs)	27 (±7)	28 (±5)	27 (±7)
Height (cm)	180 (±9)	182 (±8)	179 (±5)
Body mass (kg)	83.2 (±9.8)	89.6 (±7.4)	84.3 (±11.6)
Gym sessions (per week)	0 (±0)	4 (±1)	4 (±1)
Hand dominance	R: n=8 L: n=1	R: n=7 L: n=2	R: n=7 L: n=2
Lateral pinch (kg)	8.7 (±1.5)	9.7 (±1.2)	8.7 (±1.5)

Values presented are as means ± standard deviation

3.1 Pain VAS

A significant interaction for time and group was found for pain (VAS) ($F=11.27$, $p< 0.01$). Pairwise Comparisons revealed no significant change in the Placebo group from baseline at any post-intervention time-point ($p>0.05$). The UT_{EXP} group increased significantly in reported pain immediately post-intervention (2.92/10; $p<0.01$) and this represented the peak pain response. Pain remained elevated up to 20 minutes post-intervention ($p<0.01$), before decreasing to levels not significantly different from baseline ($p>0.05$) at 60 minutes post-intervention. The WL_{EXP} group also reported a highly significant increase in pain immediately post-intervention (4.92/10; $p<0.01$) and this was the peak pain response. Pain remained elevated across all times points ($p<0.01$). Maximum pain values were significantly higher in the WL_{EXP} (4.92/10) vs UT_{EXP} (2.92/10) group ($p=0.02$).

3.2 Blood lactate

A significant interaction for time and group was found for blood lactate (mmol/L) ($F=26.31$, $p<0.01$). Pairwise Comparisons revealed no significant change in the Placebo group from baseline at any post-intervention time-point ($p>0.05$). Both experimental groups showed a highly significant increase ($p<0.01$) in blood lactate concentration at the first post-intervention (3 minutes post) and 10 minutes post-intervention time-points before returning to levels not significantly different from baseline by 20 minutes post-intervention ($p>0.05$). Peak blood lactate concentrations ($UT_{EXP:}$ 2.2mmol/L; $WL_{EXP:}$ 2.4mmol/L) occurred at 3 minutes post-intervention for both experimental groups and response magnitude was not significantly different between these groups ($p>0.05$). See Figure 1.

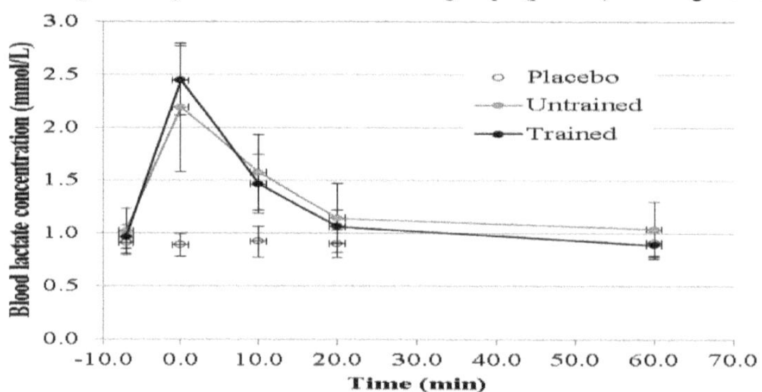

Figure 1. Blood lactate concentration over time

There was no difference in blood lactate concentration among the three groups at baseline (-7 min; $p>0.05$). **WL_{PLA}:** Lactate concentration did not change from baseline across time ($p>0.05$).

UT_{EXP} and **WL_{EXP}:** Lactate concentration increased ($p<0.01$) by 3 min post-exercise, remained elevated at 10 min post-exercise ($p<0.01$), and decreased to levels not different from baseline by 20 min post-exercise ($p>0.05$). Peak concentrations (3 min post: $UT_{EXP:}$ 2.2mmol/L; $WL_{EXP:}$ 2.4mmol/L) were not different between these two groups ($p>0.05$).

3.3 Helper/inducer T lymphocytes (CD4+CD3+)

A significant interaction for time and group was found for CD4+CD3+ lymphocytes ($F=4.42$, $p<0.01$). Pairwise Comparisons revealed no significant change in the Placebo group from baseline at any post-intervention time-point ($p>0.05$). In the UT_{EXP} group, lymphocyte count increased from baseline at 20 minutes post-intervention by 20.78% and this change was highly significant ($p<0.01$). From 20-60 minutes post-intervention, lymphocyte count decreased back towards baseline count and this was also highly significant ($p<0.01$). Lymphocyte count at the final time-point (60 minutes post-intervention) was not significantly different from baseline ($p>0.05$).

In the WL_{EXP} group, lymphocyte count did not significantly change between baseline and 20 minutes post-intervention ($p>0.05$). Lymphocyte count did elevate from 20-60 minutes post-intervention and this change was significant ($p=0.01$). Lymphocyte count at the final time-point was elevated above baseline by 19.06% and this difference was highly significant ($p<0.01$). See Figure 2.

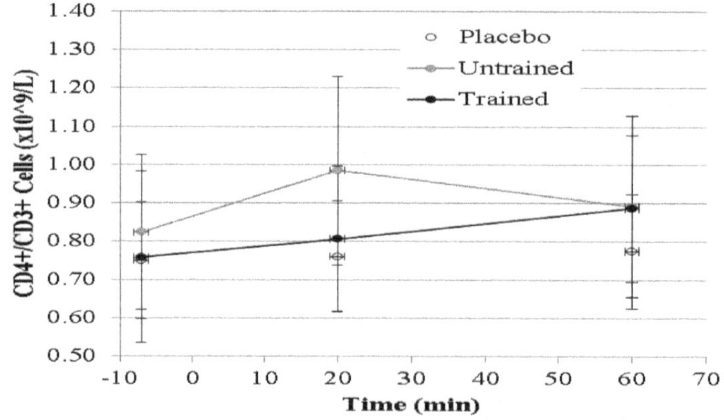

Figure 2. CD4+CD3+ T lymphocyte count over time

There was no difference in CD4+CD3+ cell count among the three groups at baseline (-7 min; $p>0.05$).

WL_{PLA}: Lymphocyte count did not change from baseline across time ($p>0.05$).

UT_{EXP}: Lymphocyte count had increased by 20 min post-exercise (Δ20.78%; $p<0.01$), then decreased from 20-60 min post ($p<0.01$). At 60 min post-exercise, lymphocyte count was not different from baseline ($p>0.05$).

WL_{EXP}: Lymphocyte count had not changed by 20 min post-exercise ($p>0.05$) but increased from 20-60 min post-exercise ($p=0.01$). At 60 min post-exercise, lymphocyte count was elevated above baseline (Δ19.06%; $p<0.01$).

3.4 Suppressor/cytotoxic T lymphocytes (CD8+CD3+)

A significant interaction for time and group was found for CD8+CD3+ lymphocytes (F=3.1, p=0.02). Pairwise Comparisons revealed no significant change in the Placebo group from baseline at any post-intervention time-point (p>0.05).In the UT_{EXP} group, lymphocyte count increased from baseline at 20 minutes post-intervention by 15.25% and this change was highly significant (p<0.01). From 20-60 minutes post-intervention, lymphocyte count decreased back towards baseline count and this was also significant (p=0.03). Lymphocyte count at the final time-point (60 minutes post-intervention) was not significantly different from baseline (p>0.05).

In the WL_{EXP} group, lymphocyte count did not significantly change between baseline and 20 minutes post-intervention (p>0.05). Lymphocyte count did increase from 20-60 minutes post-intervention however this change did not reach significance (p>0.05). Lymphocyte count at the final time-point had elevated above baseline by 11.46% and this difference was significant (p=0.033). See Figure 3.

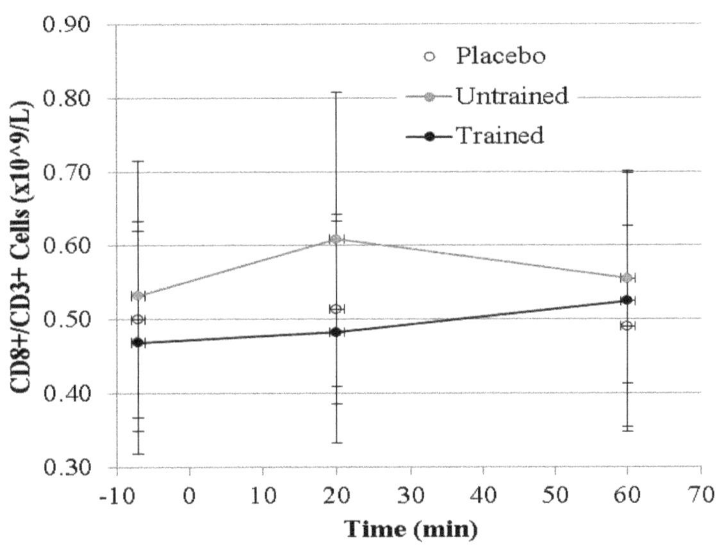

Figure 3. CD8+CD3+ T lymphocyte count over time

There was no difference in CD8+CD3+ cell count among the three groups at baseline (-7 min; p>0.05).
WL_{PLA}: Lymphocyte count did not change from baseline across time (p>0.05).
UT_{EXP}: Lymphocyte count had increased by 20 min post-exercise (Δ15.25%; p<0.01), then decreased from 20-60 min post-exercise (p=0.03). At 60 min post-exercise, lymphocyte count was not different from baseline (p>0.05).
WL_{EXP}: Lymphocyte count had not changed by 20 min post-exercise (p>0.05). Lymphocyte count did increase from 20-60 min post-exercise however this change did not reach significance (p>0.05). At 60 min post-exercise, lymphocyte count was elevated above baseline (Δ11.46%, p=0.033).

3.5 B lymphocytes (CD19+)

No interaction of time and group was found for CD19+ lymphocytes (F=1.72, p=0.16) however there was a main effect of time (F=6.86, p<0.01). Pairwise comparisons revealed no significant change in the Placebo group from baseline at any post-intervention time-point (p>0.05). In the UT_{EXP} group, lymphocyte count increased from baseline at 20 minutes post-intervention by 18.11% and this change was significant (p=0.013). From 20-60 minutes post-intervention, lymphocyte count decreased back towards baseline count however this change did not reach significance (p>0.05). Lymphocyte count at the final time-point (60 minutes post-intervention) was not significantly different from baseline (p>0.05). In the WL_{EXP} group, lymphocyte count did not significantly change between baseline and 20 minutes post-intervention (p>0.05). Lymphocyte count increased from 20-60 minutes post-intervention and this change was significant (p=0.031). Lymphocyte count at the final time-point was elevated above baseline by 28.87% and this difference was highly significant (p<0.01). See Figure 4.

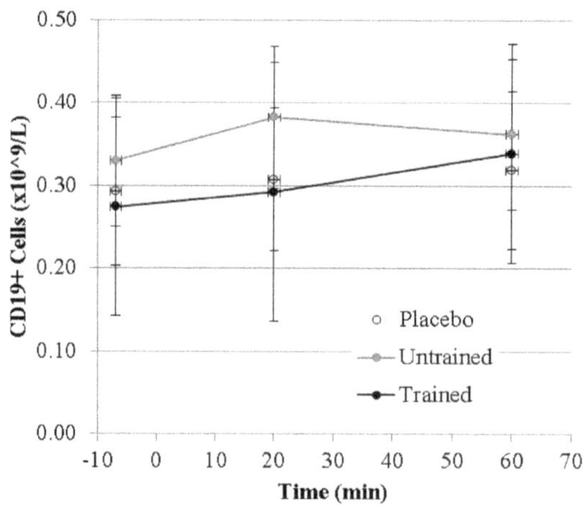

Figure 4. CD19+ B lymphocyte count over time

There was no difference in CD19+ cell count among the three groups at baseline (-7 min; $p>0.05$).
WL_{PLA}: Lymphocyte count did not change from baseline across time ($p>0.05$).
UT_{EXP}: Lymphocyte count had increased by 20 min post-exercise (Δ18.11%; $p=0.013$). A decrease occurred from 20-60 min post-exercise but did not reach significance ($p>0.05$). At 60 min post-exercise, lymphocyte count was not different from baseline ($p>0.05$).
WL_{EXP}: Lymphocyte count had not changed by 20 min post-exercise ($p>0.05$) but increased from 20-60 min post-exercise ($p=0.031$). At 60 min post-exercise, lymphocyte count was elevated above baseline (Δ28.87%; $p<0.01$).

3.6 Natural Killer lymphocytes (CD56+ and or CD16+)

No significant interactions were found for time and groups for CD56+/CD16+ lymphocytes ($F=0.23$, $p=0.92$). Additionally, no significant changes in lymphocyte count from baseline occurred across time for any of the three groups ($p>0.05$). See Figure 5.

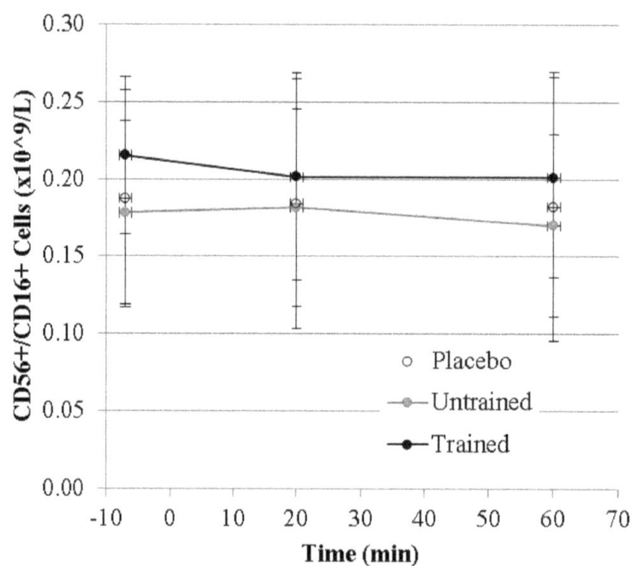

Figure 5. CD56+/CD16+ NK lymphocyte count over time

There was no difference in CD56+/CD16 cell count among the three groups at baseline (-7 min; $p>0.05$).
No changes in lymphocyte count from baseline occurred across time for any of the three groups ($p>0.05$).

3.7 Blood lactate - lymphocyte correlation

No correlation was found between change in blood lactate concentration and change in lymphocyte count: CD4+CD3+ (UT_{EXP} $r=0.11$, $p=0.78$; WL_{EXP} $r=0.16$, $p=0.68$), CD8+CD3+ (UT_{EXP} $r=0.03$, $p=0.93$; WL_{EXP} $r=0.64$, $p=0.07$), CD19+ (UT_{EXP} $r=-0.05$, $p=0.89$; WL_{EXP} $r= 0.21$, $p=0.60$) or CD56+/16+ cell counts (UT_{EXP} $r=0.20$, $p=0.76$; WL_{EXP} $r=-0.01$, $p=0.99$). The relationship observed between blood lactate concentration and CD8+CD3+ cell count in WL_{EXP} is illustrated in Figure 6; nonetheless this relationship was not statistically significant.

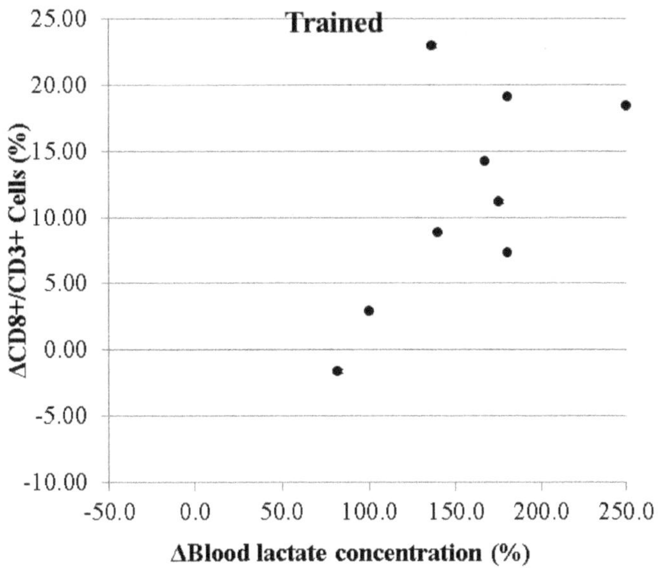

Figure 6. Blood lactate concentration & CD8+CD3+ lymphocyte correlation (WL_{EXP})
The relationship observed between changes in blood lactate concentration and changes in CD8+CD3+ cell count in WL_{EXP} ($r=0.64$) is illustrated. Nonetheless, this relationship was not significant ($p>0.05$).

4. Discussion

The present study is the first to demonstrate that a micro-dose of resistance-exercise can significantly elevate circulating B lymphocyte and T lymphocyte counts. Additionally, lymphocyte response profiles were related to the physical aptitude of subjects, and not blood lactate levels. No relationship was found between change in lymphocyte counts (CD4+CD3+ and CD8+CD3+ T cells; CD19+ B cells; CD56+/16+ NK cells) and change in blood lactate concentration for either of the experimental groups. This latter finding disproved our hypothesis that an increase in circulating lymphocyte count is related to an increase in blood lactate concentration. Functionally, these findings indicate that B and T cell trafficking in males is affected by even the smallest of physical exertions. Moreover, cell mobilisation is not regulated by mild elevations in cellular energy demand or anaerobic energy expenditure (Fernandez et al., 2006; Wirtz et al., 2014) however is influenced by physical aptitude of the host.

The present study utilised a micro-dose exercise approach which was brief in duration, low in intensity and anaerobically based (evidenced by increases in blood lactate as hypothesised). This experimental approach was considered critical in order to minimise the potential influence of exercise intensity and duration on the study results (Freidenreich & Volek, 2012; Walsh et al., 2011) so that potential relationships between blood lactate, physical aptitude and lymphocyte homeostasis could be better studied. It was also necessary to investigate the effects of a low-dose resisted exertion on lymphocyte subpopulations.

In the present study, the placebo group did not change for any measured variable across any time-points as expected. For reported pain levels, the significant increase seen for the UTEXP and WL_{EXP} groups indicates that a low intensity, short duration exercise protocol can be highly challenging beyond the physical, even in a well-trained athletic population. Moreover, the pain elevation was shortly lived (< 20 minutes) in the untrained individuals, whereas the response was maintained for at least 60 minutes (final time-point) in the weightlifters. Of note, the weightlifters reported a significantly higher peak pain response compared with the untrained group. As peak blood lactate concentrations between groups were not significantly different, a psychological phenomenon may be responsible for this result. Well trained athletes are known to place higher expectations on oneself than non-athletes (Dunn, Gotwals, & Causgrove Dunn, 2005; Gould, Dieffenbach, & Moffett, 2002) which can be associated with perfectionistic concerns, fear of failure, mental stress and elevated anxiety (Conroy, Willow, & Metzler, 2002; Stoeber et al., 2011). These alterations in psychological state are known to increase one's perception of pain (Loggia, Schweinhardt, Villemure, & Bushnell, 2008; Rhudy & Meagher, 2000) and likely explain the results of this present study. The magnitude of peak pain reported in this study for the weightlifting subjects (4.92/10) was a novel and unexpected finding considering the micro-dose nature of the exercise protocol. This is evidence that low-intensity, short-duration exercise can be highly demanding depending on the subject population and the targeted muscle groups.

Blood lactate concentrations increased significantly in both experimental groups at 3 minutes post-exercise and had normalised by 20 minutes post-exercise, indicating a similar production and clearance rate between experimental groups. The timing of the peak concentration (3 minutes post-exercise) was consistent with previously reported temporal profiles in larger-dose studies (Goodwin et al., 2007; Vucetic et al., 2015). Interestingly, lactate profiles between experimental groups were similar and may be explained by the involvement of the thumb muscle in activities of daily living, thus providing a training effect in the untrained group. Importantly, these findings indicated that the exercise-intervention challenged each experimental group to a similar level, both physically and anaerobically. The blood lactate profile demonstrated in the present study is a novel and meaningful finding alone. These results show that short duration exercise at a low physical intensity (35% and 50% of MVC) can measurably increase anaerobic energy expenditure in specific skeletal muscle (Fernandez et al., 2006; Wirtz et al., 2014). For example, a large muscle exercising at 35% MVC may be below lactate threshold for that tissue, however for the small muscle group around the thumb, this same relative intensity was above the lactate threshold. These results show how a low physical intensity of exercise can have meaningful metabolic consequences for specific myocytes. Extrapolating the results of the present study to a practical example, gripping an unloaded barbell would not be considered challenging for a trained athlete, however the coach should now consider the metabolic implications for the smaller gripping muscles, those in the thumb and hand. Additionally, we have shown that a small muscle group exertion can produce high levels of pain, thus researchers and clinicians should view exercise intensity in a broader scope than just the physical.

In relation to lymphocyte subpopulations, no significant change was seen for the CD56+/CD16+ cells. This negative result was inconsistent with the literature (Freidenreich & Volek, 2012), however as the first measurement was not taken until 20 minutes post-exercise, a response may have occurred and returned to baseline prior to this point. As this study is the first to investigate natural killer cell responses to such a short duration, micro-dose of resistance-exercise, further research should measure natural killer cell counts at more acute post-exercise time-points. Conversely, CD4+CD3+ cells, CD8+CD3+ cells and CD19+ cells all demonstrated a characteristic response pattern to exercise associated with training status. In the UTEXP group, the cell count (circulating) for these cell types had significantly increased at the first post-intervention time-point (20 minutes post-intervention) then significantly decreased back to values not different from baseline by the final time-point. In contrast, a completely different response profile was observed for the WL_{EXP} group. In the WL_{EXP} group, the same cell types showed a delayed increase. No significant increase was seen at the first post-intervention time-point, however cell counts were significantly elevated above baseline at the final time-point.

To reiterate, untrained individuals showed an early increase then a decrease in lymphocyte count, whereas weightlifting trained individuals showed no early increase followed by a delayed increase. Of note, the magnitude in lymphocyte responses were smaller than previously reported data related to high-dose exercise protocols (Freidenreich & Volek, 2012; Walsh et al., 2011), suggesting that a dose-response relationship does exist for exercise-associated lymphocytosis. However, the lymphocyte responses observed in the present study provide strong evidence that exercise intensity and duration alone do not dictate the response to exercise, as both experimental groups undertook a common exercise protocol yet responded uniquely. Another major finding of the present study is the lack of correlation between blood lactate and lymphocyte subpopulation count as previously reported in females (Miles et al., 2003). This disagreement between previous observations and those of the present study are likely explainable though differences in study design. The earlier study (Miles et al., 2003) found that high lactate responders (≥11.92 mmol/L) showed significantly greater lymphocyte count elevations than lower lactate responders (≤7.62 mmol/L). In contrast, the present study's low dose exercise protocol induced lower levels of lactate production (≤2.4mmol/L) despite significant lymphocyte count elevation. Additionally, the present study employed all-male subjects whereas Miles and associates (2003) used only females. Also, the results previously reported (Miles et al., 2003) were based on performance of a high-dose multiple-joint (squat) exercise protocol. In consideration of potential inter-individual biomechanical differences (Frank et al., 2013; Solomonow & Krogsgaard, 2001), standardisation of exercise performance and thus reliability of study results cannot be guaranteed in this latter study. Conversely, the present study utilised a highly controllable exercise intervention with strict standardisation of body positioning, skeletal joint and muscle involvement (Mathiowetz et al., 1985; Punsola-Izard et al., 2012; Towles, Hentz, & Murray, 2008). Finally, the present study included both well-trained and untrained subjects whereas the previous study recruited previously-untrained subjects only. If lymphocyte redistribution was related to mild elevations in blood lactate concentration, strong correlations should have been calculated for both experimental groups for each of the four lymphocyte subpopulations (which was not the case). Importantly, blood lactate did not differ significantly between weightlifting trained and untrained individuals in the present study. That is, peak concentrations and temporal profiles were not significantly different between experimental groups, however their lymphocyte responses to resistance-exercise where markedly different. A unique lymphocyte response relative to training status was hypothesised, however this was based upon anticipated differences in anaerobic response between groups, which was not seen. This is novel evidence that mild elevations of blood lactate cannot alone explain the selective redistribution of lymphocytes into the circulation (in males). As the present study used a common exercise protocol which exerted all subjects to a similar level of anaerobic glycolytic activity, and considering that blood lactate was cleared at a similar rate, the only significant difference between the groups was the training status variable. From another perspective, the relationship between high blood lactate levels and lymphocyte counts in females (Miles et al., 2003) contrasted with the present study's findings give rise to the notion that lymphocytes may react to lactate above a certain threshold only. Future studies should investigate this suggestion through a stringently controlled exercise protocol which employs multiple anaerobic-doses.

Since blood lactate is associated with exercise-induced catecholamine changes (Pullinen, Nicol, MacDonald, & Komi, 1999) and lymphocytes unlike other leukocytes are uniquely sensitivity to catecholamines (Benschop, Schedlowski, Wienecke, Jacobs, & Schmidt, 1997; Landmann, 1992), it may be that catecholamines and not blood lactate are responsible for the characteristic lymphocyte profiles observed in the present study. This is plausible since resistance-training is known to increase the magnitude of catecholamine release during exercise (Kraemer et al., 1999). Future researchers are encouraged to investigate if catecholamines are mechanistically responsible for the relationship between lymphocyte counts and training status post low-dose resistance-exercise. Additionally, lymphocyte functionality should now be examined post low-dose exercise to determine if the associated lymphocytosis carries clinically relevant implications.

5. Conclusion

The results of our study provide original evidence that significant changes to B and T lymphocyte homeostasis can occur in the absence of high intensity, high volume exercise. Moreover, resistance-exercise induced lymphocytosis cannot be explained by blood lactate when elevations are only mild. This finding does not rule out a potential relationship between blood lactate and lymphocyte trafficking, however suggests another mechanism may be involved at low exercise doses. Until the functional implications of these exercise-induced lymphocyte responses are determined, exercise-professionals are advised to recognise that any dose of resistance-exercise may affect lymphocyte trafficking. Whilst the influence of exercise intensity and duration on leukocyte responses to resistance-exercise have been extensively reported in the literature, our findings demonstrate that B and T lymphocytes specifically, respond to a low-dose of resistance-exercise in a characteristic manner relative to the physical aptitude of the host.

References

Azeem, K., & Kumar, R. (2011). Effects of weight training on power performance. *Journal of Physical Education and Sport, 11*(2), 124-126.

Benschop, R. J., Schedlowski, M., Wienecke, H., Jacobs, R., & Schmidt, R. E. (1997). Adrenergic control of natural killer cell circulation and adhesion. *Brain, Behavior and Immunity, 11,* 321-332. http://dx.doi.org/10.1006/brbi.1997.0499

Bush, J. A., Kraemer, W. J., Mastro, A. M., Triplett-McBride, N. T., Volek, J. S., Putukian, M., Sebastianelli, W. J., & Knuttgen, H. G. (1999). Exercise and recovery responses of adrenal medullary neurohormones to heavy resistance-exercise. *Medicine and Science in Sports and Exercise, 31*, 554-559. http://dx.doi.org/10.1097/00005768-199904000-00010

Carlson, L. A., Headley, S., DeBruin, J., Tuckow, A. T., Koch, A. J., & Kenefick, R. W. (2008). Carbohydrate supplementation and immune responses after acute exhaustive resistance-exercise. *International Journal of Sport Nutrition and Exercise Metabolism, 18*(3), 247-259.

Conroy, D. E., Willow, J. P., & Metzler, J. N. (2002). Multidimensional fear of failure measurement: The Performance Failure Appraisal Inventory. *Journal of Applied Sport Psychology, 14*(2), 76-90. http://dx.doi.org/10.1080/10413200252907752

Dohi, K., Mastro, A. M., Miles, M. P., Bush, J. A., Grove, D. S., Leach, S. K., Volek, J. S., Nindl, B. C., Marx, J. O., Gotshalk, L.A., Putukian, M., Sebastianelli, W. J., Kraemer, W. J. (2001). Lymphocyte proliferation in response to acute heavy resistance exercise in women: influence of muscle strength and total work. *European Journal of Applied Physiology, 85*(3-4), 367-373. http://dx.doi.org/10.1007/s004210100388

Douris, P., Southard, V., Ferrigi, R., Grauer, J., Katz, D., Nascimento, C., Podbielski, P. (2006). Effect of phototherapy on delayed onset muscle soreness. *Photomedicine and Laser Surgery, 24*(3), 377-382. http://dx.doi.org/10.1089/pho.2006.24.377

Dunn, J. G. H., Gotwals, J. K., & Causgrove Dunn, J. (2005). An examination of the domain specificity of perfectionism among intercollegiate student-athletes. *Personality and Individual Differences, 38*(6), 1439-1448. http://dx.doi.org/10.1016/j.paid.2004.09.009

Fernandez, J., Mendez-Villanueva, A., Pluim, B. M. (2006). Intensity of tennis match play. *British Journal of Sports Medicine, 40*(5), 387-391. http://dx.doi.org/10.1136/bjsm.2005.023168

Fess, E. E., & Moran, C. (1981). *Clinical assessment recommendations.* American Society of Hand Therapists. Indianapolis.

Frank, C., Kobesova, A., & Kolar, P. (2013). Dynamic neuromuscular stabilization & sports rehabilitation. *International Journal of Sports Physical Therapy, 8*(1), 62–73.

Freidenreich, D. J., & Volek, J. S. (2012). Immune responses to resistance-exercise. *Exercise Immunology Review, 18,* 8-41.

Gleeson, M. J. (2007). Immune function in sport and exercise. *Journal of Applied Physiology, 103*(2), 693-699. http://dx.doi.org/10.1152/japplphysiol.00008.2007

Goodwin, M. L., Harris, J. E., Hernández, A., & Gladden, B. L. (2007). Blood lactate measurements and analysis during exercise: A guide for clinicians. *J of Diabetes, Science and Technology, 1*(4), 558–569. http://dx.doi.org/10.1177/193229680700100414

Gould, D., Dieffenbach, K., & Moffett, A, (2002). Psychological characteristics and their development in Olympic champions. *Journal of Applied Sport Psychology, 14*(3), 172-204. http://dx.doi.org/10.1080/10413200290103482

Hawker, G. A., Mian, S., Kendzerska, T., & French, M. (2011). Measures of Adult Pain, Visual Analog Scale for Pain (VAS Pain), Numeric Rating Scale for Pain (NRS Pain), McGill Pain Questionnaire (MPQ), Short-Form McGill Pain

Questionnaire (SF-MPQ), Chronic Pain Grade Scale (CPGS), Short Form-36 Bodily Pain Scale (SF-36 BPS), and Measure of Intermittent and Constant Osteoarthritis Pain (ICOAP). *Arthritis Care and Research, 63*(11), S240–S252. http://dx.doi.org/10.1002/acr.20543

Jensen, M. P., Karoly, P., & Braver, S. (1986). The measurement of clinical pain intensity: a comparison of six methods. *Pain, 27*(1), 117–126. http://dx.doi.org/10.1016/0304-3959(86)90228-9

Kraemer, W. J., Fleck, S. J., Maresh, C. M., Ratamess, N. A., Gordon, S. E., Goetz, K. L., Harman, E. A., Frykman, P. N., Volek, J. S., Mazzetti, S. A., Fry, A. C., Marchitelli, L. J., & Patton, J. F. (1999). Acute hormonal responses to a single bout of heavy resistance-exercise in trained power lifters and untrained men. *Canadian Journal of Applied Physiology, 24,* 524-537.

Landmann, R. (1992). Beta-adrenergic receptors in human leukocyte subpopulations. *European Journal of Clinical Investigation, 22*(Suppl 1), 30-36.

LeBien, T. W., & Tedder, T. F. (2008). B lymphocytes: how they develop and function. *Blood, 112*(5), 1570–1580. http://dx.doi.org/10.1182/blood-2008-02-078071

Luckheeram, R. V., Zhou, R., Verma, A. D., & Xia, B. (2012). *CD4⁺T cells: differentiation and functions*. Clinical and Developmental Immunology, 2012, 925135. http://dx.doi.org/10.1155/2012/925135

Loggia, M. L., Schweinhardt, P., Villemure, C., Bushnell, M. C. (2008). Effects of psychological state on pain perception in the dental environment. *Journal (Canadian Dental Association), 74*(7), 651-656.

Mathiowetz, V., Kashman, N., Volland, G., Weber, K., Dowe, M., & Rogers, S. (1985). Grip and pinch-strength: normative data for adults. *Archives of Physical Medicine and Rehabilitation, 66*(2), 69-74.

Mathiowetz, V., Vizenor, L., & Melander, D. (2000). Comparison of Baseline Instruments to the Jamar Dynamometer and the B&L Engineering Pinch Gauge. *Occupational Therapy Journal of Research, 20*(3),147-162. http://dx.doi.org/10.1177/153944920002000301

Mathiowetz. V., Weber, K., Volland, G., & Kashman, N. (1984). Reliability and validity of grip and pinch-strength evaluations. *The Journal of Hand Surgery, 9*(2), 222-226.

Mayhew, D. L., Thyfault, J. P., & Koch, A. J. (2005). Rest-interval length affects leukocyte levels during heavy resistance-exercise. *Journal of Strength and Conditioning Research, 19,* 16-22. http://dx.doi.org/10.1519/00124278-200502000-00004

Miles, M. P., Kraemer, W. J., Nindl, B. C., Grove, D. S., Leach, S. K., Dohi, K., Marx, J. O., Volek, J. S., & Mastro, A. M. (2003). Strength, workload, anaerobic intensity and the immune response to resistance exercise in women. *Acta Physiologica Scandinavica, 178*(2), 155-163. http://dx.doi.org/10.1046/j.1365-201x.2003.01124.x

Mosser, D. M., & Edwards, J. P. (2008). Exploring the full spectrum of macrophage activation. *Nature Reviews Immunology, 8,* 958-969. http://dx.doi.org/10.1038/nri2788

Pollock, M. L., Franklin, B. A., Balady, G. J., Chaitman, B. L., Fleg, J. L., Fletcher, B., Limacher, M., Piña, I. L., Stein, R. A., Williams, M., & Bazzarre, T. (2000). Resistance-exercise in individuals with and without cardiovascular disease: benefits, rationale, safety, and prescription. An advisory from the committee on exercise, rehabilitation, and prevention, council on clinical cardiology, American Heart Association. *Circulation, 101,* 828-833. http://dx.doi.org/10.1161/01.cir.101.7.828

Pullinen, T., Nicol, C., MacDonald, E., & Komi, P. V. (1999). Plasma catecholamine responses to four resistance exercise tests in men and women. *European Journal of Applied Physiology and Occupational Physiology, 80,* 125-131. http://dx.doi.org/10.1007/s004210050568

Punsola-Izard, V., Salas-Gómez, D., Sirvent-Rivalda, E., & Esquirol-Caussà, J. (2012). Functional patterns of thumb key pinch and their influence on thumb strength and stability. *Hand Therapy, 17*(4), 78-86. http://dx.doi.org/10.1258/ht.2012.012016

Pyne, D. B., Boston, T., Martin, D.T., & Logan, A. (2000). Evaluation of the Lactate Pro blood lactate analyser. *European Journal of Applied Physiology, 82*(1-2), 112-116. http://dx.doi.org/10.1007/s004210050659

Ranisavljev, I., & Vladimir, I. (2010). Modalities of training parameter alternation in nowadays strength training practice. *Journal of Physical Education and Sport, 29*(4), 41-46.

Rhudy, J. L., & Meagher, M. W. (2000). Fear and anxiety: divergent effects on human pain thresholds. *Pain, 84*(1), 65-75. http://dx.doi.org/10.1016/s0304-3959(99)00183-9

Schulz, K. F., Chalmers, I., Hayes, R. J., & Altman, D. G. (1995). Empirical evidence of bias: Dimensions of methodological quality associated with estimates of treatment effects in controlled trials. *Journal of the American Medical Association, 273*(5), 408-412. http://dx.doi.org/10.1001/jama.273.5.408

Sellwood, K. L., Brukner, P., Williams, D., Nicol, A., & Hinman, R. (2007). Ice-water immersion and delayed-onset muscle soreness: a randomised controlled trial. *British Journal of Sports Medicine, 41*(6), 392–397. http://dx.doi.org/10.1136/bjsm.2006.033985

Solomonow, M., & Krogsgaard, M. (2001). Sensorimotor control of knee stability. A review. *Scandinavian Journal of Medicine and Science in Sports, 11*(2), 64-80. http://dx.doi.org/10.1034/j.1600-0838.2001.011002064.x

Sonnet, C., Lafuste, P., Arnold, L., Brigitte, M., Poron, F., Authier, F. J., Chretien, F., Gherardi, R. K., & Chazaud, B. (2006). Human macrophages rescue myoblasts and myotubes from apoptosis through a set of adhesion molecular systems. *Journal of Cell Science, 119,* 2497-2507. http://dx.doi.org/10.1242/jcs.02988

Spurway, N. C. (1992) Aerobic exercise, anaerobic exercise and the lactate threshold. *British Medical Bulletin, 48*(3), 569-91.

Stoeber, J. (2011). The dual nature of perfectionism in sports: Relationships with emotion, motivation, and performance. *International Review of Sport and Exercise Psychology, 4*(2), 128-145s. http://dx.doi.org/10.1080/1750984x.2011.604789

Szlezak, A. M., Tajouri, L., Keane, J., Szlezak, S. L., Minahan, C. (2015). Micro-dose of resistance-exercise: effects of sub-maximal thumb exertion on leukocyte redistribution and fatigue in trained male weightlifters. *Journal of Physical Education and Sport, 15*(3), 365-377. http://dx.doi.org/10.7752/jpes.2015.03055

Towles, J. D., Hentz, V. R., & Murray, W. M. (2008). Use of intrinsic thumb muscles may help to improve lateral pinch function restored by tendon transfer. *Clinical Biomechanics, 23*(4), 387–394. http://dx.doi.org/10.1016/j.clinbiomech.2007.11.008

Vucetic, V., Mozek, M., & Rakovac, M. (2015). Peak blood lactate parameters in athletes of different running events during low-intensity recovery after ramp-type protocol. *Journal of Strength and Conditioning Research, 29*(4):1057-1063. http://dx.doi.org/10.1519/jsc.0000000000000725

Walsh, N. P., Gleeson, M., Shephard, R. J., Gleeson, M., Woods, J. A., Bishop, N. C., Fleshner, M., Green, C., Pedersen, B. K., Hoffman-Goetz, L., Rogers, C. J., Northoff, H., Abbasi, A., & Simon, P. (2011). Position statement. Part one: Immune function and exercise. *Exercise Immunology Reviews, 17*, 6-63.

Wirtz, N., Wahl, P., Kleinöder, H., Mester, J. (2014). Lactate Kinetics during Multiple Set Resistance Exercise. *Journal of Sports Science and Medicine, 13*(1), 73–77.

16

Wnt and β-Catenin Signaling and Skeletal Muscle Myogenesis in Response to Muscle Damage and Resistance Exercise and Training

Dan Newmire
Exercise Physiology and Biochemistry Laboratory
Department of Kinesiology
Texas Woman's University, Denton, Texas, USA
304 Administration Drive, Denton, TX 76204
E-mail: dnewmire@twu.edu

Darryn S. Willoughby (Corresponding author)
Exercise and Biochemical Nutrition Laboratory
Department of Health, Human Performance, and Recreation
Baylor University, Waco, Texas, USA
1312 South 5th Street, Waco, TX, USA
E-mail: darryn_willoughby@baylor.edu

Abstract

The factors that regulate skeletal muscle hypertrophy in human adults in response to resistance training (RT) has largely focused on endogenous endocrine responses. However, the endocrine response to RT as having an obligatory role in muscle hypertrophy has come under scrutiny, as other mechanisms and pathways seem to also be involved in up-regulating muscle protein synthesis (MPS). Skeletal muscle myogenesis is a multifactorial process of tissue growth and repair in response to resistance training is regulated by many factors. As a result, satellite cell-fused myogenesis is a possible factor in skeletal muscle regeneration and hypertrophy in response to RT. The Wnt family ligands interact with various receptors and activate different downstream signaling pathways and have been classified as either canonical (β-catenin dependent) or non-canonical (β-catenin independent). Wnt is secreted from numerous tissues in a paracrine fashion. The Wnt/β-catenin signaling pathway is a highly-regulated and intricate pathway that is essential to skeletal muscle myogenesis. The canonical Wnt/β-catenin pathway may influence satellite cells to myogenic commitment, differentiation, and fusion into muscle fibers in response to injury or trauma, self-renewal, and normal basal turnover. The current literature has shown that, in response mechanical overload from acute resistance exercise and chronic resistance training, that the Wnt/β-catenin signaling pathway is stimulated which may actuate the process of muscle repair and hypertrophy in response to exercise-induced muscle damage. The purpose of this review is to elaborate on the Wnt/β-catenin signaling pathway, the current literature investigating the relationship of the Wnt/β-catenin pathway and its effects on myogenesis is response to muscle damage and resistance exercise and training.

Keywords: skeletal muscle, hypertrophy, myogenesis, cell signaling, protein synthesis, resistance training

1. Introduction

Skeletal muscle accounts for 30-40% and 40–50 % of an adult female's and male's body mass, respectively (Fu, Wang, & Hu, 2015). Adult, fully-differentiated muscle is considered stable under normal conditions. Perturbations such as age influences a muscle mass loss of ~1.9 and 1.1 kg/decade, respectively, in men and women (Janssen, Heymsfield, Wang, & Ross, 2000), and diseases such as cancer cachexia, COPD, and sarcopenia (Agustí et al., 2002; Thomas, 2007) contribute to muscle wasting. In contrast, exercise such as resistance training is known to influence skeletal muscle mass gain (Tesch, 1988). The factors that regulate skeletal muscle hypertrophy in human adults in response to resistance training (RT) has largely focused on endogenous endocrine responses such as testosterone, growth hormone (GH), and insulin growth factor-1 (IGF-1) (Hasani-Ranjbar, Soleymani Far, Heshmat, Rajabi, & Kosari, 2012; R. R. Kraemer & Castracane, 2015; W. J. Kraemer, Duncan, & Volek, 1998; W. J. Kraemer et al., 1999; Madarame, Sasaki, & Ishii, 2010; Uchida et al., 2009). However, the endocrine response to RT has recently been met with scrutiny as having an obligatory role in muscle hypertrophy due to an observed transient flux and minimized impact on strength and muscle protein synthesis (MPS) outcomes (West, Burd, Staples, & Phillips, 2010; West & Phillips, 2010). Similarly, another area largely researched is the anabolic intramuscular signaling of mTORC1, as its constituent up- and down-stream signaling intermediates [e.g., protein kinase A (Akt) and ribosomal protein S6 kinase (p70S6K)] are purported to stimulate MPS and protein accretion in response to RT. (Adegoke, Abdullahi, & Tavajohi-Fini, 2012; Drummond, Dreyer, Fry, Glynn, & Rasmussen, 2009; Hornberger, Sukhija, & Chien, 2006; Walker et al., 2011). Furthermore, the associated relationship of cell signaling and MPS has also been met with opposition due to a recent study demonstrating no correlations between the phosphorylation of the signaling proteins measured [Akt, mTORC1, eukaryotic initiation factor 4E binding protein-1 (4E-BP1), and p60S6K] and changes in muscle volume or lean body mass (LBM). Moreover, measurements of MPS 6 hr following a single bout of resistance exercise were not predictive of muscle hypertrophy following 16 wk of resistance training (Mitchell et al., 2014).

A differing trend of research has focused on observing satellite cell-fused myogenesis as a possible factor in skeletal muscle regeneration and hypertrophy in response to RT. Satellite cells (SC) are mitotically quiescent and reside in a '*stem cell niche*' between the basal lamina and the sarcolemma of their associated muscle fibers. SC's become activated into myogenic progenitor cells (MPC's), then proliferate and differentiate into nascent myoblasts, which then fuse to multinucleated myotubes and fuse into existing damaged muscle fibers, thereby donating their myonuclei to promote skeletal muscle repair for self-renewal and/or hypertrophy (Bellamy et al., 2014; Charge & Rudnicki, 2004; Yin, Price, & Rudnicki, 2013). It has been suggested that myogenesis is stimulated by Paired box gene 3 and 7 expression (Pax3/7) (Le Grand & Rudnicki, 2007; Relaix, Rocancourt, Mansouri, & Buckingham, 2005) and the basic helix-loop-helix family of transcription factors known as the myogenic regulatory factors (MRF's), MyoD, Myf5, myogenin, and MRF4. Both Pax3/7 and MRF's are required for the progression of skeletal myoblasts through the process of myogenesis (Karalaki, Fili, Philippou, & Koutsilieris, 2009; Le Grand & Rudnicki, 2007). Once the SC's are activated, they leave their *'niche'* and move outside of the basal lamina with the primary function to initiate the cycling and co-expression of Pax7 and MyoD (Le Grand & Rudnicki, 2007). The intricate process and interactions of both Pax3/7 and MRFs in myogenesis is beyond this article and can be read in depth in other reviews (Bryson-Richardson & Currie, 2008; Charge & Rudnicki, 2004; Karalaki et al., 2009; Le Grand & Rudnicki, 2007; Yin et al., 2013).

Otto, et al (2006) investigated the identity of molecules that may control the development of the satellite cells during embryogenesis and observed that members of the Wnt family of signaling proteins were robust effectors of Pax7 expression. They concluded that the canonical Wnt signaling pathway and its intracellular response of β-catenin directly activated satellite cell proliferation by way of translocation to the nucleus resulting in an increase in the expression of Pax7 (Otto et al., 2008; Otto, Schmidt, & Patel, 2006). The Wnt family proteins are seemingly indispensable regulators of MPC commitment into myoblasts and self-renewal during postnatal myogenesis (Bentzinger, Wang, & Rudnicki, 2012).

In constructing this mini-review, the online scientific database, PubMed, (www.ncbi.nlm.nih.gov/pubmed) was utilized and studies performed within the past 10 years were primarily utilized. The following sections of this review are to elaborate on the Wnt/β-catenin signaling pathway, the current literature investigating the relationship of the Wnt/β-catenin pathway, and its effects on myogenesis in response to muscle damage and resistance exercise and training. Re

2. Wnt and β-Catenin Signaling and Skeletal Muscle Myogenesis

2.1 Wnt/β-catenin Dependent Signaling Pathway

The wingless-type, mouse mammary tumor virus (MMTV) integration site family (Wnt) signaling ligands are a large family of glycoproteins. These proteins are evolutionarily-conserved secreted cysteine-rich proteins related to the genes *Drosophila wingless* (*wg*) and mouse *Int1* (subsequently named *Wnt1)*, and in mammals, most notably humans, there are 19 conserved genes related to the Wnt family. The name '*Wnt*' is derived from a combination *wingless* and *Int1* genes due to their homology amongst them. The *Int1* gene was originally identified as an oncogene that became activated by the MMTV and influenced the formation of mammary carcinomas. The Wnt family ligands interact with various receptors and activate different downstream pathways. As shown in Figure 1, these pathways have been classified as either canonical (β-catenin dependent) or non-canonical (β-catenin independent) signaling pathways. The β-catenin dependent pathway is activated by a secreted extracellular Wnt ligand that binds to one of seven known transmembrane Frizzled receptors (Fzd), and its co-receptors are known as low-density lipoprotein receptor-related proteins 5 and 6 (LRP5/6)(Baarsma, Konigshoff, & Gosens, 2013; Brack et al., 2009; Niehrs & Acebron, 2010; Julia von Maltzahn, Chang, Bentzinger, & Rudnicki, 2012). Once the Fzd receptor has been activated, it then switches on an intracellular signaling cascade by activating the disheveled proteins (Dvl) and heterotrimeric G-proteins (α, β and γ subunits), which are required for downstream signaling. In conjunction with the phosphorylation of LRP5/6 proteins, this cascade results in the inactivation of the '*degredation complex*' of proteinsm which consists of adenomatosis polyposis coli (APC), axin, serine-threonine kinase of glycogen synthase kinase-3β (GSK-3β), and casein kinase-1 (CK-1) (Li et al., 2012; Tanneberger et al., 2011; Yokoyama, Markova, Wang, & Malbon, 2012). Inactivation of this complex liberates unphosphorylated β-catenin to accumulate in the cytosol and sequentially translocate into the nucleus for gene transcription. When Wnt ligand signaling is unavailable, the degradation complex remains activated and the key effector of canonical Wnt signaling of β-catenin is targeted and phosphorylated by GSK-3β and CK-1α for proteaosomal degradation by β-transducin repeat containing E3 ubiquitin protein ligase (β–TrCP E3 ligase) and subsequent proteolysis by the ubiquitin–proteasome pathway (Angers & Moon, 2009; Baarsma et al., 2013; C. Gao, Xiao, & Hu, 2014; Logan & Nusse, 2004). However, when β-catenin has translocated and associates in the nucleus, it functions as a transcriptional co-activator with the T-cell factor/lymphoid enhancer factor-1 (TCF/LEF) family of transcription factors and induces canonical gene transcription to induce Wnt/β-catenin target gene expression that modulates numerous biological processes such as myogenesis (Abu-Elmagd et al., 2010; Han, Jin, Seto, & Yoon, 2011).

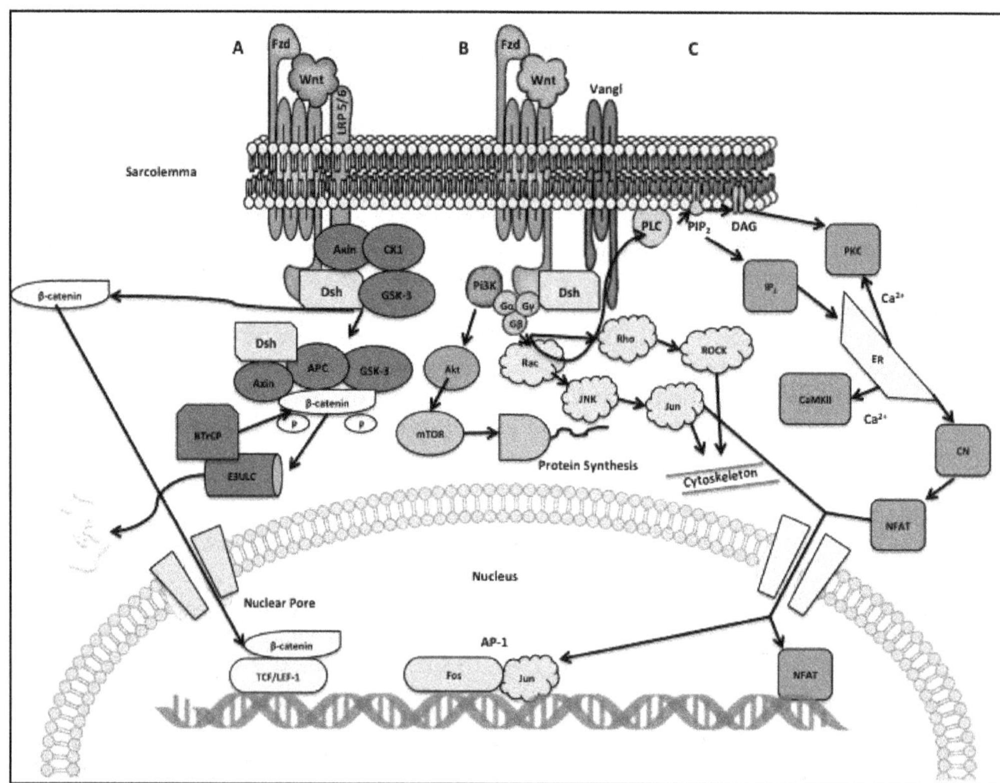

Figure 1. Canonical and Non-Canonical Wnt/β-Catenin Signaling Pathways

Canonical

The Wnt/β-catenin signaling pathway consists of adenomatous polyposis coli (APC) and axin which are scaffold proteins that form the β-catenin degradation complex. Phosphorylation of β-catenin occurs by the degradation complex kinases, glycogen synthase kinase 3 (GSK-3) and casein kinase 1α (CK-1α), which form the signal for proteolysis of β-catenin by a β-transducin repeat containing E3 ubiquitin protein ligase (β–TrCP E3 ligase) and then subsequent proteolysis by the ubiquitin–proteasome pathway. Wnt binding activation of the Frizzled (Fzd) and co-receptor low-density lipoprotein receptor-related protein 5 (LRP5), G-proteins (α, β and γ subunits), and dishevelled (Dvl) proteins are activated and lead to the recruitment of axin to the LRP5 or LRP6. This inhibits the degradation complex, influences the accumulation of β-catenin translocation to the nucleus and association with transcription factors, lymphoid enhancer factor (LEF) and T-cell factor (TCF), where it acts as a co-activator to actuate transcription.

Non-Canonical

A) Planar cell polarity (PCP) signaling is independent of β-catenin and LDL-receptor-related protein (LRP5/6), does not require T-cell factor (TCF) molecules, and leads to the activation of the small RAS homologue gene-family member of GTPases, Rho and Rac. This activates the stress kinase jun N-terminal kinase (JNK) and RHO-associated coiled-coil-containing protein kinase 1 (ROCK) and leads to cytoskeleton remodeling and changes in cell adhesion and motility. **B**) Wnt-Calcium (Ca^{2+}) signaling is modulated by G proteins and phospholipases which leads to increases in cytoplasmic free Ca^{2+} and the activation of protein kinase C (PKC), calcium calmodulin mediated kinase II (CAMKII), and calcineurin. **C**) The activation of phospholipase (PLC) by dishevelled (Dvl) leads to the cleavage of phosphatidylinositol-4,5-bisphosphate (PIP_2) into inositol trisphosphate (IP3) and diacylglycerol (DAG) and, concurrent with calcium, activates PKC. IP3 binds to membrane receptors and leads to an accumulation of cytoplasmic free Ca^{2+}. This influences an increased gene transcription of activator protein 1 (AP1) and nuclear factor of activated T cells (NFAT). Figure 1 modified from Angers & Moon, (2009).

2.2 Wnt Non-Canonical Signaling Pathways

In contrast to canonical Wnt/β-catenin gene transcription there is also a non-canonical signaling pathway that is independent of β-catenin gene transcription. The signaling event is through Fzd receptors either in conjunction with or independent of LRP co-receptors. The downstream effectors of Wnt signaling have been purported to activate of c-Jun-N-terminal kinase (JNK)-dependent or calcium- dependent signaling pathways. Similarly, this non-canonical pathway has also been suggested to activate of PCP (planar-cell-polarity), Ras-related protein 1 (rap1), atypical protein kinase C (aPKC), mechanistic target of rapamycin (mTOR), protein kinase A (PKA), and phosphatidylinositide 3-kinase (PI3K) (Baarsma et al., 2013; Gomez-Orte, Saenz-Narciso, Moreno, & Cabello, 2013; Logan & Nusse, 2004; Semenov, Habas, Macdonald, & He, 2007; Yokoyama et al., 2012). The Wnt/PCP signaling influences the regulation of tissue morphogenesis and cell division by way of regulating cellular functions, including cell polarity, cell migration, and orientation during development. This pathway modulates and coordinates, in a sequential fashion, the cellular behaviors in a variety of cells (De Calisto, Araya, Marchant, Riaz, & Mayor, 2005; B. Gao, 2012; Nishita, Endo, & Minami, 2013; Segalen & Bellaiche, 2009). Additionally it has been shown, that in differentiated myofibers, Wnt- regulated signaling of Wnt7a binding to the Fzd7 receptor directly activated the Akt/mTOR pathway. The (mechanistic target of rapamycin) mTOR pathway, more specifically mTOR complex 1 (mTORC1), is suggested to be the master regulator of cell growth and proliferation by directly influencing protein synthesis (Laplante & Sabatini, 2009). Interestingly, the activation of Akt/mTOR occurred independent of IGF-1 receptor activation, which suggests that the non-canonical Wnt pathway may activate muscle protein synthesis (MPS) through mTOR-mediated signaling (J. von Maltzahn, Bentzinger, & Rudnicki, 2012).

As seen in Table 1, the Wnt family members and components are characterized by the pathway they influence (canonical or non-canonical), the cell type, and the specific receptors that are expressed by the cell (Baarsma et al., 2013). The canonical and non-canonical pathways are considered as separate, thereby having differing actions. However, there are data suggesting cross-talk between pathways by way of Dickkopf (Dkk), a soluble secreted protein that binds to LRP and mediates its internalization. These multifaceted proteins may promote or inhibit certain actions of LRP receptors to influence Wnt/β-catenin signaling (van Amerongen & Nusse, 2009). This interaction suggests that the canonical and non-canonical pathways might be far more interactive than previous thought.

Table 1. The various ligands, receptors, components, and Wnt family members involved in the Wnt signaling pathway

Components and function	Family members
Wnt ligands	Wnt-1 (Wg), Wnt-2, Wnt-2B, Wnt-3, Wnt-3A, Wnt-4, Wnt-5A, Wnt-5B, Wnt-6, Wnt-7A, Wnt-7B, Wnt-8A, Wnt-8B, Wnt-9A, Wnt-9B, Wnt-10A, Wnt-10B, Wnt-11, Wnt-16
Alternative ligands	Norrin and R-spondin
Extracellular modulators	Secreted Frizzled related proteins (sFRP), Wnt-inhibitory factor (WIF-1), Dickkopfs (Dkk)
Fzd receptors	Fzd1, Fzd2, Fzd3 Fzd4, Fzd5, Fzd6, Fzd7, Fzd8, Fzd9, Fzd10
LRP receptors	Low-density lipoprotein receptor related proteins 5 and 6 (LRP5/6)
Alternative receptors	Ror2, Ryk and PTK7
Signaling intermediates	Dishevelleds: Dvl1, Dvl2, Dvl3
β-Catenin destruction complex	Axin, adenomatosis polyposis coli (APC), glycogen synthase kinase-3 (GSK-3), casein kinase-1 (CK-1), protein phosphatases (PP1 and PP2A)
Cellular trafficking and distribution	Cadherins, pygopus (Pygo) and legless (Lgs/BCL-9)
Effector	β-catenin (Armadillo)
Transcription factors	T-cell factor (TCF-1, TCF-3, TCF-4), lymphoid enhancer factor (LEF-1)
Intracellular modulators	Nemo-like kinase (NLK), Groucho/Transducin-like enhancer of split (TLE) inhibitor of β-catenin and TCF4 (ICAT), Chibby (Cby)

Modified from Baarsma (2013).

2.3 Wnt Secretion and Distribution

Wnt proteins are ~40 kDa in size and have been suggested to go through post-translational modification (PTM). These proteins are submitted through a process of glycosylation that plays a role in Wnt folding, secretion, and acylation via lipid modification by a mono-unsaturated fatty acid (palmitoleic acid), which attaches to a conserved serine. The lipid modification is suggested to positively influence Wnt secretory and signaling processes (Hausmann & Basler, 2006; Mann & Beachy, 2004; Takada et al., 2006; Willert & Nusse, 2012; Zhai, Chaturvedi, & Cumberledge, 2004). This lipid modification has shown to be regulated by an endoplasmic reticulum (ER) protein, porcupine enzyme (Porcn), which is a dedicated and highly-conserved component of the Wnt secretory pathway, and only found in Wnt secreting cells. Porcn, a multi-pass transmembrane O-acyltransferase, is essential for Wnt palmitoylation and maturation. Porcn is also required for serine-dependent acylation for Wnt3a transport from the ER for secretion. This PTM action suggests that Wnt proteins require a specific lipid modification for proper intracellular transport during the secretory process (Clevers & Nusse, 2012; Nusse & Varmus, 2012; Takada et al., 2006). The next step in the process of intracellular translocation of Wnt ligands is to be carried and released by exosome similar "*sorting vesicles*" named evenness interrupted (Evi) and Wntless (WLS), which bind to and escort Wnt. Evi/WLS bind to the Wnt protein in the ER, sequentially translocates to the plasma membrane for exocytosis, and then returns to the ER through the Golgi apparatus (Koles et al., 2012; Korkut et al., 2009). Lastly, the intracellular trafficking complex known as the retromer is required for Wnt signaling. The main function of the retromer complex involves the retrograde transport of Wnt translocating carrier proteins, Evi and WLS, back to the Golgi apparatus. It has been proposed that the retromer retrieves endosomal Evi/WLS, which is otherwise targeted and tagged for degradation in lysosomes. This helps with the re-utilization or "*recycling*" of Wnt transporters. When Evi/WLS are degraded in lysosomes, Wnt secretion becomes impaired (Eaton, 2008; Yu et al., 2014). The impairment of Wnt cell signaling has been found to be significantly detrimental to the growth and development of mammals during embryonic development. In the mouse model, the genetic knockout of numerous Wnt protein and their corresponding Fzd have resulted an early embryonic fatality and deleterious effects on multiple tissues (Julia von Maltzahn et al., 2012). Of these tissues, Wnt has an influence on myogenesis and has been proposed to be a major contributor of skeletal muscle development and regeneration (Bentzinger et al., 2012).

2.4 Wnt Signaling in Adult Skeletal Muscle Myogenesis

In contrast to embryonic myogenesis, adult myogenesis is stable under normal conditions with only periodic fusion of satellite cells to compensate for skeletal muscle turnover induced by typical '*daily wear and tear'*. Additionally, myofiber tissue regeneration is activated in response to numerous stressors such as weight bearing, exercise-induced muscle damage, stretching, and electrical stimulation (Le Grand & Rudnicki, 2007; Polesskaya, Seale, & Rudnicki, 2003). This stress induces myogenic regeneration and requires a template in the process of myogenic regeneration. The extracellular matrix scaffolding at the basal lamina or basement membrane is superior to the sarcolemma, and is pertinent in the regeneration process. SCs are mitotically quiescent (G_0 phase) and once activated become MPCs and are responsible for muscle regeneration, compensatory hypertrophy, and increasing the myonuclear number during normal adult muscle turnover and growth (Bentzinger et al., 2012; Ciciliot & Schiaffino, 2010). SCs are largely self-sufficient as a source for muscle regeneration. Collins et al. (2005) transplanted intact myofibers into radiation-ablated muscles and observed a that a very small number of SCs, when associated with one transplanted myofiber, generated over 100 hundred new myofibers which contained thousands of myonuclei. Moreover, these SC's vigorously self-renewed and re-populated the transplanted muscle (Collins et al., 2005). This dynamic environment coined "*stem cell niche*" is a process in which adult mammalian skeletal muscle tissue SC's can both replicate themselves for self-renewing re-population for future needs and/or activate to MPC's and differentiate into myoblasts. These myoblasts then fuse with each other to form multi-nucleated myotubes, which then form into adult muscle fibers and contribute to enhanced myonucleation, as well as the repair of the damaged fibers (Karalaki et al., 2009; Yin et al., 2013).

Stimulating the onset of myogenesis is a multifactorical process. However, it has been shown that Wnt signaling is indispensable in adult myogenesis. Polesskaya, et al. (2003) investigated an adult SC culture model using a hematopoietic restricted cell marker of $CD45^+$ with both injured and non-injured muscle fibers. Wnts5a and 5b genes were expressed in proliferating myogenic cells, but not in differentiated myotubes while Wnt7a was expressed in the myotube. In conjunction, all three Wnt genes expressed were observed to implement myogenic commitment of adult muscle SC regeneration of injured skeletal muscle. Similarly, β-catenin was highly expressed in this same experiment relative to the uninjured skeletal muscle tissue, which supports the influence of the canonical Wnt pathway as a factor in adult muscle myogenesis (Polesskaya et al., 2003). Additionally, it was found that Wnt4 was influenced by a member of the transforming growth factor beta (TGF-β) superfamily known as myostatin (Mstn), which may act as a specific inhibitor of skeletal muscle growth. Mstn is suggested to inhibit muscle growth by way of down regulating myogenic proliferation and differentiation. However, if Mstn is mutated or inhibited hyper-muscularity is promoted (Grobet et al., 1997; Joulia-Ekaza & Cabello, 2007; Williams, 2004). Non-canonical Wnt4 has been proposed to stimulate the proliferation of myogenic SC's while inhibiting Mstn signaling, which down-regulates cell proliferation (Steelman, Recknor, Nettleton, & Reecy, 2006). Jones et al. (2015), using a cell culture model, reported an alternative pathway of Wnt-stimulated myogenesis. They showed that when Wnt3a stimulated the canonical β-catenin pathway, myogenin became active and, therefore, activated follistatin (FS). FS is also a member of the TGF-β family and has a potent inhibitory effect on Mstn and the other TGF-β family member, activin A (ActA). Collectively, both Mstn and ActA have been purported to inhibit skeletal muscle myogenic differentiation and skeletal muscle hypertrophy (Gilson et al., 2009; Jones et al., 2015; Wang & McPherron, 2012). Additionally, it has been proposed that Wnt4 also activates the canonical Wnt/β-catenin pathway during myogenic differentiation that has been observed to inhibit the expression of Mstn and the regulating pathways of Mstn (Bernardi et al., 2011; Terada, Misao, Katase, Nishimatsu, & Nohno, 2013).

2.5 Canonical Wnt/β-catenin Signaling and Resistance Training

Skeletal muscle hypertrophy in response to resistance training is a highly- recognized and sought after goal. The process of muscle protein accretion and muscle mass gain is influenced by multiple factors. A more novel area of research is observing how RT influences Wnt signaling and its signaling components on skeletal muscle hypertrophy. Armstrong and Esser (2005) used a synergistic rodent ablation of the plantaris muscle after mechanical overload. The mass differences between day 0 (control) and day 7 demonstrated a 67 % increase in plantaris mass (assessed by muscle wet-weight), and comparatively after 14 days of overload, resulted in a 139 % increase in plantaris mass. They attributed this to β-catenin activation and its down stream components Fzd1, Dvl1, and Lef1. Furthermore, the Wnt-stimulated β-catenin/Lef1 targets, c-Myc, Cyclin D1, and Pitx2, were activated during skeletal muscle mechanical overload. Both c-Myc and Cyclin D1 were associated with cell-cycle regulation and in response to muscular hypertrophic growth; both showed increased gene expression in conjunction with muscular overload (Armstrong & Esser, 2005; Serrano, Baeza-Raja, Perdiguero, Jardi, & Munoz-Canoves, 2008). Another rodent model that used eccentrically-based downhill running (DHR) on a treadmill, found significant muscle damage in the soleous at 3, 5, and 6 days following the bout of DHR. Furthermore, soleus injury was significantly highest at day 6 compared to day 2 following DHR. Wnt3a, β-catenin, Lef1, and GSK3β gene and protein expression were measured in the gastrocnemius at the same time points. It was observed that there was no difference in Wnt3a nor β-catenin differences between control groups. However, they did observe a 4.2-fold and 5.0-fold increase in Lef1 mRNA expression and an inhibition of GSK3β at day 5 and 6, respectively. In response to the proposed outcome that other Wnt family members 5a, 5b, 7a, and 7b may have had an effect, although unmeasured, the authors felt that Wnt3a was the more viable measure based on previous literature in its relation to skeletal muscle repair (Amin et al., 2014). Similarly in another form of muscle tissue unrelated to resistance training, cardiac injury from pressure/volume overload induces a the Wnt/β-catenin pathway for cardiac myogenesis. In response to cardiac injury, Wnt/β-catenin signaling is suggested to indirectly influence cardiac remodeling, regulation of hypertrophy, and protection of cardiomyocytes from apoptosis (Ozhan & Weidinger, 2015). A novel topic that deserves much more research and elaboration is the human resistance training model which causes skeletal muscle damage and its relationship with Wnt signaling-induced myogenesis. Leal et al. (2011) reported from an eight-week training study that the intramuscular mRNA expression levels of Wnt1 increased 6.4-fold in response to strength training (ST) and 24.9-fold with power training (PT). There was a significant increase in β-catenin mRNA expression in response to training, but not between PT and ST groups. Additionally, PT had a 34.1-fold increase in transcription factor Lef1 mRNA expression compared to a 7.3- fold increase from ST. Lastly, Cyclin D1 expression only responded to PT with a 7.7-fold increase compared to control (Leal et al., 2011). Recently, Spillane et al. (2015) investigated a human resistance exercise model that compared a single bout of lower-body resistance exercises (LB) to a bout of upper- and lower body-resistance exercises (ULB), and observed the responses of serum testosterone concentrations and its effects on muscle testosterone, DHT, androgen receptor (AR) protein content, and AR–DNA binding. More importantly, they additionally determined serum Wnt4 concentrations and skeletal muscle β-catenin and the influence that Wnt/β-catenin signaling may have on AR-DNA binding. Their results showed no differences in serum free and total testosterone between resistance exercise bouts. Furthermore, intramuscular indices of testosterone and DHT showed no increases at any measured time point. Interestingly, the ULB bout exhibited the greatest increase of serum Wnt4 at 0.5, 1, and 2 h following the exercise bout compared to LB, along with a greater total intramuscular β-catenin elevation at 3 and 24 h post-exercise. Moreover, they observed an increased in total AR protein at 3 h post-exercise for the ULB bout, followed by a diminished amount at 24 hr post-exercise. In addition, AR-DNA binding was increased at both 3 and 24 h following the ULB bout (Spillane, Schwarz, & Willoughby, 2015). The authors suggest that, regardless of the response of serum free and total testosterone in LB and ULB resistance exercise bouts, the canonical Wnt4/β-catenin signaling may influence the increase in androgen ligand binding to the respective androgen receptors (AR), and the subsequent AR–DNA binding may upregulate the skeletal muscle protein synthetic response. This research corroborates with previous literature using prostate cells suggesting that the AR mediates translocation of Wnt stimulated β-catenin into the nucleus when exposed to exogenous androgen (Mulholland, Cheng, Reid, Rennie, & Nelson, 2002).

3. Conclusion

Skeletal muscle hypertrophy in response to resistance training is a multifaceted phenomenon that has yet to be fully or consistently elucidated by one singular cell signaling pathway or mechanism. It has been observed that the canonical Wnt/β-catenin signaling pathway influences skeletal muscle myogenesis, is indispensable, and highly-critical in skeletal muscle repair and hypertrophy in response to injury or damage. However, it is also apparent that skeletal muscle myogenesis is a multifactorial process that is influenced and regulated by many differing factors. The Wnt/β-catenin signaling pathway offers another area of research that may continue to reveal the dynamics of interconnected cell signaling pathway regulating skeletal muscle hypertrophy. Additionally, Wnt may offer a possible plasma biomarker in which to investigate responses to resistance training in various populations. Moreover, Wnt/β-catenin signaling may be a crucial biomarker to consider in sarcopenic populations in association with disease and or age in regards to time course and physical activity. However, further research requires further elucidation of Wnt/β-catenin signaling on adult human skeletal muscle tissue myogenesis and hypertrophy in conjunction with muscle damaging exercise such as resistance training.

Acknowledgements

The authors declare no conflicts of interest.

References

Abu-Elmagd, M., Robson, L., Sweetman, D., Hadley, J., Francis-West, P., & Munsterberg, A. (2010). Wnt/Lef1 signaling acts via Pitx2 to regulate somite myogenesis. *Developmental Biology, 337*(2), 211-219. doi:10.1016/j.ydbio.2009.10.023

Adegoke, O. A., Abdullahi, A., & Tavajohi-Fini, P. (2012). mTORC1 and the regulation of skeletal muscle anabolism and mass. *Applied Physiology, Nutrition, and Metabolism, 37*(3), 395-406. doi:10.1139/h2012-009

Agustí, A. G., Sauleda, J., Miralles, C., Gomez, C., Togores, B., Sala, E., . . . Busquets, X. (2002). Skeletal muscle apoptosis and weight loss in chronic obstructive pulmonary disease. *American Journal of Respiratory and Critical Care Medicine, 166*(4), 485-489.

Amin, H., Vachris, J., Hamilton, A., Steuerwald, N., Howden, R., & Arthur, S. T. (2014). GSK3beta inhibition and LEF1 upregulation in skeletal muscle following a bout of downhill running. *Journal of Physiological Sciences, 64*(1), 1-11. doi:10.1007/s12576-013-0284-5

Angers, S., & Moon, R. T. (2009). Proximal events in Wnt signal transduction. *Nature reviews Molecular cell biology, 10*(7), 468-477.

Armstrong, D. D., & Esser, K. A. (2005). Wnt/beta-catenin signaling activates growth-control genes during overload-induced skeletal muscle hypertrophy. *American Journal of Physiology: Cell Physiology, 289*(4), C853-859. doi:10.1152/ajpcell.00093.2005

Baarsma, H. A., Konigshoff, M., & Gosens, R. (2013). The WNT signaling pathway from ligand secretion to gene transcription: molecular mechanisms and pharmacological targets. *Pharmacology & Therapeutics, 138*(1), 66-83. doi:10.1016/j.pharmthera.2013.01.002

Bellamy, L. M., Joanisse, S., Grubb, A., Mitchell, C. J., McKay, B. R., Phillips, S. M., . . . Parise, G. (2014). The acute satellite cell response and skeletal muscle hypertrophy following resistance training. *PloS One, 9*(10), e109739. doi:10.1371/journal.pone.0109739

Bentzinger, C. F., Wang, Y. X., & Rudnicki, M. A. (2012). Building Muscle: Molecular Regulation of Myogenesis. *Cold Spring Harbor Perspectives in Biology, 4*(2).

Bernardi, H., Gay, S., Fedon, Y., Vernus, B., Bonnieu, A., & Bacou, F. (2011). Wnt4 activates the canonical beta-catenin pathway and regulates negatively myostatin: functional implication in myogenesis. *American Journal of Physiology: Cell Physiology, 300*(5), C1122-1138. doi:10.1152/ajpcell.00214.2010

Brack, A. S., Murphy-Seiler, F., Hanifi, J., Deka, J., Eyckerman, S., Keller, C., . . . Rando, T. A. (2009). BCL9 is an essential component of canonical Wnt signaling that mediates the differentiation of myogenic progenitors during muscle regeneration. *Developmental Biology, 335*(1), 93-105. doi:10.1016/j.ydbio.2009.08.014

Bryson-Richardson, R. J., & Currie, P. D. (2008). The genetics of vertebrate myogenesis. *Nature Reviews: Genetics, 9*(8), 632-646. doi:10.1038/nrg2369

Charge, S. B., & Rudnicki, M. A. (2004). Cellular and molecular regulation of muscle regeneration. *Physiological Reviews, 84*(1), 209-238. doi:10.1152/physrev.00019.2003

Ciciliot, S., & Schiaffino, S. (2010). Regeneration of mammalian skeletal muscle. Basic mechanisms and clinical implications. *Current Pharmaceutical Design, 16*(8), 906-914. Retrieved from http://www.ncbi.nlm.nih.gov/pubmed/20041823

Clevers, H., & Nusse, R. (2012). Wnt/beta-catenin signaling and disease. *Cell, 149*(6), 1192-1205. doi:10.1016/j.cell.2012.05.012

Collins, C. A., Olsen, I., Zammit, P. S., Heslop, L., Petrie, A., Partridge, T. A., & Morgan, J. E. (2005). Stem cell function, self-renewal, and behavioral heterogeneity of cells from the adult muscle satellite cell niche. *Cell, 122*(2), 289-301. doi:10.1016/j.cell.2005.05.010

De Calisto, J., Araya, C., Marchant, L., Riaz, C. F., & Mayor, R. (2005). Essential role of non-canonical Wnt signalling in neural crest migration. *Development, 132*(11), 2587-2597. doi:10.1242/dev.01857

Drummond, M. J., Dreyer, H. C., Fry, C. S., Glynn, E. L., & Rasmussen, B. B. (2009). Nutritional and contractile regulation of human skeletal muscle protein synthesis and mTORC1 signaling. *J Appl Physiol (1985), 106*(4), 1374-1384. doi:10.1152/japplphysiol.91397.2008

Eaton, S. (2008). Retromer retrieves wntless. *Developmental Cell, 14*(1), 4-6. doi:10.1016/j.devcel.2007.12.014

Fu, X., Wang, H., & Hu, P. (2015). Stem cell activation in skeletal muscle regeneration. *Cellular and Molecular Life Sciences, 72*(9), 1663-1677.

Gao, B. (2012). Wnt regulation of planar cell polarity (PCP). *Current Topics in Developmental Biology, 101*, 263-295. doi:10.1016/B978-0-12-394592-1.00008-9

Gao, C., Xiao, G., & Hu, J. (2014). Regulation of Wnt/β-catenin signaling by posttranslational modifications. *Cell Biosci, 4*(1), 13.

Gilson, H., Schakman, O., Kalista, S., Lause, P., Tsuchida, K., & Thissen, J. P. (2009). Follistatin induces muscle hypertrophy through satellite cell proliferation and inhibition of both myostatin and activin. *American Journal of Physiology: Endocrinology and Metabolism, 297*(1), E157-164. doi:10.1152/ajpendo.00193.2009

Gomez-Orte, E., Saenz-Narciso, B., Moreno, S., & Cabello, J. (2013). Multiple functions of the noncanonical Wnt pathway. *Trends in Genetics, 29*(9), 545-553. doi:10.1016/j.tig.2013.06.003

Grobet, L., Martin, L. J., Poncelet, D., Pirottin, D., Brouwers, B., Riquet, J., . . . Georges, M. (1997). A deletion in the bovine myostatin gene causes the double-muscled phenotype in cattle. *Nature Genetics, 17*(1), 71-74. doi:10.1038/ng0997-71

Han, X. H., Jin, Y. R., Seto, M., & Yoon, J. K. (2011). A WNT/beta-catenin signaling activator, R-spondin, plays positive regulatory roles during skeletal myogenesis. *Journal of Biological Chemistry, 286*(12), 10649-10659. doi:10.1074/jbc.M110.169391

Hasani-Ranjbar, S., Soleymani Far, E., Heshmat, R., Rajabi, H., & Kosari, H. (2012). Time course responses of serum GH, insulin, IGF-1, IGFBP1, and IGFBP3 concentrations after heavy resistance exercise in trained and untrained men. *Endocrine, 41*(1), 144-151. doi:10.1007/s12020-011-9537-3

Hausmann, G., & Basler, K. (2006). Wnt lipid modifications: not as saturated as we thought. *Developmental Cell, 11*(6), 751-752. doi:10.1016/j.devcel.2006.11.007

Hornberger, T. A., Sukhija, K. B., & Chien, S. (2006). Regulation of mTOR by mechanically induced signaling events in skeletal muscle. *Cell Cycle, 5*(13), 1391-1396. Retrieved from http://www.ncbi.nlm.nih.gov/pubmed/16855395

Janssen, I., Heymsfield, S. B., Wang, Z., & Ross, R. (2000). Skeletal muscle mass and distribution in 468 men and women aged 18–88 yr. *Journal of Applied Physiology, 89*(1), 81-88.

Jones, A. E., Price, F. D., Le Grand, F., Soleimani, V. D., Dick, S. A., Megeney, L. A., & Rudnicki, M. A. (2015). Wnt/β-catenin controls follistatin signalling to regulate satellite cell myogenic potential. *Skelet Muscle, 5*(1), 14.

Joulia-Ekaza, D., & Cabello, G. (2007). The myostatin gene: physiology and pharmacological relevance. *Current Opinion in Pharmacology, 7*(3), 310-315. doi:10.1016/j.coph.2006.11.011

Karalaki, M., Fili, S., Philippou, A., & Koutsilieris, M. (2009). Muscle regeneration: cellular and molecular events. *In Vivo, 23*(5), 779-796. Retrieved from http://www.ncbi.nlm.nih.gov/pubmed/19779115

Koles, K., Nunnari, J., Korkut, C., Barria, R., Brewer, C., Li, Y., . . . Budnik, V. (2012). Mechanism of evenness interrupted (Evi)-exosome release at synaptic boutons. *Journal of Biological Chemistry, 287*(20), 16820-16834. doi:10.1074/jbc.M112.342667

Korkut, C., Ataman, B., Ramachandran, P., Ashley, J., Barria, R., Gherbesi, N., & Budnik, V. (2009). Trans-synaptic transmission of vesicular Wnt signals through Evi/Wntless. *Cell, 139*(2), 393-404. doi:10.1016/j.cell.2009.07.051

Kraemer, R. R., & Castracane, V. D. (2015). Endocrine alterations from concentric vs. eccentric muscle actions: a brief review. *Metabolism, 64*(2), 190-201. doi:10.1016/j.metabol.2014.10.024

Kraemer, W. J., Duncan, N. D., & Volek, J. S. (1998). Resistance training and elite athletes: adaptations and program considerations. *Journal of Orthopaedic and Sports Physical Therapy, 28*(2), 110-119. doi:10.2519/jospt.1998.28.2.110

Kraemer, W. J., Hakkinen, K., Newton, R. U., Nindl, B. C., Volek, J. S., McCormick, M., . . . Evans, W. J. (1999). Effects of heavy-resistance training on hormonal response patterns in younger vs. older men. *J Appl Physiol (1985), 87*(3), 982-992. Retrieved from http://www.ncbi.nlm.nih.gov/pubmed/10484567

Laplante, M., & Sabatini, D. M. (2009). mTOR signaling at a glance. *Journal of Cell Science, 122*(20), 3589-3594.

Le Grand, F., & Rudnicki, M. A. (2007). Skeletal muscle satellite cells and adult myogenesis. *Current Opinion in Cell Biology, 19*(6), 628-633.

Leal, M. L., Lamas, L., Aoki, M. S., Ugrinowitsch, C., Ramos, M. S., Tricoli, V., & Moriscot, A. S. (2011). Effect of different resistance-training regimens on the WNT-signaling pathway. *European Journal of Applied Physiology, 111*(10), 2535-2545. doi:10.1007/s00421-011-1874-7

Li, V. S., Ng, S. S., Boersema, P. J., Low, T. Y., Karthaus, W. R., Gerlach, J. P., . . . Clevers, H. (2012). Wnt signaling through inhibition of beta-catenin degradation in an intact Axin1 complex. *Cell, 149*(6), 1245-1256. doi:10.1016/j.cell.2012.05.002

Logan, C. Y., & Nusse, R. (2004). The Wnt signaling pathway in development and disease. *Annual Review of Cell and Developmental Biology, 20*, 781-810. doi:10.1146/annurev.cellbio.20.010403.113126

Madarame, H., Sasaki, K., & Ishii, N. (2010). Endocrine responses to upper- and lower-limb resistance exercises with blood flow restriction. *Acta Physiologica Hungarica, 97*(2), 192-200. doi:10.1556/APhysiol.97.2010.2.5

Mann, R. K., & Beachy, P. A. (2004). Novel lipid modifications of secreted protein signals. *Annual Review of Biochemistry, 73*, 891-923. doi:10.1146/annurev.biochem.73.011303.073933

Mitchell, C. J., Churchward-Venne, T. A., Parise, G., Bellamy, L., Baker, S. K., Smith, K., . . . Phillips, S. M. (2014). Acute post-exercise myofibrillar protein synthesis is not correlated with resistance training-induced muscle hypertrophy in young men. *PloS One, 9*(2), e89431.

Mulholland, D. J., Cheng, H., Reid, K., Rennie, P. S., & Nelson, C. C. (2002). The androgen receptor can promote beta-catenin nuclear translocation independently of adenomatous polyposis coli. *Journal of Biological Chemistry, 277*(20), 17933-17943. doi:10.1074/jbc.M200135200

Niehrs, C., & Acebron, S. P. (2010). Wnt signaling: multivesicular bodies hold GSK3 captive. *Cell, 143*(7), 1044-1046. doi:10.1016/j.cell.2010.12.003

Nishita, M., Endo, M., & Minami, Y. (2013). [Regulation of cellular responses by non-canonical Wnt signaling]. *Clinical Calcium, 23*(6), 809-815. doi:CliCa1306809815

Nusse, R., & Varmus, H. (2012). Three decades of Wnts: a personal perspective on how a scientific field developed. *EMBO Journal, 31*(12), 2670-2684. doi:10.1038/emboj.2012.146

Otto, A., Schmidt, C., Luke, G., Allen, S., Valasek, P., Muntoni, F., . . . Patel, K. (2008). Canonical Wnt signalling induces satellite-cell proliferation during adult skeletal muscle regeneration. *Journal of Cell Science, 121*(Pt 17), 2939-2950. doi:10.1242/jcs.026534

Otto, A., Schmidt, C., & Patel, K. (2006). Pax3 and Pax7 expression and regulation in the avian embryo. *Anatomy and Embryology, 211*(4), 293-310. doi:10.1007/s00429-006-0083-3

Ozhan, G., & Weidinger, G. (2015). Wnt/β-catenin signaling in heart regeneration. *Cell Regen (Lond), 4*(1).

Polesskaya, A., Seale, P., & Rudnicki, M. A. (2003). Wnt signaling induces the myogenic specification of resident CD45+ adult stem cells during muscle regeneration. *Cell, 113*(7), 841-852. Retrieved from http://www.ncbi.nlm.nih.gov/pubmed/12837243

Relaix, F., Rocancourt, D., Mansouri, A., & Buckingham, M. (2005). A Pax3/Pax7-dependent population of skeletal muscle progenitor cells. *Nature, 435*(7044), 948-953.

Segalen, M., & Bellaiche, Y. (2009). Cell division orientation and planar cell polarity pathways. *Seminars in Cell & Developmental Biology, 20*(8), 972-977. doi:10.1016/j.semcdb.2009.03.018

Semenov, M. V., Habas, R., Macdonald, B. T., & He, X. (2007). SnapShot: Noncanonical Wnt Signaling Pathways. *Cell, 131*(7), 1378. doi:10.1016/j.cell.2007.12.011

Serrano, A. L., Baeza-Raja, B., Perdiguero, E., Jardi, M., & Munoz-Canoves, P. (2008). Interleukin-6 is an essential regulator of satellite cell-mediated skeletal muscle hypertrophy. *Cell Metab, 7*(1), 33-44. doi:10.1016/j.cmet.2007.11.011

Spillane, M., Schwarz, N., & Willoughby, D. S. (2015). Upper-body resistance exercise augments vastus lateralis androgen receptor-DNA binding and canonical Wnt/beta-catenin signaling compared to lower-body resistance exercise in resistance-trained men without an acute increase in serum testosterone. *Steroids, 98*, 63-71. doi:10.1016/j.steroids.2015.02.019

Steelman, C. A., Recknor, J. C., Nettleton, D., & Reecy, J. M. (2006). Transcriptional profiling of myostatin-knockout mice implicates Wnt signaling in postnatal skeletal muscle growth and hypertrophy. *FASEB Journal, 20*(3), 580-582. doi:10.1096/fj.05-5125fje

Takada, R., Satomi, Y., Kurata, T., Ueno, N., Norioka, S., Kondoh, H., . . . Takada, S. (2006). Monounsaturated fatty acid modification of Wnt protein: its role in Wnt secretion. *Developmental Cell, 11*(6), 791-801. doi:10.1016/j.devcel.2006.10.003

Tanneberger, K., Pfister, A. S., Kriz, V., Bryja, V., Schambony, A., & Behrens, J. (2011). Structural and functional characterization of the Wnt inhibitor APC membrane recruitment 1 (Amer1). *Journal of Biological Chemistry, 286*(22), 19204-19214. doi:10.1074/jbc.M111.224881

Terada, K., Misao, S., Katase, N., Nishimatsu, S., & Nohno, T. (2013). Interaction of Wnt Signaling with BMP/Smad Signaling during the Transition from Cell Proliferation to Myogenic Differentiation in Mouse Myoblast-Derived Cells. *International Journal of Cell Biology, 2013*, 616294. doi:10.1155/2013/616294

Tesch, P. A. (1988). Skeletal muscle adaptations consequent to long-term heavy resistance exercise. *Medicine & Science in Sports & Exercise, 20*(5 Suppl), S132-134.

Thomas, D. R. (2007). Loss of skeletal muscle mass in aging: examining the relationship of starvation, sarcopenia and cachexia. *Clinical Nutrition, 26*(4), 389-399.

Uchida, M. C., Crewther, B. T., Ugrinowitsch, C., Bacurau, R. F., Moriscot, A. S., & Aoki, M. S. (2009). Hormonal responses to different resistance exercise schemes of similar total volume. *Journal of Strength and Conditioning Research, 23*(7), 2003-2008. doi:10.1519/JSC.0b013e3181b73bf7

van Amerongen, R., & Nusse, R. (2009). Towards an integrated view of Wnt signaling in development. *Development, 136*(19), 3205-3214.

von Maltzahn, J., Bentzinger, C. F., & Rudnicki, M. A. (2012). Wnt7a-Fzd7 signalling directly activates the Akt/mTOR anabolic growth pathway in skeletal muscle. *Nature Cell Biology, 14*(2), 186-191. doi:10.1038/ncb2404

von Maltzahn, J., Chang, N. C., Bentzinger, C. F., & Rudnicki, M. A. (2012). Wnt signaling in myogenesis. *Trends in Cell Biology, 22*(11), 602-609.

Walker, D. K., Dickinson, J. M., Timmerman, K. L., Drummond, M. J., Reidy, P. T., Fry, C. S., . . . Rasmussen, B. B. (2011). Exercise, amino acids, and aging in the control of human muscle protein synthesis. *Medicine & Science in Sports & Exercise, 43*(12), 2249-2258. doi:10.1249/MSS.0b013e318223b037

Wang, Q., & McPherron, A. C. (2012). Myostatin inhibition induces muscle fibre hypertrophy prior to satellite cell activation. *Journal of Physiology, 590*(Pt 9), 2151-2165. doi:10.1113/jphysiol.2011.226001

West, D. W., Burd, N. A., Staples, A. W., & Phillips, S. M. (2010). Human exercise-mediated skeletal muscle hypertrophy is an intrinsic process. *International Journal of Biochemistry and Cell Biology, 42*(9), 1371-1375. doi:10.1016/j.biocel.2010.05.012

West, D. W., & Phillips, S. M. (2010). Anabolic processes in human skeletal muscle: restoring the identities of growth hormone and testosterone. *Phys Sportsmed, 38*(3), 97-104. doi:10.3810/psm.2010.10.1814

Willert, K., & Nusse, R. (2012). Wnt proteins. *Cold Spring Harbor Perspectives in Biology, 4*(9), a007864. doi:10.1101/cshperspect.a007864

Williams, M. S. (2004). Myostatin mutation associated with gross muscle hypertrophy in a child. *New England Journal of Medicine, 351*(10), 1030-1031; author reply 1030-1031. Retrieved from http://www.ncbi.nlm.nih.gov/pubmed/15352277

Yin, H., Price, F., & Rudnicki, M. A. (2013). Satellite Cells and the Muscle Stem Cell Niche. *Physiological Reviews, 93*(1), 23-67.

Yokoyama, N., Markova, N. G., Wang, H. Y., & Malbon, C. C. (2012). Assembly of Dishevelled 3-based supermolecular complexes via phosphorylation and Axin. *J Mol Signal, 7*(1), 8. doi:10.1186/1750-2187-7-8

Yu, J., Chia, J., Canning, C. A., Jones, C. M., Bard, F. A., & Virshup, D. M. (2014). WLS retrograde transport to the endoplasmic reticulum during Wnt secretion. *Developmental Cell, 29*(3), 277-291. doi:10.1016/j.devcel.2014.03.016

Zhai, L., Chaturvedi, D., & Cumberledge, S. (2004). Drosophila wnt-1 undergoes a hydrophobic modification and is targeted to lipid rafts, a process that requires porcupine. *Journal of Biological Chemistry, 279*(32), 33220-33227. doi:10.1074/jbc.M403407200

17

The Size and Strength Development in Elite Youth Ice Hockey Players

Jeff R. Leiter (Corresponding author)
Pan Am Clinic Foundation, 75 Poseidon Bay, Winnipeg R3M 3E4, Canada
E-mail: jleiter@panamclinic.com

Dean M. Cordingley
Pan Am Clinic Foundation, 75 Poseidon Bay, Winnipeg R3M 3E4, Canada
E-mail: dcordingley@panamclinic.com

Adam J. Zeglen
Focus Fitness, 3969 Portage Ave, Winnipeg R3K 1W4, Canada
E-mail: azeglen@truenorth.mb.ca

Glenn D. Carnegie
Focus Fitness, 3969 Portage Ave, Winnipeg R3K 1W4, Canada
E-mail: glenn.carnegie@canucks.com

Peter B. MacDonald
Pan Am Clinic, 75 Poseidon Bay, Winnipeg R3M 3E4, Canada
E-mail: pmacdonald@panamclinic.com

Abstract

Background: Ice hockey is a fast, physical sport that requires high levels of muscular strength, muscular endurance and agility. **Objectives:** This study was conducted to create a profile including: anthropometric measurement, muscular strength, muscular endurance, lower body jump height and distance, and agility characteristics for elite youth hockey players. **Methods:** Pre-season off-ice testing results were retrospectively reviewed from a human performance database. Variables included height, weight, body fat percentage, grip strength, push-ups/bench press, supine rows, the plank test, vertical jump, standing long jump, hip adductor and abductor strength, and the 5-10-5 shuttle, and. One-way ANOVAs (1group x 4 time) and Tukeys post-hoc tests were performed to determine changes in the immediately successive age group ($p<0.05$). **Results:** Participants included male Bantam-(age: 13-14) and Midget-(age: 15-17) AAA ice-hockey players (n=260). Age categories were grouped as 13 years old (yo)(n=75), 14 yo (n=70), 15 yo (n=58), and 16-17 yo (n=57). Increases between successive age groups were observed in the following variables: weight (13, 14, 15 and 16-17 yo), height (13 and 14 yo), left and right grip strength (13, 14, 15, and 16-17 yo), bench press (15 and 16-17 yo), left and right hip abduction (14, 15, and 16-17 yo), and vertical and standing long jump (13, 14, and 15 yo). Total time for the 5-10-5 shuttle run test decreased from 13 to 14yo, and 14 to 15 yo. **Conclusion:** Changes with age in off-ice performance variables of elite amateur hockey players should be recognized, followed, and addressed during player development to maximize the potential for elite performance and reduce the risk of injury.

Keywords: Athletic Performance, Training, Physical Fitness

1. Introduction

1.1 Introduce the problem

Ice hockey involves aggressive play at fast speeds, requiring near maximal heart rates (Jackson, Snydmiller, Game, Gervais, & Bell, 2016), with a high frequency and magnitude of physical contact (Cox, Miles, Verde & Rhodes, 1995; Montgomery, 2006). The majority of injuries in ice hockey are a result of a collision between two players (Azuelos, Pearsall, Turcotte & Montgomery, 2004) and can be related to the discrepancy in size, strength and speed of the competitors (Montgomery, 2006), especially at the amateur level (Emery et al., 2011). During youth development, there can be a wide range of size, strength and skill levels amongst peers, and this variance may increase the risk of injury in youth hockey. At the time of data collection, Hockey Canada allowed body-checking beginning at the age of 12 (Peewee level). Hockey Canada since revised the rule for the start of the 2013-2014 season such that body-checking is not allowed until the age of 13 (Bantam level) (Hockey Canada, 2014). Physical development with respect to size and strength is important for these players to resist injuries (Gledhill & Jamnik, 2007) and maximize performance, especially when transitioning to an older age group with players that may be larger, stronger and faster.

1.2 Review of literature

Prior to the NHL entry draft an athletic profile of each player is obtained through a combined series of standardized tests (referred to as a 'Combine') that evaluate the player's physical stature and physiological fitness level (Gledhill & Jamnik, 2007). These tests include anthropometric measures (height, weight, body composition) and assessments of anaerobic and aerobic fitness, muscular power, muscular strength, muscular endurance and flexibility (Gledhill & Jamnik, 2007). These tests were adopted and adapted for youth hockey players included in our study to establish size and strength profiles for each age group. National Hockey League (NHL) players have become heavier, taller and stronger (Montgomery, 2006) allowing them to optimize power for skating and shooting and maintain aggressive play while being less prone to injuries (Gledhill & Jamnik, 2007). The size and athletic profile of NHL players are well documented and understood; there is a paucity of literature in youth hockey players. While age, division of play, body checking (Emery & Meeuwisse, 2006), and position (Grant et al., 2015) can contribute to an increased risk of injury, the effects of body size and strength differences on injury rates in youth hockey have not been addressed. The purpose of this study was to investigate size and fitness differences amongst elite youth hockey players in successive age groups from 13-17 years. To our knowledge, this is the most comprehensive assessment of size and fitness differences by age category in elite youth hockey.

2. Methods

2.1 Participants

Participants included Bantam- (age: 13-14) and Midget- (age: 15-17) AAA hockey players (n=260) from 14 teams preparing to compete in the 2012-2013 season. All staff members were trained in the proper methodology for each test. At a pre-season meeting parents/guardians were informed that de-identified data could be used for research purposes and inclusion of this data was voluntary and were given the opportunity to exclude the data of their dependant(s). Ethical approval was received from the local research ethics board and the local hockey organization. All parents/guardians were informed that de-identified data from league testing could be used for research purposes. All parents/guardians were notified that inclusion of data was voluntary and could exclude the data of their dependant(s).

2.2 Experimental Design

This is a retrospective study in which our human performance database was reviewed for all AAA (13-17 year old hockey players who participated in a pre-season testing combine prior to the 2012-2013 season. Personal identifiers were removed for each athlete.

2.3 Procedures

Body mass was measured to the nearest 0.1 kg in shorts only using a calibrated electronic scale (Taylor, HoMedics Group Canada, Toronto, Ontario). Height was measured to the nearest 0.1 cm (Seca 700, Seca Precision for Health, Hamburg, Germany). Body fat was determined using skin folds at 7 sites (chest, triceps, subscapular, suprailiac, abdomen, front thigh and midaxillary) using skin-fold calipers (Chattanooga Baseline Skinfold Caliper, Chattanooga Group, Vista, CA) and body fat % was calculated (Siri, 1961). This method has had R values reported between 0.888 and 0.918 (Jackson & Pollock, 1978). All skinfolds were performed by the same experienced tester to ensure consistency between athletes.

Grip strength was used to assess upper body strength. Players were instructed to stand erect with elbows extended and arms to the side and squeeze the hydraulic grip dynamometer (Jamar hand dynamometer, Sammons Preston Rolyan, Bolingbrook, Il) with as much force as possible (Canadian Society for Exercise Physiology, 2003). Players performed three repetitions for each arm, alternating between arms after each repetition. The maximum force of each hand was recorded. Upper body muscular endurance was assessed with push-ups for Bantam players (age 13-14) and bench press for Midget players (age 15-17). The Bantam players were instructed to lay prone on the floor with hands positioned under each shoulder. For the 'push-up' phase, players were instructed to extend at the elbow into a push-up position. For the 'downward' phase, players were instructed to touch their chest against a 4 cm tall piece of foam. The test was stopped when players reached complete fatigue and/or could no longer maintain form during the upward or downward phase of the push-up. The Midget players performed a bench press with a resistance of 52.3 kgs (115 lbs) to assess upper body strength. Each player was instructed to perform as many repetitions as possible to a maximum of 25. During the 'downward' phase of all repetitions, the players were required to touch the bar to their chest. During the 'push' phase the players were instructed to reach full extension at the elbow joint. Feet were required to remain on the floor and the lower back/buttocks of the athlete were required to stay in contact with the bench.

Lower body strength was determined with hip abduction and adduction strength. Players were tested lying supine on an athletic therapy table. A hand-held dynamometer (DFX 2 Series Digital Force Gauge, Largo, FL) was placed 5 cm proximal to the medial (Adduction test) or lateral (Abduction test) malleoli of the ankle (Figure 1). A series of three, two second maximal isometric contractions were performed for the abductors and then adductors of each leg with 30 seconds of recovery between each contraction. Players alternated between legs after each repetition. The maximum value of each test was recorded to the nearest 0.1 kg of force.

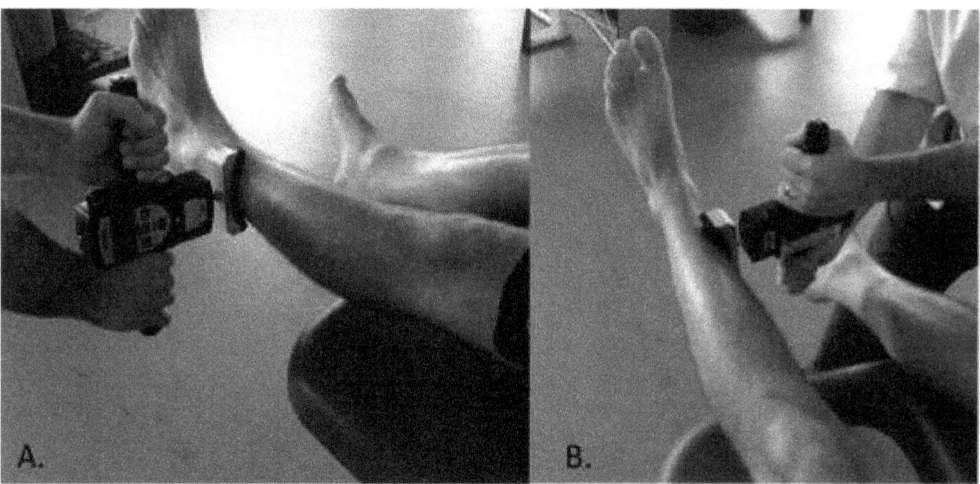

Figure 1. A. Force gauge placement for hip abduction strength testing. B. Force gauge placement for hip adduction strength testing

Upper back endurance was determined with supine rows. A barbell was placed on a squat rack (34.5 cm from the ground), and the player positioned themselves under the bar with hands shoulder width apart and a pronated grip on the bar. Feet were placed shoulder width apart on the floor with knees flexed to 90 degrees and hips and trunk in a neutral position. When instructed, the player pulled until the chest of the athlete contacted the bar and then returned to the starting position with shoulders flexed and elbows extended. When a player could no longer touch the bar with their chest, the test was stopped and the number of repetitions recorded. Abdominal muscle and core endurance was assessed using a front plank. The athletes were instructed to have elbows and forearms on the ground with upper arms perpendicular to the ground. The athlete had to maintain a neutral spine and hold the position for as long as possible (up to 120 seconds). The length of time was recorded until the form of the athlete waivered or maximal fatigue was reached. Lower body vertical jump height and standing long jump distance was assessed. Vertical jump was measured to the nearest 0.5 inch (1.27 cm) using a Vertec Jump Trainer (Sports Imports, Columbus, OH). A standing reach height was first established. The athletes reached with their dominant hand to displace the highest bar (vane) possible on the Vertec while keeping their feet together and flat on the floor. Players then stood directly beneath the Vertec and performed a counter movement vertical jump attempting to touch the highest vane possible. Each player performed 3 repetitions and the highest height was recorded.

Standing long jump was measured to the nearest 0.5 cm using a cloth tape measure attached to the floor. The athletes stood with toes behind the start of the tape measure and were instructed to jump as far as possible. The distance traveled was measured to the heel that landed closest to the start line. Players performed three jumps and the longest distance was recorded. Multi-directional agility and speed were assessed with a 5-10-5 shuttle test. Three cones were placed along a straight line, five yards (4.57 meters) apart. Players started with their feet straddling the center cone and sprinted to the cone on his right or left side. The player touched the cone, then sprinted in the opposite direction to touch the far cone and finally reversed direction and sprinted to the centre cone. In total, the player covered 20 yards (18.3 meters). The test was performed four times, two times with the player going to the right first and two times with the player going to the left first. The fastest time for each direction was used in analysis.

2.3.1Data and Statistical analysis

A one-way (1 group x 4 time) ANOVA was performed to determine an overall test of significance for the mean differences of all age groups. If a significant main effect was found, a Tukeys HSD (honestly significant difference) test was performed to identify which differences were significant. The alpha level was set at $p<0.05$ to signify a significant difference for all analyses. SPSS 20.0 (IBM Corporation, Armonk, NY) was used to perform statistical analyses.

3. Results

3.1 Anthropometric measures

The number of athletes in each age category was Bantams: 13 yo (n=75), 14 yo (n=70), and Midgets: 15 yo (n=58), 16-17 yo (n=57). All athletes were male. Anthropometric means are summarized (height, Figure 2; weight, Figure 3; body fat % and BMI, Table 1). Percentile data for height, weight and body fat percentage are presented (Table 2). The weight of athletes significantly increased with every successive age group, 13 to 14 ($p<0.001$), 14 to 15 ($p=0.005$), 15 to 16 ($p=0.013$) (Figure 3). The only increase in height was found between the 13 and 14 yo ($p<0.001$). There was no associated change in body fat with these physical changes, however BMI increased from ages 13 to 14 ($p=0.024$) and 14 to 15 ($p=0.012$), but not 15 to 16 ($p=0.204$; Table 1).

Table 1. Anthropometric and athletic profile measures according to age

Age (yrs)	13	14	15	16-17
n=	75‡	70#	58&	57†
Body Fat (%)	9.3 (3.5)	9.3 (3.5)	9.8 (3.7)	11.0 (3.5)
Body Mass Index (kg/m2)	20.6 (2.1)	21.7 (1.9)*	22.9 (2.5)*	23.7 (2.2)
Push-ups (reps)	25.0 (9.9)	25.0 (12.8)	n/a	n/a
Bench-press (reps)	n/a	n/a	9.78(5.8)	17.0(7.8)*
Supine row (reps)	18.5 (7.2)	19.9 (8.0)	22.0 (6.7)	23.1 (8.1)
Plank (s)	112.6 (16.8)	114.6 (15.3)	116.2 (13.0)	118.2 (8.5)
Vertical jump (cm)	43.9 (7.9)	47.5 (6.1)*	52.8 (8.9)*	53.3(10.16)
5-10-5 shuttle (s)	5.5 (0.3)	5.3 (0.2)*	5.2 (0.2)*	5.1 (0.2)
Adduction left leg (kg)	14.6 (3.3)	15.8 (3.2)	16.6 (3.3)	19.2 (3.4)*
Adduction right leg (kg)	14.6 (3.3)	16.1 (3.5)	17.5 (3.7)	19.0 (3.2)
Abduction left leg (kg)	14.6 (2.9)	15.3 (2.4)	16.9 (3.2)*	19.0 (3.3)*
Abduction right leg (kg)	14.8 (3.1)	15.5 (2.7)	17.0 (3.7)*	19.5 (2.9)*
Left/Right leg Adduction	1.00 (0.11)	0.99 (0.12)	0.96 (0.13)	1.0 (0.11)
Left/Right leg Abduction	0.99 (0.09)	1.00 (0.12)	1.01 (0.12)	0.98 (0.09)
Ad/Abduction left leg	1.01 (0.16)	1.03 (0.16)	1.00 (0.16)	1.02 (0.16)
Ad/Abduction right leg	0.99 (0.17)	1.05 (0.17)	1.05 (0.18)	0.98 (0.11)

Data represented as means (SD). Each age category was compared to the immediately successive age group. * indicates a significant difference, $p<0.05$.

‡ For supine rows one athlete did not complete this test due to injury

For push-ups, supine rows and 5-10-5 shuttle run, two athletes did not complete each test and one athlete did not complete vertical jump.

& For vertical jump, plank, and left hip adduction and abduction, one athlete did not complete the tests while two athletes did not complete the 5-10-5 shuttle, five did not complete supine rows and 7 did not complete bench press due to injuries.

† For bench press, standing long jump, vertical jump and 5-10-5 shuttle run, one athlete did not complete these tests while two athletes did not complete the supine rows due to injury.

Table 2. Percentiles for anthropometric measures

		Percentile						
	Age (yrs)	5	10	25	50	75	90	95
Height (cms)	13	154.0	160.0	162.6	165.1	172.7	180.0	180.8
	14	165.0	167.6	170.1	175.0	179.0	182.9	185.4
	15	166.0	167.6	172.7	177.8	182.9	185.4	186.1
	16-17	167.8	172.5	175.3	180.3	185.4	189.7	193.0
Weight (kgs)	13	45.9	47.5	51.9	56.3	62.1	69.8	77.1
	14	55.4	57.0	61.6	65.5	71.4	76.3	83.0
	15	59.4	61.0	64.6	68.5	79.6	85.7	94.7
	16-17	62.9	66.6	72.1	75.8	81.1	89.4	96.8
Body Fat (%)	13	16.5	15.2	11.2	8.3	6.9	5.4	4.7
	14	16.9	14.4	11.7	8.2	7.0	5.8	5.5
	15	19.4	15.6	11.8	9.1	7.1	6.0	5.3
	16-17	18.0	15.9	13.3	10.7	8.3	6.8	6.2

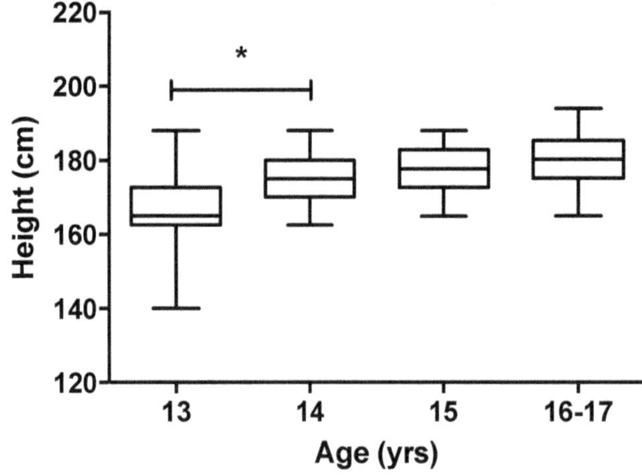

Figure 2. Changes in height (cm) between age groups of elite youth hockey players. * indicates a significant difference, p<0.05.

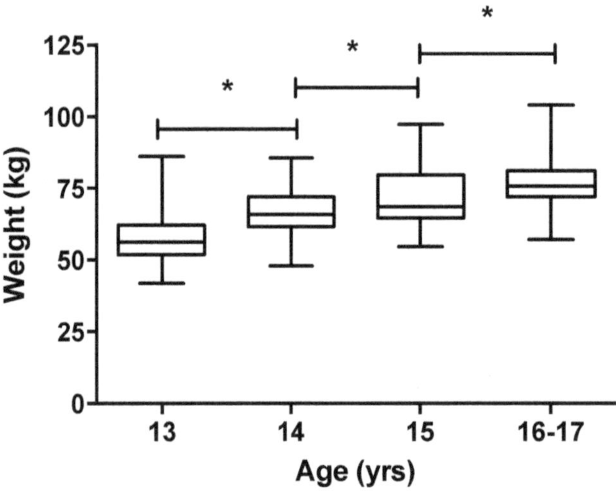

Figure 3. Changes in body weight (kg) between age groups of elite youth hockey players. * indicates a significant difference, p<0.05.

3.2 Fitness measures

Grip strength increased significantly with all successive age groups for both the left- and right-hand (Figure 4). There was no difference between the 13 and 14 yo athletes who performed push-ups to fatigue (p=0.98), but there was a difference between the 15 and 16 yo athletes (Midget players) for bench press repetitions to fatigue (p<0.001; Table 1). Since Bantam (push-up) and Midget (115 lbs bench press) players were instructed to use different resistance exercises a statistical comparison between the 14 and 15 yo was not performed.

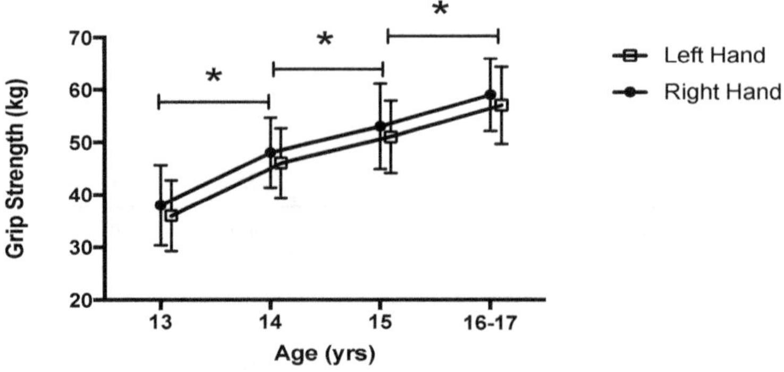

Figure 4. Changes in left and right hand grip strength (kg) between age groups of elite youth hockey players. * indicates a significant difference, p<0.05.

With respect to lower body strength, hip abduction strength increased in both the left and right legs between the 14 and 15 yo (p=0.019 and p=0.032, respectively) and 15 to 16 yo (p=0.001 and p=<0.001, respectively). The only increase in hip adduction strength was observed in the left legs of the 15 to 16 year-olds (p<0.001). The ratio of adductor to abductor strength of the right and left legs of all age groups demonstrated that adductor strength was at least 98% of abductor strength. However, 21 players (9%) had an adductor to abductor strength ratio less than 0.80 in at least one leg, and seven (3%) in both legs suggesting an adductor muscle imbalance. All hip ab/adduction ratios are summarized in Table 1.

3.3 Jump height and distance

The distance a player was able to achieve performing the standing long jump test increased from the ages of 13 to 14 (p<0.001) and 14 to 15 years (p<0.001), but not from 15 to 16 years (p=0.867;Figure 5). Similarly, vertical jump scores increased in the younger age groups, but not the 15 to 16 yo groups (p=0.99).

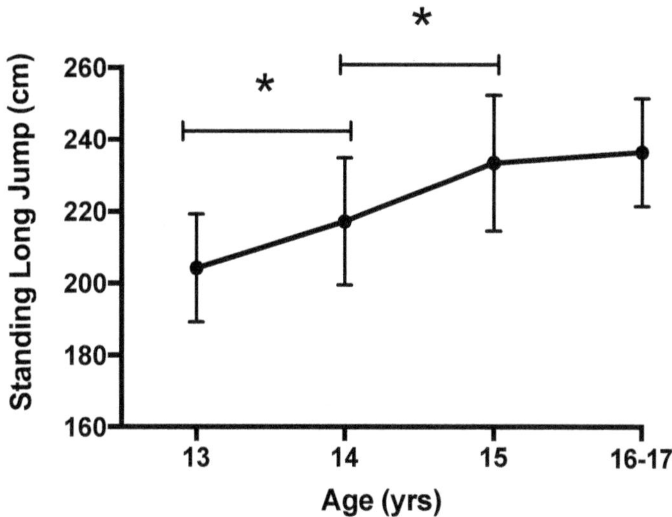

Figure 5. Changes in standing long jump distance (cm) between age groups of elite youth hockey players. * indicates a significant difference, p<0.05.

3.4 Agility measures

Time to complete the 5-10-5 shuttle run decreased as the athletes increased in age from 13 to 14 (p<0.001) and 14 to 15 (p=0.006). Although performance times continued to improve between the 15 and 16 yo athletes significance was not reached (p=1.0).

3.5 Muscular endurance

There were no changes observed in upper back, abdominal or core endurance results between successive age groups (Table 1).

4. Discussion

The most important finding of this study was that the greatest changes in size and strength occur between the ages of 13- and 15- years of age. Since this is a period of development where body-checking is introduced and skill levels may demonstrate the greatest variability, size and strength may factor in to injury risk more so than at the later ages. To our knowledge, this is the most comprehensive assessment of size and strength of elite youth hockey players to date.

The height of players increased in succeeding age groups from 13 to 14 years of age which corresponds to the onset of puberty for males (Rogol, Roemmich & Clark, 2002). In 1984-1985, Regnier et al.(1989) reported that the average height of 13-14 year old players (n=58) was 164.5 (6.14) compared to 167.6 (8.4) in our study. There was an increase in body mass between all age groups in our study. Bantam and Midget athletes in our study demonstrated ranges in mass of 96.14 lb (43.7 kgs) and 108.46 lb (49.3) respectively. Emery and Meeuwisse (2006) reported body mass ranges for Pee Wee, Bantam and Midget as high as 130 lb, 130 lb and 115 lb respectively (Emery & Meeuwisse, 2006). This large discrepancy in the mass of players within the same age group has been theorized to contribute to increased injury risk. At the University level of competition, Grant and colleagues (2015) demonstrated that for each 5 kg increase in body mass, injury rate increased by a factor of 1.3 and for players with a BMI > 25 kg/m^2, the risk of injury was 2.1 times higher than players with a BMI < 25 kg/m^2. Of our athletes, 9% (n=23) presented with a BMI > 25 kg/m^2 potentially putting them at a higher risk of injury. Conversely, smaller players (i.e. < 37 kg) have been shown to be at a greater risk of injury in Pee Wee(Emery et al., 2010), but there is no association between body mass and injury risk at the Bantam level(Emery et al., 2011). A limitation in the youth hockey studies is that strength and body fat percentage were not measured, which is a potential reason for the discrepancy between studies.

The increase in body mass in each age group did not result in a change in body composition with the average body fat recorded at 9.8% for all players. Since body fat percentage remained consistent despite an increase in mass; this ensured an optimal strength/mass ratio. In theory, an optimal strength/mass ratio would allow players to move their own body weight as fast and efficiently as possible. Although body fat percentage is an indicator of optimal strength/mass ratio, it has not been shown to be a predictor of injury risk(Grant et al., 2015). Over time, the athlete has changed with the ultimate goal of optimizing size and strength. Quinney et al.(2008) longitudinally tracked NHL athletes over a 26 year period (1979 to 2005) and found an increase in body mass without a concurrent change in body composition, indicating body mass gains are due to lean body mass and not fat mass. Montgomery (2006) noted that NHL players with the Montreal Canadiens hockey team in the year 2003 were on average 17 kg heavier and 10 cm taller than players in 1917, which he attributed to changes in nutrition, strength and conditioning and the recruiting processes. Increases in body mass have also been observed in the National Football League (1972-1998)(Snow, Millard-Stafford & Rosskopf, 1998; Wilmore & Haskell, 1972) and the general Canadian population (1981-1996)(Tremblay, Katzmarzyk & Willms, 2002). It appears that the trend for heavier and taller athletes with optimal strength/mass ratios could be due to changes in training habits, nutrition as well as micro-evolution of the entire population.

When compared to normative data for the same aged youth(Mathiowetz, Wiemer, & Federman, 1986) grip strength was considerably higher in our study suggesting that elite youth hockey players incur greater demands on upper body strength than the average adolescent. Unpublished data from our lab demonstrates that the average grip strength of NHL players is 67.8 kg and 68.8 kg for the left and right hands, respectively. Although the average grip strength of NHL players is greater than all groups tested in our study, this is an attainable value based on the chronological trends of our sample. In addition to sport, grip strength is a useful measure to predict mortality later in life. Males with higher grip strength in the middle years of life have a lower long-term mortality risk, even when education, occupation, age, physical activity, smoking, and body height are taken into account(Rantanen et al., 2000). There was no change in mean number of push-ups between 13 and 14 year olds, however there was a significant difference between 15 and 16 year olds (bench press). Interestingly, Grant and colleagues (2015) demonstrated that for every increase in 5 reps of barbell bench press (84.1 kg), injury risk increased by 1.3 times in University players. It is likely that stronger players play a more physical style and engage in body contact more often, which would increase the risk of injury. Although a statistical comparison was not employed between the 14 and 15 year olds due to the difference in tests (push-up vs. bench press), estimated comparisons were performed unsatisfactorily. During the push-up down phase (elbows flexed and shoulders extended), players supported approximately 75% of body weight and 69% during the upward phase (elbows extended and shoulders flexed)(Suprak, Dawes, & Stephenson, 2011). Therefore, it can be estimated that the 13 and 14 year old players moved a maximum resistance of 43.5 and 50.2kg, respectively, based on average body weight for each group. This is similar to the 52.3 kg (115 lbs) of resistance used for the bench press test in the 15 and 16 year old age groups. However, since the 14 year olds performed a mean of 25 push-ups, indicating they are in the 95th percentile for their age group(Catley & Tomkinson, 2011) while the 15 year olds performed an average of only 9.78 bench press reps, statistical comparison of muscle isolation exercises (i.e. bench press) with total body exercises (i.e. push ups) is not recommended. Hip adductor and abductor strength are is paramount for the sport of ice hockey. Activation of the adductor and abductor muscle groups is required to perform a skating motion,(de Koning, de Groot, & van Ingen Schenau, 1991) and is positively correlated with skating speed(Chang, Turcotte, & Pearsall, 2009). Muscle imbalances in hip ad/abductor strength may predispose a hockey player to muscle strains of the adductor musculature. Tyler and colleagues (2001) reported that a hockey player is 17 times more likely to sustain an adductor strain if adductor strength is less than 80% of the abductor strength of the ipsilateral leg. Our research identified 9% of players with a ratio less than 80% in at least one leg and 3% in both legs. Specific training programs should be designed for these players to balance muscle strength and reduce the risk of adductor strains, due to the debilitating nature of this injury and the risk or re-injury (2.6 times greater in players that have had an adductor injury)(Emery, Meeuwisse & Powell, 1999).

Both standing long jump and vertical jump increased between the 13 and 14 year olds and the 14 and 15 year olds. The results observed with our athletes (vertical jump, 49.3 ± 8.6 cm; standing long jump, 221.4 ± 21.3 cm) are similar to those previously observed for 36 elite hockey players 15-22 years of age (vertical jump, 51.4 ±6.7 cm; standing long jump, 210 ±19 cm)(Farlinger, Kruisselbrink, & Fowles, 2007). Players also showed an improvement in 5-10-5 agility shuttle run performance each year up to and including 15 years of age. The physical maturation and increased musculoskeletal fitness level of the athletes aged 13-15 are consistent with males experiencing the onset of puberty at age 13(Rogol et al., 2002). Although athletes at this age are going through many physical changes, it is agreed that physical training does not inhibit growth and development if appropriate nutrient intake is achieved(Rogol et al., 2002). With respect to injuries, this manuscript addresses a limitation in most epidemiological manuscripts investigating injuries in youth hockey players. Although this study did not address injury rates, our results do address not only size, but also fitness differences that have not been thoroughly investigated in youth hockey players.

4.1 Practicle applications

Athletic profiles of elite youth ice hockey players change between succeeding age groups. Strength training may help eliminate any large physiological jumps between age groups. Understanding how strength, power, endurance and agility develops in youth can not only assist the hockey community with creating appropriate training programs, but also provide public health organizations with valuable information when developing activity guidelines for youth in general.

5. Conclusion

This study demonstrated that there are many strength and size changes that take place between immediately succeeding age groups, which could make it challenging for an athlete to transition to the next age group in elite sports. The normative data set has potential implications on training programs with the creation of bench marks at each age to help assess an athlete's anthropometric characteristics, musculoskeletal fitness and agility.

Acknowledgments

Financial assistance was provided by the Pan Am Clinic Foundation. The authors would also like to acknowledge Focus Fitness for their assistance with all testing and the use of their space, Treny Sasyniuk for support with the writing of this manuscript, and all participants and the AAA hockey organization for their support. The authors have no conflict of interest to report.

References

Azuelos, Y.H., Pearsall, D.J., Turcotte, R., & Montgomery, D.L. (2004). A review of ice hockey injuries: location, diagnosis, mechanism. In Pearsall, D.J. & Ashare, A.B. (Eds.), Safety in ice hockey (Vol. 4, pp. 59–67). West Conshohcken, Penn.: American Society for Testing and Materials International.

Canadian Society for Exercise Physiology. (2003). The Canadian physical activity, fitness and lifestyle approach: CSEP-Health & Fitness Program's Health-Related Appraisal and Counselling Strategy. (3rd ed.). Ottawa, ON.

Catley, M. J., & Tomkinson, G. R. (2011). Normative health-related fitness values for children: analysis of 85347 test results on 9-17-year-old Australians since 1985. *British Journal of Sports Medicine, 47(*2), 98–108.

Chang, R., Turcotte, R., & Pearsall, D. (2009). Hip adductor muscle function in forward skating. *Sports Biomechanics, 8*(3), 212–222. http://doi.org/10.1080/14763140903229534

Cox, M. H., Miles, D. S., Verde, T. J., & Rhodes, E. C. (1995). Applied physiology of ice hockey. *Sports Medicine (Auckland, NZ), 19*(3), 184.

de Koning, J. J., de Groot, G., & van Ingen Schenau, G. J. (1991). Coordination of leg muscles during speed skating. Journal of Biomechanics, 24(2), 137–146.

Emery, C. A., Kang, J., Shrier, I., Goulet, C., Hagel, B. E., Benson, B. W., Meeuwisse, W. H. (2010). Risk of injury associated with body checking among youth ice hockey players. *JAMA, 303*(22), 2265–2272.

Emery, C. A., & Meeuwisse, W. H. (2006). Injury Rates, Risk Factors, and Mechanisms of Injury in Minor Hockey. The American Journal of Sports Medicine, 34(12), 1960–1969. http://doi.org/10.1177/0363546506290061

Emery, Carolyn A., Meeuwisse, Willem H., & Powell, John W. (1999). Groin and Abdominal Strain Injuries in the National Hockey League. *Clinical Journal of Sport Medicine, 9*(3), 151–156.

Emery, C., Kang, J., Shrier, I., Goulet, C., Hagel, B., Benson, B., Meeuwisse, W. (2011). Risk of injury associated with bodychecking experience among youth hockey players. Canadian Medical Association Journal, 183(11), 1249–1256.

Farlinger, C. M., Kruisselbrink, L. D., & Fowles, J. R. (2007). Relationships to skating performance in competitive hockey players. Journal of Strength and Conditioning Research, 21(3), 915.

Gledhill, N., & Jamnik, V. (2007). Detailed assessment protocols for NHL entry draft players. York University, Toronto.

Grant, J. A., Bedi, A., Kurz, J., Bancroft, R., Gagnier, J. J., & Miller, B. S. (2015). Ability of preseason body composition and physical fitness to predict the risk of injury in male collegiate hockey players. *Sports Health: A Multidisciplinary Approach, 7(*1), 45–51.

Hockey Canada. (2014). Referee's Case Book/Rule Combination 2014-2015. Hockey Canada. Retrieved from http://cdn.agilitycms.com/hockey-canada/Hockey-Programs/Officiating/Downloads/rulebook_casebook_e.pdf

Jackson, A. S., & Pollock, M. L. (1978). Generalized equations for predicting body density of men. *British Journal of Nutrition, 40*(03), 497–504.

Jackson, J., Snydmiller, G., Game, A., Gervais, P., & Bell, G. (2016). Movement Characteristics and Heart Rate Profiles Displayed by Female University Ice Hockey Players. *International Journal of Kinesiology and Sports Science, 4*(1). http://doi.org/10.7575/aiac.ijkss.v.4n.1p.43

Mathiowetz, V., Wiemer, D. M., & Federman, S. M. (1986). Grip and pinch strength: norms for 6-to 19-year-olds. The American Journal of Occupational Therapy, 40(10), 705–711.

Montgomery, D. L. (2006). Physiological profile of professional hockey players-a longitudinal comparison. *Applied Physiology, Nutrition, and Metabolism, 31(*3), 181–185.

Quinney, H. A., Dewart, R., Game, A., Snydmiller, G., Warburton, D., & Bell, G. (2008). A 26 year physiological description of a National Hockey League team. *Applied Physiology, Nutrition, and Metabolism, 33*(4), 753–760.

Rantanen, T., Harris, T., Leveille, S. G., Visser, M., Foley, D., Masaki, K., & Guralnik, J. M. (2000). Muscle strength and body mass index as long-term predictors of mortality in initially healthy men. *The Journals of Gerontology Series A: Biological Sciences and Medical Sciences, 55*(3), M168–M173.

Regnier, G., Boileau, R., Marcotte, G., Desharnais, R., Larouche, R., Bernard, D., Boulanger, D. (1989). Effects of Body-Checking in the Pee-Wee (12 and 13 Years Old) Division in the Province of Quebec. In C. R. Castaldi & E. F. Hoerner (Eds.), Safety in Ice Hockey (Vol. 1, pp. 84–94). Philadelphia, PA: ASTM International.

Rogol, A. D., Roemmich, J. N., & Clark, P. A. (2002). Growth at puberty. *Journal of Adolescent Health, 31*(6), 192–200.

Siri, W.E. (1961). Body composition from fluid space and density. In Techniques for measuring body composition (J. Brozek and A. Henschel, pp. 223–224). Washington D.C.: National Academy of Sciences.

Snow, Teresa K., Millard-Stafford, Mindy, & Rosskopf, Linda B. (1998). Body Composition Profile of NFL Football Players. *Journal of Strength and Conditioning Research, 12*(3), 146–149.

Suprak, D. N., Dawes, J., & Stephenson, M. D. (2011). The effect of position on the percentage of body mass supported during traditional and modified push-up variants. The Journal of Strength & Conditioning Research, 25(2), 497–503.

Tremblay, M.S., Katzmarzyk, P.T., & Willms, J.D. (2002). Temporal trends in overweight and obesity in Canada, 1981-1996. *International Journal of Obesity, 26*(4), 538–543.

Tyler, T. F., Nicholas, S. J., Campbell, R. J., & McHugh, M. P. (2001). The association of hip strength and flexibility with the incidence of adductor muscle strains in professional ice hockey players. The American Journal of Sports Medicine, 29(2), 124–128.

Wilmore, J.H., & Haskell, W.L. (1972). Body composition and endurance capacity of professional football players. *Journal of Applied Physiology, 33*(5), 564–567.

18

The Effect of Concurrent Aerobic and Anaerobic Exercise on Stress, Anxiety, Depressive Symptoms, and Blood Pressure in Renal Transplant Female Patients

Elham Shakoor

Department of Sport Physiology, School of Physical Education and Sport Sciences, Shiraz University, Shiraz, Iran

E-mail: eli_shakoor@yahoo.com

Mohsen Salesi (Corresponding author)

Department of Sport Physiology, School of Physical Education and Sport Sciences, Shiraz University, Shiraz, Iran

E-mail: mhsnsls@gmail.com

Maryam Koushki

Department of Sport Physiology, School of Physical Education and Sport Sciences, Shiraz University, Shiraz, Iran

E-mail: koushkie53@yahoo.com

Enayatollah Asadmanesh

Department of Sport Physiology, School of Physical Education and Sport Sciences, Shiraz University, Shiraz, Iran

E-mail: e_asadmanesh@yahoo.com

Darryn S. Willoughby

Department of Health, Human Performance, and Recreation, Exercise and Biochemical Nutrition Laboratory, Baylor University, Waco, TX, USA

Email: darryn_willoughby@baylor.edu

Ahmad Qassemian

Department of Sport Physiology, School of Physical Education and Sport Sciences, Shiraz University, Shiraz, Iran

Email: ahmadqassemian@gmail.com

Abstract

Background: Prevalence of stress, anxiety, depressive symptoms, and high blood pressure are known to be important issues among renal transplant patients. **Objective:** The main purpose of this study was to evaluate the effect of selected exercises on blood pressure, stress, anxiety, depressive symptoms, and blood pressure among renal transplant patients. **Method:** Thirty two women patients (aged, 20-50 years) with 2 to 3 years post renal transplantation history were voluntarily and objectively recruited. Participants were randomly divided into two groups, exercise (n=16) and control (n=16). The exercise group performed 10 weeks of exercise 3 days per week, and for 60-90 minutes per session. The control group involved no exercise. The DASS21 questionnaire was used to collect psychological data, and blood pressure was measured before and after 10 weeks of exercise. Data analysis was conducted using dependent and independent t-tests. **Results:** Concurrent exercise significantly reduced anxiety, stress, depressive symptoms, and systolic blood pressure in the exercise group only (p=0.000). **Conclusion:** Ten weeks of low-intensity exercise can be an effective measure to improve the stress, anxiety, depressive symptoms, and blood pressure in renal transplant patients. Our results suggest that a regular pattern of selected exercises can be effective on stress, anxiety, depressive symptoms, and blood pressure and may be beneficial for renal transplant patients.

Keywords: Selected exercise, Stress, Anxiety, Depressive symptoms, Renal transplant

1. Introduction

End-stage renal failure is an irreversible progressive renal dysfunction in which the body's ability to maintain fluid and electrolyte balance is lost, leading to uremia or azotemia (Rigatto et al. 2000). The number of people suffering from end-stage renal disease is increased by 6% annually, and 25,000 patients have been reported in Iran (Mahdavi-Mazdeh 2012). End-stage chronic renal failure patients cannot survive without replacement therapy (Rigatto et al. 2000). In Iran, 52.7% of patients undergo hemodialysis (Kargarfard et al., 2015) and 45.5% benefit from renal transplantation (Mousavi, Soleimani, and Mousavi 2014). With regard to problems like dialysis machine dependence, anxiety and high cost patients often prefer to undergo renal transplantation to survive (Painter et al. 2002; Sorensen et al. 2012; Boostani and Ghorbani 2014). Renal transplantation is currently an effective method in the treatment of advanced chronic renal failure (Spitzer and Avner 2012). Despite the benefits of renal transplantation, patients are confronted with a host of new problems after transplantation (Boostani and Ghorbani 2014).

Despite the benefits of kidney transplantation, it is associated with specific complications and can lead to social and psychological problems (Masoudi Alavi, Sharifi, and Aliakbarzadeh 2009). The prevalence of psychiatric illnesses before and two months after transplantation has been reported to be 11.1% and 36.1%, respectively. Depression and anxiety are reported to be common among patients with renal failure (Masoudi Alavi, Sharifi, and Aliakbarzadeh 2009). In the study of Dobbels et al (2008) concerning depression in renal transplant recipients, which was performed on 47,899 patients, 3,360 patients were depressed after 3 years (Dobbels et al. 2008). In a study conducted in Tehran, the rate of depression in patients with renal transplantation was reported similar to dialysis patients (Masoudi Alavi, Sharifi, and Aliakbarzadeh 2009). Hypertension is among the health problems (Kargarfard et al., 2016) of renal transplant patients, which is a common complication after renal transplantation (Kasiske et al. 2000). The prevalence of hypertension after renal transplantation in combination with cyclosporine is 60-80% (Magee and Milford 2004). In another study, the prevalence of hypertension has been reported to be 90% after renal transplantation (Budde et al. 1997). Recent studies have indicated that lifestyle can be effective in development of stress, anxiety and psychological pressures, which influence hypertension (Sadeghi et al., 2016; Sadeghi, Shariat, Asadmanesh, & Mosavat, 2013).

There is a clear relationship between sport and leisure activity with resilience and stress (Ma et al. 2013). A recent study (Pooranfar et al. 2014) found that 10 weeks of exercise training improved the quality and quantity of sleep, as well as a number of sleep-related physiological parameters (Shakoor, koushki Jahromi, & Sadeghi, 2015; Shariat, Kargarfard, & Sharifi, 2012) in renal transplant recipients, and would be an effective approach to treat sleep-related disorders (Shariat et al., 2015)in renal transplant recipients. Another study found significant beneficial effects of regular exercise on physical fitness, walking capacity, cardiovascular dimensions (e.g. blood pressure and heart rate), health-related quality of life (Afzalpour et al., 2016), and some nutritional parameters in adults with chronic kidney disease (Heiwe and Jacobson 2011). On the other hand , there is considerable evidence of numerous beneficial effects of physical activity on the health of patients with renal disease (Johansen 2005), which can reduce symptoms of anxiety and depressive symptoms, and promoting mood and feelings of well-being (Mazzoni et al. 2014). Given the above facts, the objective of present study was to evaluate the impact of a 10-week concurrent aerobic and anaerobic exercise program on stress, anxiety, depressive symptoms and hypertension in renal transplant patients.

2. Methods

2.1 Study design and participation

This study utilized a randomized control trial research design. The current study involved an experimental pretest-posttest design with test and control groups. Fifty women patients admitted to Nemazee Hospital in Shiraz, Iran with age range of 20 to 50 years satisfying the conditions of entry into the study (2 to 3 years after renal transplantation) were selected based on targeted purposive sampling, and were randomly divided into exercise (n= 17) and control (n= 17) groups. After selection, all participants read and signed an informed consent form. All participants then completed a questionnaire before examination by a physician to check the medical condition and exclusion criteria. All participations did not consume dietary supplements (e.g. proteins, carbohydrates, amino acids) at least three months before this study (Shariat et al. 2015). The exclusion criteria included cardiovascular problems and chronic diseases (e.g. heart disease, stroke, diabetes, cancer) The inclusion criteria included the ability to walking and low-intensity running on treadmill, and the ability to pedal on cycle ergometer (Ulubay et al. 2006). The participants were not allowed to participate in other physical activity exercises during the study, and both groups were advised to continue with a normal sleep pattern of approximately 8 hours per night for the duration of the experimental study period. This study was in agreement with the principle of Helsinki Declaration and approved by the ethical committee in the Shiraz Medical University, in Iran. Finally, two participants (one in exercise and one in control group) did not finish the intervention due to personal reasons. Therefore, the final sample was 32 females, 16 in the exercise group and 16 in the control group. The progress through the phases of screening, enrolment, allocation, post-testing, and data analysis is illustrated in Figure 1.

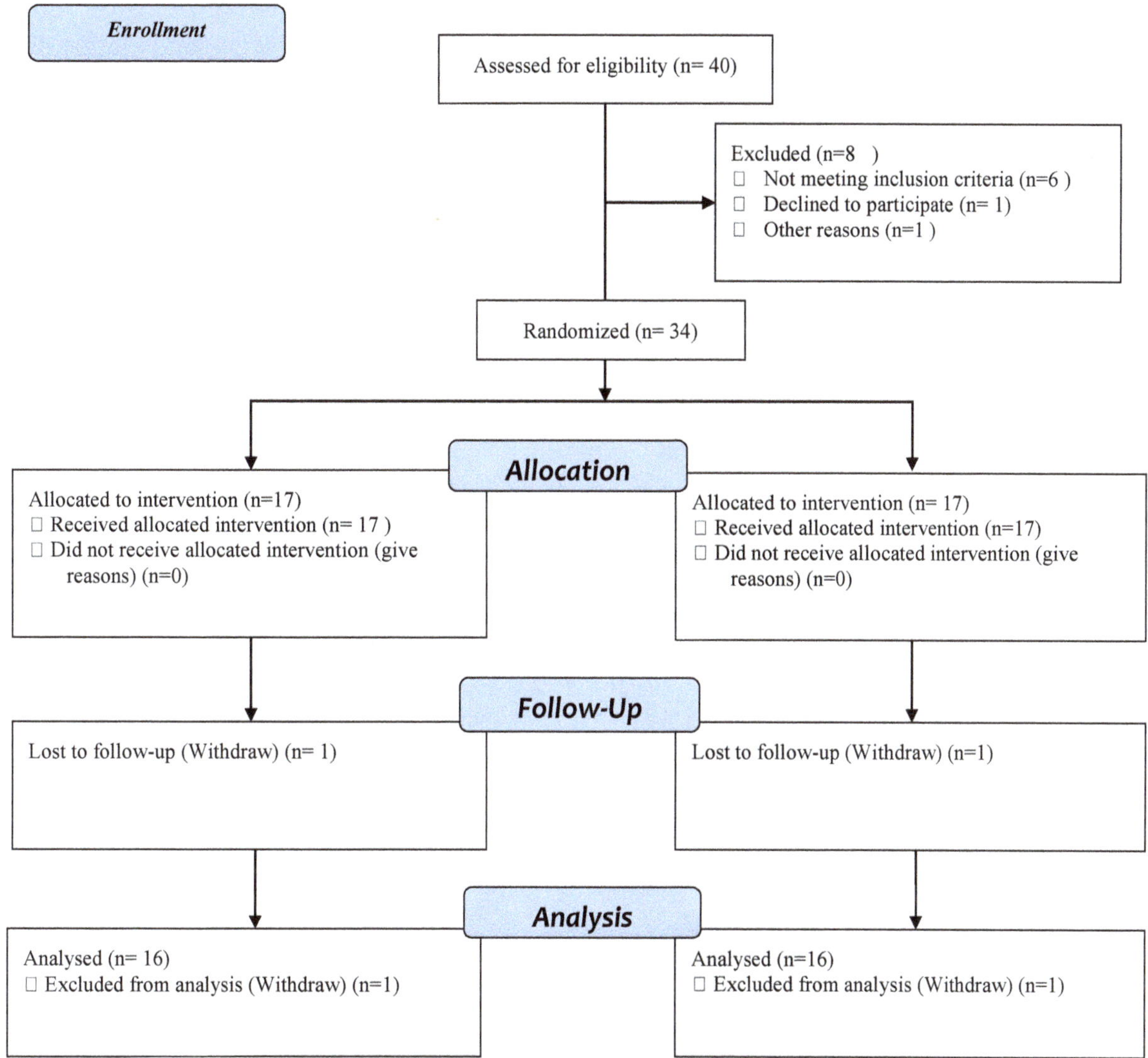

Figure 1. Flow diagram of the progress through the phases of a parallel randomized trial

2.2 The exercise protocol

The test group participants participated in an exercise program for ten weeks. The exercise program was designed by an experienced coach of conditioning under supervision of a certified strength and conditioning specialist (CSCS) with regard to the physical condition of patients in terms of the type, intensity, frequency, and repetition of the exercise after a pilot study verifying the safety, efficiency and simplicity (Gordon et al. 2005; Shariat et al. 2015). The experimental group performed the exercise program for 10 weeks, three sessions per week for 60-90 minutes. Each session included a 15-minute warm-up, 20 minutes of aerobic exercise, 20 minutes of resistance exercise, and a 10-minute cool-down including running with a slow pace followed by stretching and light exercises (Johansen 2005). The control group did not participate in any exercise during the 10-week period. Before and after the exercise protocol Research variables (depressive symptoms, anxiety and stress, and plod pressure) were measured.

The participants performed the main workout for 35-55 minutes between 10 to 12 am in a circuit consisting of 9-17 stations, with 3-6 circles per session, 1-2 minutes of rest between each station, and 3-5 minutes of rest between circles (Pooranfar et al. 2014; Painter et al. 2003) which was a combination of aerobic exercises using a bicycle ergometer (Nautilus, Vancouver, WA, USA), treadmill (Nautilus, Vancouver, WA, USA) and resistance exercises with free weights (Iron Grip Barbell Company, Santa Ana, CA, USA). The aerobic exercise was done on a stationary bicycle or treadmill with 40-70% maximum heart rate and the resistance exercise involved 45- 65% intensity of 1 maximum repetition (1RM). The aerobic exercise was performed with mild- to moderate-intensity corresponding to 40- 60% maximum VO2. After 10 minutes of general warm-up exercises and stretching, the resistance exercise group participants started the testing session. The aerobic exercises were performed for 30 minutes with an increase of 10 minutes in duration every 4 weeks during 10 weeks (Baria et al. 2014; Shakoor et al. 2015).

2.3 Data collection procedure

On the first day of the sampling process, blood pressures of the participants were measured by a sport physiologist after 5 minutes in the sitting position. Blood pressures were also taken 30 minutes before exercise and after 10 weeks of exercise training. The DASS-21 questionnaire (depressive symptoms, anxiety and stress scale (DASS-21), a valid and reliable questionnaire to measure depressive symptoms (Johansen 2005), was completed by each participants, under the supervision of researcher before the exercise protocol and after 10 weeks of exercise. DASS21 is a self-test questionnaire for depressive symptoms, anxiety and stress. It consists of 21 questions in three equal parts (7 items each) concerning each of the indexes under consideration (Salehi Fadardi 2009).

2.4 Statistical analysis

To evaluate the changes in Stress, Anxiety, Depressive symptoms and blood pressure (Systolic and Diastolic) across the experiments, a two way repeated-measure ANOVA with a within-participants factor (pre and post-test) and a between-participants factor (experiment and control) was performed. Analysis of data was performed with the Statistical Package for Social Scientists (SPSS) version 20 (IBM, New York, USA). The Levene test was employed to check sphericity, and normal distribution was verified using the Kolmogorov-Smirnov adaptation test. An α-level of < 0.05 was accepted as statistically significant.

3. Results

The distribution of dependent variables in both groups was subjected to normality testing. Table 1 shows the result of within participants and the interaction. According to the results for all research variables, there were significant differences between pre- and post-test for all variables.

Table1. Result of ANOVA within – between participants effects

Variable	Source	MS	F	p value	$\eta 2$
Stress	test	141.016	25.528	<0.001	0.460
	test * group	165.766	30.008	<0.001	0.500
Anxiety	test	107.641	44.104	<0.001	0.595
	test * group	92.641	37.958	<0.001	0.559
Depression	test	112.891	39.8	<0.001	0.570
	test * group	102.516	36.142	<0.001	0.546
Systolic	test	189.063	3.017	0.093	0.091
	test * group	1806.25	28.828	<0.001	0.490
Diastolic	test	19.141	0.406	0.529	0.013
	test * group	478.516	10.146	0.003	0.253

According to the result of analysis variance, the interaction effect was significant for all variables hence mean comparisons between pre and post-test was performed for all variables separately (Table 2). The results revealed a significant difference between pre and post-test for the exercise group only, while there was no significant difference between pre and post-test for the control group.

Table 2. Bonferroni post hoc test for comparing between and within groups

		Pre test	between groups diff**	Post test	between groups diff	within groups diff*
Variable	**Groups**		**P value**		**P value**	**P value**
Systolic	exercise	124.4± 9.1	0.463	110.3± 9	<0.001	<0.001
	control	126.6± 7.5		133.8± 7.4		.055
Diastolic	exercise	75.9± 11.7	0.271	71.6± 7.9	<0.001	.082
	control	80.3± 7.4		86.9± 7.7		.091
Stress	exercise	11.7± 3.6	0.262	5.5± 2.9	0.001	<0.001
	control	10.1± 4.1		10.4± 4.3		0.766
Anxiety	exercise	7.5± 3.7	0.607	2.5± 2.6	0.009	<0.001
	control	6.7± 5		6.5± 5.1		0.737
Depression	exercise	8.9± 3.8	0.391	3.8± 2.4	0.009	<0.001
	control	7.6± 4.7		7.5± 4.8		0.835

*comparison between pre and posttest, ** comparison between control and exercise, Data is expressed as means ±standard deviations

4. Discussion

The results showed that a round of physical activity including aerobic and anaerobic exercise can reduce systolic blood pressure, stress, anxiety and depressive symptoms in renal transplant patients. One goal of this study was to evaluate the effect of exercise on blood pressure in renal transplant patients. As these patients are usually overweight and have high blood pressure, exercise can be useful to reduce their blood pressure. The results of this study showed that performing 10 weeks of concurrent exercise has a significant effect in reduction of systolic blood pressure. However, with respect to the studies on other participants, the results of our study were consistent with the following studies. Christen and Johansson (Johansen 2005) reported reduced blood pressure after an aerobic exercise in patients with chronic renal failure. In addition, physical activity reduces systolic blood pressure in patients with hypertension. However, Miller et al (Miller et al. 2002) found no significant difference in blood pressure after 6 months of physical activity in hemodialysis patients. The difference between our study and the mentioned studies can be probably attributed to the difference in the intensity and duration of exercise programs as well as the difference between age and sex of participants, the preparation level of participants and their health status. The aerobic exercise programs significantly reduce blood pressure of the kidney patients. some clinical advantage of aerobic and anaerobic exercise has been well-known in hypertensive and normotensive individuals (Nybo et al. 2010) as well as in CKD patients (Boyce et al. 1997). Aerobic exercise lowers blood pressure by reducing peripheral vascular resistance due to the improvement of endothelium-mediated vasodilatation, attenuation of increased sympathetic nervous system activity and vascular remodeling (Baria et al. 2014).

The exact mechanism of the effect of exercise on blood pressure reduction is unknown; although, it may be attributed to catecholamines produced by the exercise. This reaction is involved in reduced peripheral resistance to blood flow and subsequent reduction of blood pressure (Painter et al. 2003; Pooranfar et al. 2014). Physical activity can facilitate the excretion of sodium by the kidneys, resulting in reduced fluid volume and blood pressure. It seems that exercise can reduce blood pressure by increasing the number of capillaries in active skeletal muscle, increased cardiac output, reduced vascular resistance due to dilatation, decreased resistance to blood flow, improved neural regulation of blood vessels, reduced peripheral resistance, decreased heart rate during rest and activity and changes of body weight (Baria et al. 2014). Such adaptations increase the transverse cavity area and result in improved venous dilatation, such that increased blood flow during exercise can trigger the waste removal process, which can be effective in improvement and control of blood pressure (Shinn et al. 2001). In the present study, after data collection and statistical analysis, the results indicated that the level of stress, anxiety and depressive symptoms was lower in renal transplant patients of test group performing the designed exercised program during 10 weeks relative to control group. The results of our study were in line with previous studies (Painter et al. 2002; Heiwe and Jacobson 2011) which asserted that, although exercise plays a positive role in mental health, it is not effective upon anxiety, stress and depressive symptoms. Meanwhile, Hale (1997) reported that physical outdoor activities have not been accepted as an effective intervention strategy by clinical psychologists and psychiatrists. It seems that the differences between results of this research with other studies are related to factors such as the use of different protocols with various variables and exercise intensities, different physical and exercise conditions of participants, nutritional status, mental–emotional status, sex and age. Exercise reduces neural pressures and depressive symptoms in the work ambient. This phenomenon is explained by increased level of serotonin and norepinephrine during exercise activities, which result in depressive symptoms reduction (Smith and Elliott 2003). In other words, physical training affects human spirit in two ways: endorphin release and reduction of cortisol levels (the hormone secreted in blood after stress). According to physiology specialists, endorphins are natural sedative drugs causing pleasant feelings. Physical training increases the level of endorphin secretion. Some researchers concluded that physical training has a considerable effect in increasing the serotonin level (the hormone Effective in upgrading the mood) (Dunn et al. 2005). Thus, exercise seems to cause increased delivery of endorphin and serotonin to body and preservation of it for a longer period during exercise (Anderson and Shivakumar 2013). Higher consumption of antihypertensive drugs and the incidence of side effects of these medications, as well as weakening of the individuals due to gradual complications of such drugs, can be likely reasons for higher prevalence of depressive symptoms over time. the relative frequency of depression in patients treated with antihypertensive drugs was three times higher than those without high blood pressure, and patients suffering from depression are less likely to cooperate with respect to consumption of antihypertensive drugs (Johansen et al. 2012). A number of other studies support the link between depressive symptoms and high blood pressure (Johansen et al. 2012; Marmot 1985). In one study, evaluation of 508 patients over four years showed no correlation between depressive symptoms and hypertension (Shinn et al. 2001). In another study, a 20-year follow-up study showed that patients with symptoms of depression are afflicted with hypertension much more frequently than those without depression (Jonas and Lando 2000). These contradictory findings indicated that the relationship between depression and hypertension can be a bilateral multifactorial relationship, in which a number of factors play the role of predisposing factors and others the supportive role. Recognizing these factors, with the aim of intervention programs, demands further studies with strong methodologies.

5. Conclusion

The present study was designed to determine the effect of 10 weeks concurrent aerobic and anaerobic exercise program can decrease on psychological factor such as stress, anxiety and depressive symptoms reduce systolic blood pressure, in renal transplant patients. The study has gone some way towards enhancing our understanding of exercise program for especial participants or patients. A limitation of this study is that the numbers of patients and controls were relatively small. In addition this study was conducted on female and further research needs to examine.

References

Afzalpour, M. E., Bashafaat, H., Shariat, A., Sadeghi, H., Shaw, I., Dashtiyan, A. A., & Shaw, B. S. (2016). Plasma protein carbonyl responses to anaerobic exercise in female cyclists. *International Journal of Applied Exercise Physiology*, *5*(1), 53–58.

Anderson, E., and Geetha,S,. (2013). Effects of exercise and physical activity on anxiety. *Frontiers in psychiatry* 4 (27):1-4.

Baria, F., Maria A., Danilo T.A., Adriano, A., Mariana, L.R, Marco Túlio,M, and Lilian, C. (2014). Randomized controlled trial to evaluate the impact of aerobic exercise on visceral fat in overweight chronic kidney disease patients. *Nephrology Dialysis Transplantation* 29 (4):857-864.

Boostani, H., and Ali, A. (2014). The comparison of general health status between hemodialysis and kidney transplant patients in university hospitals of Ahvaz, Iran. *Journal of Renal Injury Prevention* 3 (1):27.

Boyce, M.L, Robert A.R., Pratap S.A., Carlos,R., Angelique, F., Paul.,F, Dan, S., and Chris, N. (1997). Exercise training by individuals with predialysis renal failure: cardiorespiratory endurance, hypertension, and renal function. *American Journal of Kidney Diseases* 30 (2):180-192.

Budde, K, J Waiser, L Fritsche, J Zitzmann, M Schreiber, R Kunz, and H-H Neumayer. (1997). Hypertension in patients after renal transplantation. Paper read at Transplantation Proceedings.

Dobbels, F, Melissa A.S, Jon J.S, Anne V.T, J Ross,M., and Bertram, L.K. (2008). Depressive disorder in renal transplantation: an analysis of Medicare claims. *American Journal of Kidney Diseases* 51 (5):819-828.

Dunn, A.L., Madhukar H.T., James B.K, Camillia G, C, and Heather, H. (2005). Exercise treatment for depression: efficacy and dose response. *American journal of preventive medicine* 28 (1):1-8.

Gordon, E.J, Thomas. P, Laura A.S, Peter J.M, and Ashwini R.S. (2005). Needed: tailored exercise regimens for kidney transplant recipients. *American journal of kidney diseases: the official journal of the National Kidney Foundation* 45 (4):769.

Heiwe, S, and Stefan H.J. (2011). Exercise training for adults with chronic kidney disease. *The Cochrane Library*.

Johansen, A, Jostein H, Robert S, and Ottar B. (2012). Anxiety and depression symptoms in arterial hypertension: the influence of antihypertensive treatment. The HUNT study, Norway. *European journal of epidemiology* 27 (1):63-72.

Johansen, K.L. (2005). Exercise and chronic kidney disease. *Sports Medicine* 35 (6):485-499.

Jonas, B. S, and James F.L. (2000). Negative affect as a prospective risk factor for hypertension. *Psychosomatic Medicine* 62 (2):188-196.

Kargarfard, M., Lam, E. T. C., Shariat, A., Shaw, I., Shaw, B. S., & Tamrin, S. B. M. (2016). Efficacy of massage on muscle soreness, perceived recovery, physiological restoration and physical performance in male bodybuilders. *Journal of Sports Sciences*, *34*(10), 959–965.

Kargarfard, M., Shariat, A., Shaw, B. S., Shaw, I., Lam, E. T. C., Kheiri, A., … Tamrin, S. B. M. (2015). Effects of Polluted Air on Cardiovascular and Hematological Parameters After Progressive Maximal Aerobic Exercise. Lung, 193(2), 275–281.

Kasiske,.B.L, Miguel A, William E, Robert S, Gabriel M, Robert S, David R,. (2000). Recommendations for the outpatient surveillance of renal transplant recipients. *Journal of the American Society of Nephrology* 11 (suppl 1):S1-S86.

Ma, L, Hong, L, Yueh-Min, L, Hsiang-Li, H, Lan, L, Mei-Yu, L, and Kuo-Cheng, L. (2013). The relationship between health-promoting behaviors and resilience in patients with chronic kidney disease. *The Scientific World Journal*, 12(3), 76-79.

Magee, C, and Edie, M. (2004). Clinical aspects of renal transplantation. *Brenner BM. Brenner & Rector's The kidney. 7th ed. Philadelphia: WB. Saunders, Elsevier*:2810-6.

Mahdavi-Mazdeh, M. (2012). The Iranian model of living renal transplantation. *Kidney international* 82 (6):627-634.

Marmot, M.G. 1985. Psychosocial factors and blood pressure. *Preventive medicine* 14 (4):451-465.

Masoudi, A, Khadije, Sh, and Zahra, A. (2009). Depression and anxiety in patients undertaken renal replacement therapy in Kashan during 2008. *KAUMS Journal (FEYZ)* 12 (4):46-51.

Mazzoni, D, E Cicognani, G Mosconi, V Totti, GS Roi, M Trerotola, and A Nanni Costa. (2014). Sport Activity and Health-Related Quality of Life After Kidney Transplantation. Paper read at Transplantation Proceedings.

Miller, B.W, Cheryl,L, Mary, E, Darlene, H, and Mark, A. (2002). Exercise during hemodialysis decreases the use of antihypertensive medications. *American Journal of Kidney Diseases* 39 (4):828-833.

Mousavi, S, Soleimani, A and Mousavi,M. 2014. Epidemiology of end-stage renal disease in Iran: A review article. *Saudi Journal of Kidney Diseases and Transplantation* 25 (3):697.

Nybo, L, Emil, S, Markus, D, Magni,M, Therese,H, Lene,S, Jens,B, Morten,B, Jens,J, and Per,A. (2010). High-intensity training versus traditional exercise interventions for promoting health. *Med Sci Sports Exerc* 42 (10):1951-8.

Painter, L, Lisa,H, Karen,R, Liliana,L, Steven,M, Marylin,D, Stephen,L, and Nancy,L. 2003. Effects of exercise training on coronary heart disease risk factors in renal transplant recipients. *American journal of kidney diseases* 42 (2):362-369.

Painter, P, Lisa,H, Karen,R, Liliana,L, Suzanne,D, Steven,P, Stephen,T, and Nancy,L. (2002). A randomized trial of exercise training after renal transplantation. *Transplantation* 74 (1):42-48.

Pooranfar, S, E Shakoor, MJ Shafahi, M Salesi, MH Karimi, J Roozbeh, and M Hasheminasab. (2014). The Effect of Exercise Training on Quality and Quantity of Sleep and Lipid Profile in Renal Transplant Patients: A Randomized Clinical Trial. *International journal of organ transplantation medicine* 5 (4):157.

Rigatto, C, Robert,N, Gloria,M, Ronald, G, and Patrick,S. 2000. Long-term changes in left ventricular hypertrophy after renal transplantation. *Transplantation* 70 (4):570-575.

Sadeghi, H., Hakim, M. N., Hamid, T. A., Amri, S. Bin, Razeghi, M., Farazdaghi, M., & Shakoor, E. (2016). The Effect of Exergaming on Knee Proprioception in Older Men: A Randomized Controlled Trial. Archives of Gerontology and Geriatrics.

Sadeghi, H., Shariat, A., Asadmanesh, E., & Mosavat, M. (2013). The Effects of Core Stability Exercise on the Dynamic Balance of Volleyball Players. *International Journal of Applied Exercise Physiology*, *2*(2), 1–10.

Salehi,F, J. 2009. A comparative study of anxiety, stress, and depression in physically abused and non-abused Iranian wives. *Iranian Journal of Psychiatry and Behavioral Sciences* 3.

Shakoor, E, Maryam,K., Mohsen,S, and Hassan, S. 2015. The Effects of 10 Weeks Concurrent Aerobic and Strength Exercise on Quality of Life and Resilience of Kidney Transplant Patients. *International Journal of Applied Exercise Physiology* 4 (2):1-8.

Shariat, A., Bahri Mohd Tamrin, S., Daneshjoo, A., & Sadeghi, H. (2015). The Adverse Health Effects of Shift Work in Relation to Risk of Illness/Disease: A Review. *Acta Medica Bulgarica*, *42*(1), 63–72.

Shariat, A., Kargarfard, M., & Sharifi, G. R. (2012). The effect of heavy resistance exercise on circadian rhythm of salivary cortisol in male body building athletes. *Journal of Isfahan Medical SchooL (I.U.M.S)*, *29*, 2400–2412.

Shariat, A, Kargarfard,M., Danaee, M., and Tamrin, SBM. (2015). Intensive resistance exercise and circadian salivary testosterone concentrations among young male recreational lifters. *The Journal of Strength & Conditioning Research* 29 (1):151-158.

Shinn, E., Walker,S., Kay, T., Sachik, T, and John, P. (2001). Blood pressure and symptoms of depression and anxiety: a prospective study*. *American Journal of Hypertension,* 14 (7), 660-664.

Smith, LL, and CH Elliott. 2003. Demystifying and defeating depression. *Depression for dummies. New Jersey, NJ: Wiley.*

Sorensen, E, Mark,J, Hocine, T., Tammy, S., Lena,M., Bethany,K., Kristina,L., and Daniel,E,. (2012). The kidney disease quality of life cognitive function subscale and cognitive performance in maintenance hemodialysis patients. *American Journal of Kidney Diseases,* 60 (3), 417-426.

Spitzer, A, and Ellis,D. (2012). *Inheritance of kidney and urinary tract diseases*. Vol. 9: Springer Science & Business Media.

Ulubay, G., B. Akman, S. Sezer, K. Calik, F. Eyuboglu Oner, N. Ozdemir, and M. Haberal. (2006). Factors Affecting Exercise Capacity in Renal Transplantation Candidates on Continuous Ambulatory Peritoneal Dialysis Therapy. *Transplantation Proceedings,* 38 (2), 401-405.

19

Inter-observer Reliability of a Real-time Observation Tool in Handball

Iván González-García (Corresponding author)
Faculty of Education and Sport Sciences, University of Vigo
A Xunqueira Campus, Pontevedra, Spain
E-mail: ivanglezgarcia@uvigo.es

Luis Casáis Martínez
Faculty of Education and Sport Sciences, University of Vigo
A Xunqueira Campus, Pontevedra, Spain
E-mail: luisca@uvigo.es

Jorge Viaño Santasmarinas
Faculty of Education and Sport Sciences, University of Vigo
A Xunqueira Campus, Pontevedra, Spain
E-mail: jorgeviano@uvigo.es

Miguel A. Gómez Ruano
Faculty of Physical Activity and Sport Sciences, University of Madrid
Central building, 7th floor, Madrid, Spain
E-mail: miguelangel.gomez.ruano@upm.es

Abstract

Background: The analysis of the competition in real time is currently one of the most important aspects to develop the sport. The purpose of the analysis should be creating valid and reliable knowledge for coaches to make the best decisions in a situation of competition. **Objectives:** This study was to determine the inter-observer reliability of the real-time observation tool for handball. **Methods:** Two groups of two observers each one were required to analyze the men's handball final of the London 2012 Olympic Games (average age: 23.72 ± 2.16 years; experience as handball players: 14.69 ± 1.92 years; experience as coaches: 4.64 ± 4.04 years). The process of training of the observers lasted 22 days, accounting twelve hours of work distributed in 12 training sessions. **Results:** The reliability showed a very good agreement between the independent observers (Kappa values were 0.96 and 0.90) in the registered events of both teams, and a very good agreement (Kappa values were 0.85 and 0.94) of the registered actions of the goalkeepers. The high coefficient of intra-class correlation with a value of 0.98 and the low value of the standard error with a 0.11 of the actions of the players of both teams showed a high level of inter-observer reliability. **Conclusions:** These results showed that the tool of observation in handball is reliable for registering the events of a real time match by well-trained observers. With the help of the HandballTAS and using technology, large volumes of real-time data were collected in a simple and easily usable.

Keywords: handball; reliability; performance indicators; real time; game analysis

1. Introduction

Observational analysis during teams and players′ performance is essential for the tasks design, organization, teaching methods, and improving training in team sports (Hughes & Franks, 1997; Hughes & Bartlett, 2002). Many of the studies in handball have used tools of observation for data collection during a match, such as the Handball Match Analysis Computerized Notation System (Krusinskiene & Skarbalius, 2002), the Pictorial Handball Match Statistics (Gruić, Vuleta, & Milanovič, 2006; Volossovitch & Gonçalves, 2003; Zhiwen et al., 2005), the Swiss Timing Handball

(Pokrajac, 2008; Taborsky, 2008), the Utilius vs Handball (Poehler, 2007) and the Interplay Sports Handball 2.1 (Hordvik, 2011).

Other studies in handball have validated: i) a system for observing the players´ decision making (Martín et al., 2013); ii) a tool for the study of the players and teams´ dynamics during single games (Prudente, Garganta, & Anguera, 2004); iii) a system about the observation of coaches' behaviour (Tzioumakis et al., 2009); or iv) the explosive strength of the shot from different zones of the field (Vuleta et al., 2010).

Most of the methods of performance analysis were not based on automated techniques of data entry. Human errors during the compilation of data can limit the reliability of the methods used (O´Donoghue, 2007). Validity and reliability in performance analysis is essential to meet its purposes with efficiency. However, this scientific base has not been fully established and controlled for in many of the studies (Tenga et al., 2009).

Reliability refers to the reproducibility of values of a test, assay or other measurement in repeated trial on the same individuals (Hopkins, 2000a). It is defined as a characteristic of the measurement or the experimental procedure in which the same results take place in two or more separate occasions (Kent, 1994).

The tests of reliability in the analysis of sports performance are used to assess the agreement between the observers and to guarantee the objectivity of the process of data gathering (Berry, Johnston, & Mielke, 2008; Choi, O'Donoghue, & Hughes, 2007; Cooper et al., 2007; Hughes, Cooper, & Nevill, 2004; Lames & McGarry, 2007; Nevill et al., 2002; O'Donoghue, 2007; Robinson & O'Donoghue, 2007). This is essential for the development of studies in sport contexts, bringing the validity and objectivity that are necessary in the scientific field.

Inter-observer consistency allows establishing the objectivity of the system and proving that it can be used to collect data from observations independently of the individual perception of the encoder. There are two crucial prerequisites to obtain a sufficient level of reliability of the data collected in the research. On the one hand, measuring reliability and validity among observers with a suitable instrument; and on the other hand, training the observers in a systematic and coherent way to achieve good results in these measurements (O´Donoghue, 2010).

Therefore, the aim of this study is to determine the reliability inter-observer of the real-time observation tool in handball HandballTAS (Handball Tactic Analysis System).

2. Methods

2.1 Sample

The match chosen as the subject of the current inter-observer reliability study was the men's handball final of the London 2012 Olympic Games that took place on the 12th of August, 2012 between Sweden and France. A total of 22 players from both teams were involved in the match. The criteria proposed by Heinemann (2003), by which the object of the research study is accessible using the recording of matches for the data collection, were taken into account.

The observation was carried out by four observers (average age: 23.72 ± 2.16 years). They had experience as handball players for 14.69 ± 1.92 years and experience as coaches in lower categories for 4.64 ± 4.04 years. The process of training of the observers lasted 22 days, from 14/11/2013, up to 5/12/2013 accounting twelve hours of work distributed in 12 training sessions.

In every training session the observers were subjected to the same conditions: (i) the observer is isolated in a room to keep the intra-sessional connection; and (ii) at the same time and in the same place in stable conditions and without the presence of any person with the intention to avoid interferences, with the exception of the researcher.

Four observers were required to analyze the game independently: two observer registered the team of Sweden (observer 1 and observer 2), and two observers registered the team of France (observer 3 and observer 4).

2.2 Software and taking of data

The software has been designed to register the individual actions of the players during a handball match in real time. The process to evaluate the inter-observer reliability was similar to the study of Liu et al. (2013) used to evaluate the inter-observers reliability of a live football match using Opta Sportdata. Previous research has studied the effectiveness of handball teams through record of offensive and defensive players actions (Balint & Curiţianu, 2012; Bilge, 2012; Meletakos, Vagenas, & Bayios, 2011; Rogulj, Srhoj, & Srhoj, 2004; Srhoj et al., 2001; Yamada et al., 2014).

To analyze the reliability of the software, the individual actions of the players were divided in two groups: (1) actions related to the attack: received free-throw, assist, turnover, throw-in, committed steps, committed illegal dribble, committed offensive foul, committed entering the goal area goal, throw block, caused yellow card, caused exclusion, caused disqualification, shot with opposition, and shot without opposition; (2) actions related with the defense: committed free-throw, overcome by direct opponent, steal, committed throw-in, caused steps, caused illegal dribble, caused offensive foul, caused entering the goal area, blocked shot, committed yellow card, committed exclusion, and committed disqualification. El registro de estas acciones durante un partido tiene como ventaja el aumento del conocimiento del juego y la disposición de esa información inmediatamente para que el entrenador pueda aumentar la eficacia de sus intervenciones. The record of these actions during a match has the advantage of increasing the knowledge of the game and the disposition of such information immediately in order that the coach could increase the effectiveness of their interventions.

The software is presented on a touchscreen mobile device (tablet) in order to register all events in real time as quickly and easily as possible (see Figure 1). Before beginning with the record of events, the general information of the match is annotated: name of observer, date, hour, place, championship, phase, match time and period. To take the record the individual offensive and defensive actions of systematic form every action is associated with a number of a player. If the player throws the ball, the degree of opposition (with opposition or without opposition), the result (goal, save, out or post), the location and the area of the field from where the throw occurs are noted down. All actions are associated with a numerical situation (equality, superiority, inferiority or forewarning signal passive play) at a particular time of a match.

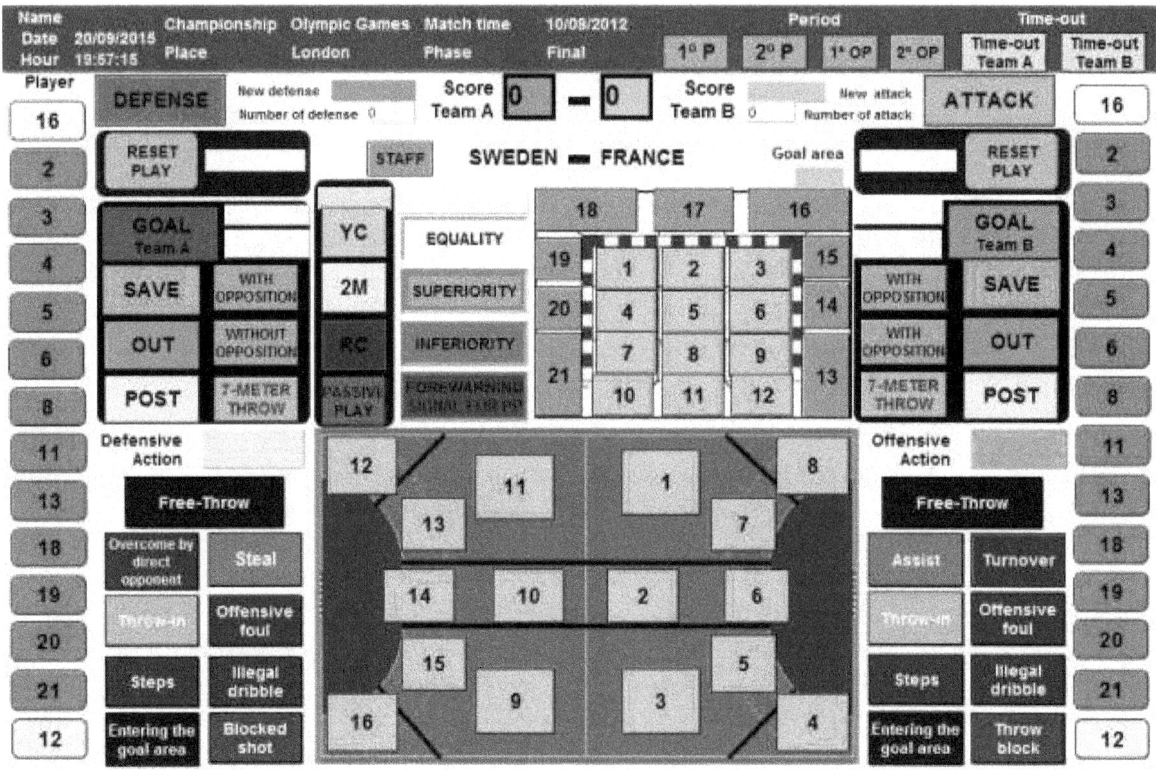

Figure 1. Buttons of the different actions of the HandballTAS

2.3 Actions registered with the tool

The following actions were defined and described in order to clarifying the data gathering:

Yellow card: Awarded by the referee to a player as a result of a fault or unsportsmanlike behavior.

Assist: Technical action of an attacking player who passes the ball to a teammate without opposition in a way that leads to score a goal.

Attack: The team has the possession of the ball in its own field or in the opponet´s field, and the attack phase begins.

Forewarning signal for passive play: The referee indicates the warning of passive play when a team does not have the intention of attacking or to throw to the goal.

Blocked shot: Technical action of a defending player who intercepts the trajectory of the ball in a throwing on goal.

Defense: The team loses the ball possession, beginning their defense phase.

Disqualification: Red card awarded by the referee to a player due to an unsportsmanlike behavior.

Illegal dribble: Offensive action in which the team loses the possession of the ball due to an infraction of the rules of the game.

Exclusion: Exclusion of a player for 2 minutes indicated by the referee due to repeated fouls, unsporting conduct, an incorrect change, or as a result of a disqualification.

Offensive foul: Infraction made by a player as a result of a foul on a defender indicated by the referee. The team loses the possession of the ball.

Throw-in: A player sends the ball out of the field of play.

Out: The throw on goal finishes out of the goal boundaries.

Goal: Throw on goal that crosses the goal line.

Free-throw: A defender commits an infraction on an attacker, and then the referees stop the game indicating a free-throw.

Equality: Game situation in which the same number of players on both teams are present on the field of play.

Inferiority: Game situation in which a smaller number of players of the team observed are present on the field of play.

Interruption: Game situation in which the attack or defense of the team observed is stopped as a result of a free-throw, out of play, a time-out or any circumstance in which the game is stopped.

Entering the goal area: Action in which a player invades the goal area.

Passive play: The referee indicates passive game when the team in possession of the ball does not change its way of attacking or does not execute a throwing after the referee has indicated the warning of passive play.

Throw block: Throwing directed to goal but neutralized following the rules by a defender before the goalkeeper can intercept it.

Shot with opposition: Action of throwing to goal following the rules with at least a defender in the shot line.

Shot without opposition: Action of throwing to goal following the rules without any defenders in the shot line.

Save: Throwing that the goalkeeper neutralizes so that the ball does not cross the goal line.

Steps: Offensive action in which the team loses the possession of the ball due to an infraction of the player with the ball. The referee indicates the steps hand-signal.

Turnover: The attacking team loses the possession of the ball and the defending team takes the possession of the ball.

Post: Shot that directly touches one of the goalposts. If the ball touches the post after a save of the goalkeeper, it is considered a goalkeeper's save. If the ball touches the goalposts and later crosses the goal line, it is considered a goal.

Steal: The defensive team recovers the possession of the ball and the offensive team loses the possession of ball.

Overcome by direct opponent: Defensive action in which the defensive player is overcome by an attacker with ball possession using a displacement, feint or fixation. Surpassing an adversary in the one to one action is considered to be overcome by the direct opponent.

Superiority: Game situation in which there is a higher number of players of the team observed on the field of play.

7-meter throw: Action of a defender against the rules that destroys a clear goal chance of an attacker. The referee then indicates the corresponding infraction.

2.4 Statistical analysis

The events of both teams and the actions of the goalkeepers were compared between the two groups of observers using the *Cohen's Kappa (k),* which determines the proportion of cases in which there is agreement among observers once excluded the proportion of cases in which the agreement between them is a consequence of chance (Robinson & O´Donoghue 2007). The *Kappa* values can range from - 1.0 to 1.0. The agreement in the interpretation of the *Kappa* value was valued as follows: <0 less than the possibility of agreement; 0.01-0.20 poor agreement; 0.21-0.40 fair agreement; 0.41-0.60 moderate agreement; 0.61-0.80 good agreement; 0.81-0.99 very good agreement (Altman, 1991; O´Donoghue, 2010; Viera & Garret, 2005).

Absolute reliability values (mean, change in the mean, standardized typical error and the intra-class correlation coefficient) of different individual actions of the players were calculated using the spreadsheet developed by Hopkins (2000b). Each team was registered by two independent observers. Therefore, there were two groups of values of absolute reliability, on the one hand Swedish players and on the other hand, French players. The results presented below were the average of the two groups. The value of the standardized typical error should be doubled and their levels of disagreement are as follows: <0.20 trivial; 0.21-0.60 small; 0.61-1.20 moderate; 1.21-2.00 large; 2.01-4.00 very large; >4.00 extremely large (Hopkins, 2000a; Smith & Hopkins, 2011).

3. Results

Table 1 shows 864 events agreed by the two groups of independent observers, 437 for Sweden and 427 for France. The *Kappa* values of the two teams' events were 0.90 and 0.96 respectively, which showed a very good agreement between independent observers.

Table 1. Agreement of team events registered by independent observers

Teams	**Agreed Events**	**Events registered by Observer 1**		**Events registered by Observer 2**		***Kappa* Value**
		Total	Disagreed	Total	Disagreed	
Sweden	437	449	3	440	12	0.96
France	427	447	20	447	20	0.90

The table 2 shows that there were 202 goalkeepers' actions observed for both groups, 98 for Johan Sjöstrand and 104 for Thierry Omeyer. The *Kappa* values of the goalkeeper's actions were 0.85 and 0.94 respectively, which also showed very good agreement between observers.

Table 2. Agreement of goalkeeper actions registered by independent observers

Players	**Agreed Events**	**Events registered by Observer 1**		**Events registered by observer 2**		***Kappa* Value**
		Total	Disagreed	Total	Disagreed	
Johan Sjostrand	98	110	2	100	12	0.85
Thierry Omeyer	104	104	5	109	0	0.94

Standardized typical errors of the different individual actions of the players from both teams were recorded by independent observers with a value of 0.11 (Table 3). The intra-class correlation index, with a value of 0.98, shows high levels of reliability.

Table 3. Reliability of the actions of the players involved in the match registered by the independent observers

Indicators	**Mean ± SD**	**Change in the mean ± confidence limits**	**Standardized typical error**	**Intra-class correlation** (ICC)
Attacking related actions	7.4 ± 8.1	0.08 ± 0.46	0.11	0.98
Defending related actions	5.1 ± 7.5	-0.48 ± 0.52	0.12	0.98
Total actions	6.3 ± 7.8	-0.14 ± 0.31	0.11	0.98

* Confidence limits of standardized typical error are the factors ×/÷ 1.35

Table 4 showed the absolute reliability of performance indicators of the players who took part in the observed match. Standardized typical errors are located in a range from 0 to 0.55, and the intra-class correlation coefficients varied from 0.77 to 1.00, showing a good level of reliability.

Table 4. Reliability of individual players' key performance indicators coded by the independent observers

Indicators	Mean ± SD	Change in the mean ± confidence limits	Standardized typical error	Intra-class correlation (ICC)
Received Free-throw	2.3 ± 2.5	0.14 ± 0.21	0.13	0.98
Assist	1.2 ± 1.5	-0.05 ± 0.23	0.23	0.95
Turnover	0.5 ± 0.9	0.00 ± 0.19	0.24	0.96
Committed throw-in	0.1 ± 0.3	0.00 ± 0.00	0.00	1.00
Committed steps	0.1 ± 0.4	0.05 ± 0.29	0.42	0.86
Committed offensive foul	0.3 ± 0.6	0.05 ± 0.14	0.26	0.96
Committed Entering the Goal Area	0.2 ± 0.4	0.05 ± 0.17	0.42	0.95
Throw block	0.1 ± 0.3	0.00 ± 0.00	0.00	1.00
Caused yellow card	0.2 ± 0.4	-0.09 ± 0.24	0.51	0.90
Caused exclusion	0.3 ± 0.5	0.00 ± 0.00	0.00	1.00
Shot with opposition	1.5 ± 2.1	0.05 ± 0.37	0.24	0.95
Shot without opposition	1.3 ± 1.7	-0.09 ± 0.20	0.18	0.97
Committed Free-throw	2.3 ± 2.4	-0.09 ± 0.30	0.21	0.96
Overcome by Direct Opponent	0.5 ± 1.1	-0.23 ± 0.33	0.34	0.92
Steal	0.5 ± 0.8	0.00 ± 0.18	0.27	0.94
Throw-in	0.1 ± 0.3	0.00 ± 0.00	0.00	1.00
Caused steps	0.1 ± 0.3	0.00 ± 0.00	0.00	1.00
Caused offensive foul	0.3 ± 0.6	0.00 ± 0.27	0.55	0.77
Caused Entering the Goal Area	0.2 ± 0.4	0.00 ± 0.23	0.54	0.82
Blocked shot	0.1 ± 0.3	0.00 ± 0.00	0.00	1.00
Committed yellow card	0.2 ± 0.4	-0.05 ± 0.16	0.36	0.94
Committed exclusion	0.3 ± 0.4	0.05 ± 0.16	0.35	0.94

* *Confidence limits of standardized typical error are the factors ×/÷ 1.35*

4. Discussion

The high *Kappa* values, intra-class correlation coefficients, and the low standardized typical errors show a high level of inter-observer reliability using the *HandballTAS*. The degree of reliability and validity among independent observers show that the instrument is suitable for the record of the actions in real time. Likewise, observers have undergone systematic and consistent training to achieve good results during the observational measurements (O´Donoghue, 2010).

Another technological tool used in handball is the one presented by Martín et al. (2011), and Martín et al. (2013) developing a program to observe decision making of the player based on the instrument validated by Oslin et al. (1998). Those authors developed and validated the *Game Performance Assessment Instrument (GPAI).* Validity and reliability are examined through three separate studies using middle school physical education specialists and their sixth-grade classes. The stability-reliability coefficient showed, as this study does, a high level of reliability. The soccer, basketball, and volleyball correlation coefficients ranged from 0.84 to 0.97, from 0.84 to 0.99, and from 0.85 to 0.97, respectively.

Lozano & Camerino (2012), designed an instrument of observation with syntactic rules and codes (Fernández et al., 2009; Jönsson et al., 2006) to know the variables involved in offensive efficiency in handball. The degree of inter-observer agreements using the Cohen's *Kappa* coefficient was of 0.95, a similar value to the present study.

It is necessary to know the actions that generate a greater disagreement by the independent observers (Liu et al., 2013). According to Bradley et al. (2007), the disagreed events mainly came from misrecognizing individual players. For example, during defensive situation it is not easy to differentiate who commits an area of goal invasion foul when there are several players inside the goal area. One of the actions with greater disagreement among the observers is the offensive foul. In addition, the intra-class correlation coefficients of committed steps, enters of goal area and caused offensive foul were the lowest ones, while their standardized typical errors were the highest ones. These findings may be due to the fact that their records were much lower compared to other actions and performance indicators.

5. Conclusion

The present study demonstrates that the method of record using the instrument of observation *HandballTAS* has a high inter-observer reliability. The statistics generated by the instrument of observation can be valid for subsequent research studies. With the help of the observational instrument and using technology, large volumes of real-time data are collected in a simple and easily notation system. The data obtained showed that only two observers are able to make valid and reliable data form using the *HandballTAS* for a handball match.

References

Altman D.G. (1991). *Practical Statistics for Medical Research.* London: Chapman & Hall.

Balint E., & Curiţianu E. (2012). The importance of anticipation in increasing the defense efficiency in high performance handball. *Bulletin of the Transilvania University of Braşov, 5 (54)* (1), 103-112.

Berry K.J., Johnston J.E., & Mielke Jr. P.W. (2008). Weighted kappa for multiple raters. *Perceptual and Motor Skills,* 107(3): 837-848.

Bilge, M. (2012). Game analysis of Olympic, World and European Championships in Men´s Handball. *Journal of Human Kinetics, 35,* 109-118.

Bradley P., O'Donoghue P., Wooster B., & Tordoff, P. (2007). The reliability of ProZone MatchViewer: A video-based technical performance analysis system. *International Journal Performance Analysis in Sport,* 7(3): 117-129.

Choi H., O'Donoghue P., & Hughes M. (2007). An investigation of inter-operator reliability tests for real-time analysis system. *International Journal of Performance Analysis in Sport,* 7(1): 49-61.

Cooper S., Hughes M., O'Donoghue P., & Nevill A.M. (2007). A simple statistical method for assessing the reliability of data entered into sport performance analysis systems. *International Journal of Performance Analysis in Sport*, 7(1): 87-109.

Fernández J., Camerino O., Anguera M.T., & Jonsson G.K. (2009). Identifying and analyzing the construction and effectiveness of offensive plays in basketball by using systematic observation. *Behavior Research Methods,* 41(3): 719-730.

Gruič I., Vuleta D., & Milanovič D. (2006). Performance indicators of teams at the 2003 Men's World Handball Championship in Portugal. *Kinesiology,* 38(2): 164-173.

Heinemann K. (2003). *Introducción a la Metodología de la Investigación Empírica en las Ciencias del Deporte.* Barcelona: Paidotribo.

Hopkins W.G. (2000a). Measures of reliability in sports medicine and science. *Sport Medicine,* 30: 1-15.

Hopkins W.G. (2000b). Reliability for consecutive pair of trials (excel spreadsheet). In: A new view of statistics. Available at Sportsci.org: Internet Society for Sport Science. Sportsci.org/resource/stats/xrely.xls; accessed on 24.01.2014

Hordvik M.M. (2011). *Læring gjennom videofeedback: Et aksjonsforskningsprosjekt om hvordan anvende video for å bidra til eget lags utvikling.* Norway: Thesis Unpublished, Department of Coaching and Psychology.

Hughes M., & Franks I. (1997). *Notational Analysis of Sport.* London: E & FN Spon.

Hughes M., Cooper S., & Nevill A. (2004). Analysis of notation data: Reliability. *Notational Analysis of Sport: System for Better Coaching and Performance in Sport,* 2: 189-205.

Hughes M.D., & Bartlett R.M. (2002). The use of performance indicators in performance analysis. *Journal of Sports Sciences,* 20(10): 739-754.

Jonsson G.K., Anguera M.T., Blanco-Villaseñor Á., Losada J.L., Hernández-Mendo A., Ardá T, ... & Castellano J. (2006). Hidden patterns of play interaction in soccer using SOF-CODER. *Behavior Research Methods,* 38(3): 372-381.

Kent M. (1994). *The Oxford Dictionary of Sports Sciences and Medicine.* Oxford: Oxford University Press.

Krusinskiene R., & Skarbalius A. (2002). Handball match analysis: Computerized notation system. *Ugdymas, Kuno Cultura, Sportas,* 3(44): 23-33.

Lames M., & McGarry T. (2007). On the search for reliable performance indicators in game sports. *International Journal of Performance Analysis in Sport,* 7(1): 62-79.

Liu H., Hopkins W., Gómez M.A., & Molinuevo J.S. (2013). Inter-operator reliability of live football match statistics from Opta Sportsdata. *International Journal of Performance Analysis in Sport,* 13: 803-821.

Lozano D., & Camerino O. (2012). Eficacia de los sistemas ofensivos en balonmano. *Apunts. Educación Física y Deportes,* 2(108): 66-77.

Martín I., Cavalcanti L.A., Chirosa L.J., & Aguilar J. (2011). El programa PROTODEBA v.1.0. Una proposta per a l´observació de la presa de decisions en hándbol. *Apunts. Educación Física y Deportes,* 2(104): 80-87.

Martín I., González A., Cavalcanti L.A., Chirosa L.J., & Aguilar J. (2013). Fiabilidad y optimización del programa PROTODEBA v 1.0 para la observación de la toma de decisiones en balonmano. *Cuadernos de Psicología del Deporte,* 13(1): 63-70.

Meletakos P., Vagenas G., & Bayios I. (2011). A multivariate assessment of offensive performance indicators in Men's Handball: Trends and differences in the World Championships. *Internacional Journal of Performance Analysis in Sport, 11*(2), 284-294.

Nevill A.M., Atkinson G., Hughes M.D., & Cooper S. (2002). Statistical methods for analysing discrete and categorical data recorded in performance analysis. *Journal of Sports Sciences,* 20(10), 829-844.

O´Donoghue P. (2010). *Research Methods for Sports Performance Analysis*. Oxon: Routledge.

O'Donoghue P. (2007). Reliability issues in performance analysis. *International Journal of Performance Analysis in Sport,* 7(1): 35-48.

Oslin J.L., Mitchell S.A., & Griffin L.L. (1998). The game performance assessment instrument (GPAI): Development and preliminary validation. *Journal of Teaching in Physical Education,* 17: 231-243.

Poehler C. (2007). The use of utilius® VS for the diagnosis of tactical modes of behaviour in team hand-ball. *Leistungssport,* 37(2): 29-32.

Pokrajak B. (2008). EHF Men´s Euro 2008 - analysis, discussion, comparison, tendencies in modern handball. *EHF Web Periodical,* 1-15.

Prudente J., Garganta J., & Anguera M.T. (2004). Desenho e validação de um sistema de observação no andebol. *Revista Portuguesa de Ciências do Desporto,* 4(3): 49-65.

Robinson G., & O'Donoghue P. (2007). A weighted kappa statistics for reliability testing in performance analysis of sport. *International Journal of Performance Analysis in Sport,* 7(1): 12-19.

Rogulj N., Srhoj V., & Srhoj L. (2004). The contribution of collective attack tactics in diffentiating handballl store efficiency. *Collegium Antropologicum, 28*(2), 739-746.

Smith T.B., & Hopkins W.G. (2011). Variability and predictability of finals times of elite rowers. *Medicine Science in Sports & Exercise,* 43: 2155-60.

Srhoj V., Rogulj N., Padovan M., & Katić R. (2001). Influence of the attack end conduction on match result in handball. *Collegium Antropologicum, 25*(2), 611-617.

Taborsky F. (2008). Cumulative indicators of team playing performance in handball (Olympic Games tournaments 2008). *EHF Web Periodical,* 1-10.

Tenga A., Kanstad D., Ronglan L., & Bahr R. (2009). Developing a new method for team match performance analysis in professional soccer and testing its reliability. *International Journal of Performance Analysis in Sport,* 9(1): 8-25.

Tzioumakis Y., Michalopoulou M., Aggelousis N., Papaioannou A., & Christodoulidis T. (2009). Youth coaches behavior assessment through systematic observation. *Inquiries in Sport & Physical Education,* 7(3): 344-354.

Viera A.J., & Garrett J.M. (2005). Understanding inter-observer agreement: The kappa statistic. *Family Medicine,* 37: 360-363.

Volossovitch A., & Gonçalves I. (2003). The significance of game indicators for winning and losing team in handball. *E. Müller, H. Schwameder, G. Zallinger, & V. Fastenbauer (Eds.), Proceedings of the 8th Annual Congress of European College of Sport Science,* Salzburg: ECSS, 335.

Vuleta D., Sporiš G., Talović M., & Jelešković E. (2010). Reliability and factorial validity of power tests for handball players. *Sport Science,* 3(1): 42-46.

Yamada E., Aida H., Fujimoto H., & Nakagawa A. (2014). Comparison of game performance among European National Women's Handball Teams. *International Journal of Sport and Health Science, 12*, 1-10.

Zhiwen L., Wei Z., Jianming L., & Jiale T. (2005). The official scouting system of International Handball Federation. In *International Association for Sport Information (Eds.), the Value of Sports Information: Toward Beijing 2008, Proceedings of the 12th IASI World Congress,* Beijing, China: 62-66.

20

Influenza A Vaccination Knowledge, Attitude, Practice of Athletes Competing in Canadian Interuniversity Sport in Calgary, Alberta

Janell Lautermilch
Faculty of Medicine, University of Calgary
2500 University Drive, Calgary, T2N 1N4, Canada
E-mail: jtlauter@gmail.com

Tak Fung
Research Consulting Services, Information Technologies, University of Calgary
2500 University Drive, Calgary, T2N 1N4, Canada
E-mail: tfung@ucalgary.ca

Andrew Stewart
Faculty of Kinesiology, University of Calgary
2500 University Drive, Calgary, T2N 1N4, Canada
E-mail: stewaraj@ucalgary.ca

Patricia K. Doyle-Baker (Corresponding Author)
Faculty of Kinesiology, University of Calgary
2500 University Drive, Calgary, T2N 1N4, Canada
E-mail: pdoyleba@ucalgary.ca

Abstract

Objective: To assess the knowledge, attitude and practice (KAP) of Canadian Interuniversity Sport (CIS) athletes regarding influenza A vaccination. **Design:** Cross-sectional survey. Setting: University of Calgary. Participants: The CIS athlete (N=450) population was sampled by convenience (n=177, mean age 20.4 ± 2.2 years) and compared to non-athlete kinesiology students (n=34, 21.06 ± 2.7 years of age). Independent variable: Vaccination history. **Main outcome measures:** A frequency analysis was employed to describe the KAP of each group. Groups were compared by χ^2 or Kruskal-Wallis analysis. **Results:** Over half of athletes were aware of influenza vaccination safety, effectiveness and side effects. Athletes were significantly more concerned about contracting the virus due to potential consequences, such as an interruption of training and infection of teammates, compared to non-athletes ($p<0.05$). Nearly one third (29.2%) of athletes reported vaccination participation. **Conclusion:** The vaccination participation of CIS athletes is low when requirements for herd immunity are considered.

Keywords*:* Athletes, university students, influenza, influenza A, knowledge, attitude, practice

1. Introduction

Influenza is a widespread acute respiratory ailment that affects the lives of millions of Canadians each year (Health Canada, 2013). The severity of the illness ranges from an asymptomatic infection to death in the most extreme cases (World Health Organization [WHO], 2011). However, most commonly, influenza infection results in an acute illness that persists for approximately one week, with malaise and cough lingering for an additional week (WHO, 2011). The World Health Organization (WHO) indicates that people at any age with immunocompromised conditions are at a higher risk for hospitalization associated with infection of the flu (WHO, 2011).

Influenza A is a known subtype of influenza and has been reported to be responsible for causing several respiratory epidemics including the recent H1N1 flu outbreak in 2009, which was highly contagious in nature (WHO, 2011). According to the WHO (2011), these recent increases in rates of influenza infection have resulted in rises in respiratory infirmity, physician appointments, hospitalizations and even deaths leading to escalating estimates in the virus's overall health burden. The influenza vaccine is associated with a decrease in respiratory symptoms, physician appointments across all age groups, hospitalizations and deaths among people at high risk, and missed work days in adults (WHO, 2011). Influenza vaccination is currently considered the most effective preventive measure available against influenza infection (Daly & Gustafson, 2011; Valenciano, Kissling & Cohen, 2011).

Athletes are a population that is under studied yet may be at an elevated risk for infection with influenza including the potential for severe outcomes of infection as a result of their increased susceptibility to immunocompromised conditions (WHO, 2011; Daly & Gustafson, 2011). Many athletes believe that physical training enhances immunity and helps prevent upper respiratory tract infection such as the common cold or "flu" (influenza) (Eichner, 1995). However, athletes are likely at an increased risk for transmission and contraction of influenza due to more frequent air travel than non-athletes, increased close contact with others through sport and are more likely to share surfaces such as workout equipment or water bottles which can act as disease vectors (Young, Fricker, Maughan & MacAuley, 1998). They are also susceptible to immunocompromised conditions as the result of high intensity training (Neiman, 1997). This acute immune suppression can be measured from 3 to 72 hours following high intensity exercise (Neiman, 1994). Due to the increased risk of contraction as a result an athlete's daily activities and immunocompromised conditions, it is recommended that athletes receive the influenza vaccine (Daly & Gustafson, 2011; Eichner, 1995; Young et al. 1998).

The researchers undertook a comprehensive literature search and found no articles that specifically explored the knowledge, practice and attitudes around the issue of influenza vaccination in the university athlete population. As a proxy measure, the literature on general university undergraduate students reports 8.0 – 44.19% engagement in the vaccine (Author, 2013). To achieve herd immunity 80% vaccination rate in healthy persons or 90% vaccination rate in high-risk groups is necessary (Plans-Rubió, 2012). Based on this information, vaccination participation is low in this university population. The purpose of this study was to investigate the knowledge, attitudes and practice of Canadian Interuniversity Sport (CIS) athletes concerning influenza A immunization. In addition, due to an increase in time allowance for the study, the responses of athletes were compared with kinesiology students to identify differences in knowledge, attitude and practice between athletes and non-athletes. It was hypothesized that there would be no difference between knowledge, attitude and practice among Canadian Interuniversity Sport (CIS) athletes and Kinesiology students with regards to influenza A immunization.

2. Methods

2.1 Participants

For the purposes of this study, an athlete was defined as an individual currently competing in the Canada Interuniversity Sport (CIS) competition. The University of Calgary CIS population was sampled by convenience. The expected response rate based on previous online survey distribution by email to university students regarding influenza vaccination was 41% (Milunic, Quilty, Super & Noritz, 2010). Therefore, the expected athlete response rate was approximately 185 (N=450). The survey was distributed using SurveyMonkey (SurveyMonkey.com) during January and February of 2014 at the University of Calgary, Alberta. The survey distribution occurred following considerable media attention regarding the Alberta Health Services influenza vaccination campaign as well as publicized deaths as a result of the H1N1 strain.

The non-athlete kinesiology students were also recruited by convenience and received the survey as a result of enrollment in an upper level Kinesiology course focusing on health (N=34). The researchers used the same online survey with wording tailored to student daily activities and therefore the expected response rate was also 41% (n=14).

2.2 Questionnaire

The questionnaire was developed according to the Ajzen framework for survey design (2002) using the Integrated Behaviour Model (IBM) which has been demonstrated in the published literature to be efficacious when applied to health behaviours (Ajzen, 2002; Godin & Kok, 1996). The survey was 19 questions (6 demographic, 13 Section 3-A, 5-B, & 5-C) and was validated through distribution to club status rowing and baseball teams at the University of Calgary (n=17) before dissemination to the survey population of varsity status teams and kinesiology students.

The study aim was to describe the proportion of CIS athletes that participate in the Alberta seasonal influenza vaccination program and the researchers used the term practice as engagement in a specific behaviour regularly. Participation was self-reported for a lifetime vaccination history in the demographic section (question 6), history of vaccination participation during their degree or athletic career in Section B (question 4) and future intentions to be vaccinated in Section B (question 5) and Section C (question 4). Appendix A provides the athlete specific survey. Non-athletes were given the same questions with language tailored to general student behavior.

A common definition of knowledge was employed, i.e. the information, understanding or awareness derived from education or experience of an individual (Merriam-Webster's Collegiate Dictionary, 2012). Section A (question 1, 2, 3) of the survey observes the participant's knowledge of the safety and effectiveness of the influenza A vaccine, awareness of potential side effects, as well as their primary source for learning about the influenza A vaccination.

Attitude is a feeling or thought process that influences an individual's behaviour (Merriam-Webster's Collegiate Dictionary, 2012). Section B (question 1, 2, 3) assesses the respondent's attitude towards the effects of the vaccine, past experience or expectation of experience of influenza vaccination, as well as intrinsic value for receiving the influenza vaccine.

Section C (question 1, 2, 3) of the survey was designed to better understand the respondent's attitude towards their risk as a result of daily behaviours, the potential individual consequences of infection with influenza and their concern for infection of others.

2.3 Outcome Measures

This cross-sectional study examined the three dependent variables of knowledge, attitude and practice as measured by responses to the survey questionnaire.

2.4 Analysis

A descriptive analysis (means and percentages) was employed to identify trends in knowledge, attitude and practice of CIS athletes regarding influenza A vaccination. The responses to each question were expressed as a percent. Using the added comparison group of non-athlete kinesiology students, a χ^2 test statistic was employed to detect differences in the responses of athletes and non-athlete kinesiology students regarding their knowledge and lifetime vaccination history. A Kruskal-Wallis test was used to show the differences in responses of athletes and non-athlete kinesiology students across the questions with a Likert scale rating. A greater mean rank was used to indicate a higher, more positive or agreeable rating on the Likert scale. The significance level for the comparison of athletes to non-athlete kinesiology students was set at $p<0.05$.

2.5 Ethical Consideration

The study received ethical approval by the Conjoint Health Research Ethics Board (REB13-1276) on January 8, 2014.

3. Results

The mean age of athletes was 20.4 ± 2.2 years and the overall response rate was 39.3%. The survey completion rate of 95.5% was based on the number of athletes (n=177) who accessed the survey. The mean age of non-athletes was 21.06 ± 2.7 years. Respondents were dropped from the analysis if questions were left blank (Athletes n=8, Non-athletes n=1). Participant characteristics are in Table 1.

Table 1. Comparison of Athlete and Non-Athlete Participant Characteristics

		Athletes		**Non-Athlete Students**	
Characteristic		n	%	n	%
Sex					
	Male	76	42.9	7	20.6
	Female	101	57.1	27	79.4
Age (years)					
	18	36	20.3	5	14.7
	19	37	20.9	4	11.8
	20	29	16.4	7	20.6
	21	26	14.7	8	23.5
	22	26	14.7	4	11.8
	23	7	4.0	1	2.9
	24	9	5.1	2	5.9
	25	5	2.8	0	0.0
	26	0	0.0	1	2.9
	27	0	0.0	1	2.9
	28	0	0.0	0	0.0
	29	0	0.0	0	0.0
	30	1	1.1	1	1.1
	Mean Age	21.06 ± 2.7		20.4 ± 2.2	
Degree					
	Undergraduate	174	98.3	34	100.0
	Graduate	3	1.7	0	0.0
Faculty					
	Arts	60	33.9	1	2.9
	Business	19	10.7	0	0.0
	Education	5	2.8	0	0.0
	Engineering	13	7.3	0	0.0
	Environmental Design	1	0.6	0	0.0
	Kinesiology	28	15.8	31	92.1
	Medicine	9	5.1	1	2.9
	Nursing	8	4.5	0	0.0
	Science	34	19.2	1	2.9
Years of Education Completed at the University Level					
	Less than 1	42	23.7	7	20.6
	1-2	49	27.7	7	20.6
	2-3	29	16.4	6	17.6
	3-4	26	14.7	11	32.4
	4-5	27	15.3	3	8.8
	Greater than 5	4	2.3	0	0.0

Over half of the athletes (54.9%) knew that the effectiveness and safety of the present influenza A vaccine had been demonstrated through scientific research and (58.3%) were aware of the potential side effects of the vaccination (Table 2). The greatest percentage of athletes (46.3%) stated media as their primary source for learning about the influenza vaccination. Slightly less athletes (41.7%) selected family physician, nurse or other health care provider as their primary source for information and 12.0% said that they had not been informed that the influenza A vaccination might be important. Kinesiology students exhibited a smaller percentage of uninformed individuals (3.0%), and a greater percentage of respondents selecting the media (60.6%) as their primary source of information. Approximately one third (36.4%) of kinesiology students indicated that their main source of information was a health care provider.

Table 2. Response Frequency Comparison by Grouping of Athletes and Kinesiology Students for Vaccination Participation History and Current Knowledge.

Question	Response	Response by Group (%)			Test Statistic		
	Yes/No	Athletes	Kinesiology Students	Total	χ^2	Degrees of Freedom (df)	p-value
In your lifetime that you can recall have you ever had the flu shot?	Yes	78.0	74.3	n = 164	0.226	1	0.635
	No	22.0	25.7	n = 48			
The effectiveness and the safety of the present influenza vaccine has been demonstrated through scientific research.	Yes	54.9	73.5	n = 121	4.505	2	0.105
	No	9.7	8.8	n = 20			
	I don't know	35.4	17.6	n = 68			
Are you aware of potential side effects, i.e. beyond the typical soreness associated with a needle, from being vaccinated with the influenza A vaccine?	Yes	58.3	73.5	n = 127	4.195	2	0.123
	No	27.4	23.5	n = 56			
	I don't know	14.3	2.9	n = 26			

*Significant at p<0.05

The χ^2 analysis comparing athletes (78.0%) to non-athlete kinesiology students (74.3%) revealed no significant difference in the self-reported previous lifetime history of vaccination participation (p>0.05) (Table 2). There were also no significant differences in the level of knowledge on the effectiveness, safety and side effects of the vaccine (p>0.05) (Table 2). The survey revealed that 54.9% of athletes and 73.5% of students stated that 'the effectiveness and safety of the present influenza A vaccine had been demonstrated through scientific research' (Table 2). Similar proportions were seen regarding awareness of the potential side effects of the vaccine.

The percentage of athletes that report to have received the vaccine more than once during their university degree/athletic career, and that intend to receive the vaccine for the remainder of their university degree/athletic career was 29.2% and 29.4%, respectively (Figure 1).

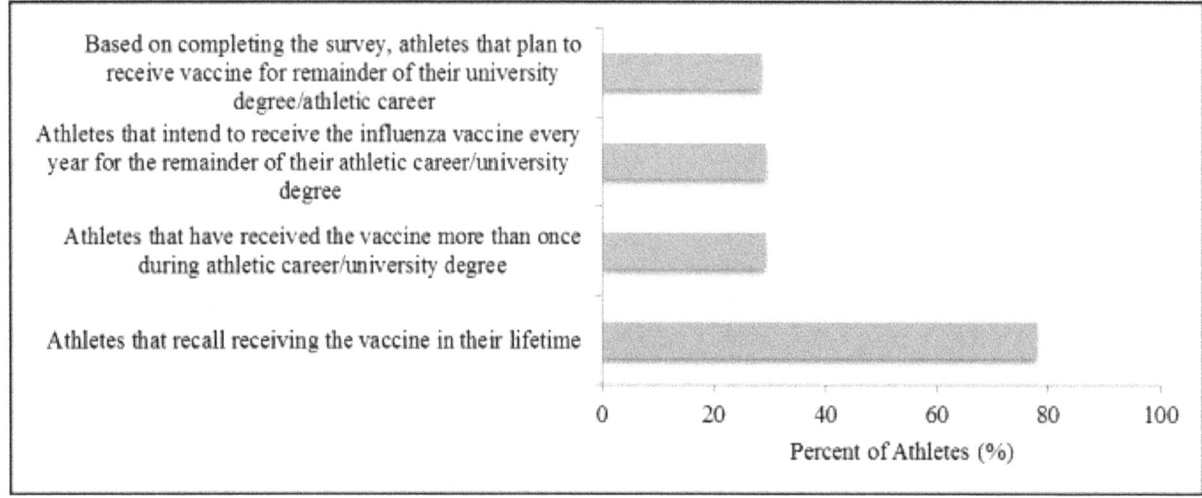

Figure 1. Comparison of history and intention of vaccination participation percentage of athletes

The percentage of Likert scaled responses for questions regarding the attitude and practice of athletes are presented in Table 3. Just over half (54.0%) of athletes reported to have never received the influenza A vaccine throughout their university degree/athletic career.

Table 3. Frequency and Percent of Likert Scaled Responses Regarding Attitude and Practice of the Influenza A Vaccination

Survey Question	Percentage of Likert Scale Rating					Total Sample
	1	2	3	4	5	
How would you rate the effects of receiving the influenza vaccine?	Harmful 2.4%	Somewhat harmful 12.4%	Neutral 32.4%	Somewhat beneficial 26.5%	Beneficial 26.5%	N=170
Based on past experience or expectation of receiving the influenza vaccine, how would you rate the experience? (Includes accessing the vaccine and receiving the vaccination.)	Unpleasant 8.2%	Somewhat unpleasant 13.5%	Neutral 52.4%	Somewhat pleasant 13.5%	Pleasant 12.4%	N=170
In terms of intrinsic value to you for the influenza vaccine, how would you rate receiving the influenza vaccine?	Worthless 8.8%	Somewhat worthless 13.5%	Neutral 30.0%	Somewhat valuable 30.0%	Valuable 17.6%	N=170
How many times have you received the influenza vaccine since the beginning of your university degree/athletic career?	Never 54.0%	Once 16.8%	I don't know 5.3%	More than once, but not every year 2.4%	Every year 16.8%	N=170
I intend to receive the influenza vaccine every year for the remainder of my university degree/athletic career.	Extremely unlikely 28.8%	Unlikely 22.4%	Undecided 19.4%	Likely 15.3%	Extremely likely 14.1%	N=170
As an athlete, my daily activities put me at an elevated risk for contraction of the influenza A virus.	Strongly disagree 5.3%	Disagree 27.8%	I don't know 24.9%	Agree 34.3%	Strongly agree 7.7%	N=169
As an athlete, I am concerned about the potential consequences, such as an interruption in training and competition, due to contraction of the influenza A virus.	Strongly disagree 4.7%	Disagree 14.8%	I don't know 8.9%	Agree 50.3%	Strongly agree 21.3%	N=169
As an athlete, I worry about transmitting the influenza A illness to my teammates.	Strongly disagree 6.5%	Disagree 14.8%	I don't know 13.0%	Agree 49.1%	Strongly agree 16.6%	N=169
After completion of this survey, I plan to receive the influenza vaccine every year for the remainder of my university degree/athletic career.	Strongly disagree 20.1%	Disagree 20.7%	I don't know 30.8%	Agree 16.0%	Strongly agree 12.4%	N=169

The Kruskal-Wallis analysis revealed a significant difference between the ratings of athletes and kinesiology students on the effects of receiving the influenza vaccine ($p<0.05$) (Table 4). Kinesiology students presented a higher, more positive, mean rank (120.40) compared to the athletes (98.92) (Table 4).

Significant differences between athletes and non-athlete students were found concerning the consequences of infection and transmission of the virus ($p<0.05$) (Table 4). The athlete group yielded a higher mean rank in accordance with higher agreeableness with statements expressing a concern for consequences such as an interruption in training or studies as well as worry for transmitting the infection to teammates and or others (Table 4). The remaining Likert scale questions explored the intrinsic value for the vaccine, experience of receiving the vaccine as well as current and past participation throughout university attendance yielded non-significant values in the comparison of athletes and non-athletes.

Table 4. Kruskal-Wallis Analysis by Group of Likert Scaled Responses Regarding Attitude and Practice of the Influenza A Vaccination

Question	**Likert Scale Response Range**	**Kruskal-Wallis Mean Rank by Group**		**Test Statistic**		
	1-5	Athletes	Non-Athlete Students	χ^2	df	p-value
How would you rate the effects of receiving the influenza vaccine?	Harmful to Beneficial	98.92	120.40	4.045	1	0.044*
		n = 170	n = 34			
Based on past experience or expectation of receiving the influenza vaccine, how would you rate the experience? (Includes accessing the vaccine and receiving the vaccination)	Unpleasant to Pleasant	103.62	96.91	0.433	1	0.510
		n =170	n = 34			
In terms of intrinsic value to you for the influenza vaccine, how would you rate receiving the influenza vaccine?	Worthless to Valuable	101.70	106.49	0.197	1	0.657
		n = 170	n = 34			
How many times have you received the influenza vaccine since the beginning of your university degree/athletic career?	Never to Every Year	96.73	104.01	0.560	1	0.454
		n =161	n = 34			
I intend to receive the influenza vaccine every year for the remainder of my university degree/athletic career.	Extremely Unlikely to Extremely Likely	101.93	105.37	0.101	1	0.750
		n = 170	n = 34			
As an athlete, my daily activities put me at an elevated risk for contraction of the influenza A virus.	Strongly Disagree to Strongly Agree	101.84	102.79	0.008	1	0.928
		n = 169	n = 34			
As an athlete, I am concerned about the potential consequences, such as an interruption in training and competition, due to the contraction of the influenza A virus.	Strongly Disagree to Strongly Agree	105.57	84.26	4.262	1	0.039*
		n = 169	n = 34			
As an athlete, I worry about transmitting the influenza A virus to my teammates.	Strongly Disagree to Strongly Agree	105.96	82.32	5.150	1	0.023*
		n = 169	n = 34			
After completion of this survey, I plan to receive the influenza vaccine every year for the remainder of my university degree/athletic career.	Strongly Disagree to Strongly Agree	101.01	106.94	0.304	1	0.581
		n = 169	n = 34			

4. Discussion

This study investigated the knowledge, attitude and practice of CIS athletes concerning the influenza vaccination utilizing a cross-sectional survey design. Information regarding the knowledge of effectiveness, safety and side effects of the vaccine, attitudes towards the effects, intrinsic values, and personal risk as well as past vaccination participation and future intentions of vaccination reception was collected. The published literature to the best of the researchers' knowledge has not yet explored these factors in an athletic population. However, CIS athletes are by definition university students in addition to their athletic roles and therefore the current literature reporting on university students is expected to be an appropriate proxy and comparison for the trends identified in this study. The results of this study are limited by the cross-sectional survey design as well as the infancy of research in this specific population.

The questions assessing the current knowledge of athletes found that approximately half of the athletes knew that the influenza A vaccine was effective and safe and these individuals were informed of the potential side effects beyond the soreness of a needle prick. This was not found to be significantly different from the knowledge level of kinesiology students ($p>0.05$) (Table 2). The percentages of athletes and kinesiology students understanding the effectiveness and safety (see Table 2) were greater than the 39.1% found in first year university students by Akan et al (2010). The greater percentage of athletes and kinesiology students demonstrating knowledge of the safety and effectiveness of the vaccine in this study could be the result of a bias in the positive direction presented by the affirmative wording of the statement

'The effectiveness and safety of the present influenza A vaccine has been demonstrated through scientific research'. The percentage of athletes (35.4%) that reported that they did not know if the vaccine had been demonstrated scientifically to be safe and effective is consistent with the findings of Naing & Tan (2011). Based on written comments provided in the comment box at the conclusion of the survey, further research is required to determine the knowledge of athletes surrounding the mechanism of the vaccine as well as the limitations of its protection in order to provide a more detailed description of the current knowledge standard.

Both the athletes (46.3%) and the kinesiology students (60.6%) reported the media as their primary source for learning about the influenza vaccination in the past year. This variation is also found in the literature with reports of 72.1% and 45% of university students stating media as their primary source for vaccine education (Akan et al., 2010; Merrill, Kelly & Cox, 2010). The variation across the literature is likely the result of the context of the survey distribution such as seasonal or pandemic outbreaks as in the case of the study by Akan et al (2010). However, this does not explain the variation between athletes and kinesiology students within this study. This is particularly interesting given that both groups were exposed to the increased media attention surrounding the availability of the flu vaccine in the city of Calgary throughout the month of January 2014. It is possible that due to the limited time of student-athletes, less attention is paid to television, the newspaper, etc.

The published research that investigated university students indicated that students who receive advice on the influenza vaccine from health care professionals were more likely to receive the vaccine (Merrill, Kelly & Cox. 2010; Rodas et al., 2012; Ramsey & Marczinski, 2011). Just under half of the athletes (41.7%), lower than the 52% reported in the literature, indicated that a family physician, nurse or other health care provider was their main source for knowledge surrounding the vaccine (Mavros et al., 2011). An important factor to consider in the future is the patient and health care provider's relationship, which could affect the individuals' reception of the vaccine. Vaccinations have been reported to occur at multiple types of patient encounter sites (Levy, Ambrose, Oleka & Lewin, 2009). Perhaps implementing changes within the system of care for athletes could improve vaccine adherence and ultimately overall health. Further studies should consider the response of athletes to education from athletic therapists and or physiotherapists, as they are often involved in the care of athletes throughout their careers.

The only significant difference found between athletes and non-athlete kinesiology students in attitude was the rating of the effects of the vaccine, with kinesiology students yielding a higher rating overall (1=Harmful, 5=Beneficial, Table 4). This difference is likely the result of the greater percentage of kinesiology students demonstrating the knowledge of the safety, effectiveness and potential side effects of the vaccine, despite the lack of significant difference found through the χ^2 analysis. However, the small sample size of kinesiology students restricted the statistical analysis and the comparison of the two groups.

A very high percentage (>70%) of athletes and kinesiology students recalled having the flu shot in their lifetime (Table 2). Respondents may have overestimated their actual vaccination rates and likely confound their answer due to confusion of the influenza vaccine with other childhood vaccinations (Rickert, Santoli, Shefer, Myrick, Yusuf, 2006). The result could also be enhanced due to a recall bias. Future questionnaires should include a specific time period.

In regards to the practice of athletes in influenza vaccination, approximately one third of athletes received the vaccine more than once throughout their athletic career and intend to continue to receive the vaccine for the remainder of their career (Figure 1). This is consistent with the literature on the university student population (24.75%) (Author, 2013). Unfortunately, the reported participation rate of university students and athletes in influenza vaccination is very low when compared to the 80% vaccination rate required for herd immunity of the average population and 90% requirement for high risk populations (Plans-Rubió, 2012). Within the scope of this study, the approximate 30% participation rate suggests a disconnect may exist between the demonstrated knowledge and seemingly positive attitude by over half of the athlete population towards the influenza vaccine.

The most revealing result of this study was the significant difference found between athletes and kinesiology students in their concern for consequences of infection with the virus and transmission to others ($p<0.05$). Compared to kinesiology students, athletes indicated a higher agreeableness (greater mean rank) with statements regarding concern for potential consequences of infection with the influenza virus (Table 4). These concerns specifically included an interruption in training and competition, and transmission of the virus to teammates. It appears that athletes are aware of the detriment to their personal training regime or competition performance as a result of a lowered level of health and are therefore concerned about contracting the virus. Furthermore, they are concerned about the general health of their teammates and the implications to team performance as a result of transmission of the virus. Despite this concern, only 42.0% of athletes agree and or strongly agree that their daily activities put them at an elevated risk for contraction of the influenza virus and only one third actually report to regularly engage in influenza vaccination behaviours. This trend implies that the athlete population is not aware of their potential increased risk for infection of the influenza virus and perhaps that they are not convinced of the preventative benefits of vaccination practices.

5. Conclusion

Athletes are at an elevated risk for contraction of the influenza virus due to repeated bouts of immune suppression, increased contact with others as well as shared surfaces through training, competition and other team activities (Young et al., 1998). The questionnaire employed in this study has identified the current trends of CIS athletes regarding their knowledge, attitude and practice of the influenza A vaccination. In addition, these trends were compared across another population of university students. The results of this study may inform the planning of future behavior change communication (BCC) strategies in this population. A BCC strategy would enhance the knowledge and awareness of the risk for influenza infection, and the adoption of preventative health behaviors, such as vaccination. Therefore, the implementation of a BCC strategy also has the potential to facilitate a greater standard of health conducive with training and competition in the CIS athlete population.

References

Ajzen I. (2002). *Constructing a TPB Questionnaire: Conceptual and Methodological Considerations*. Pp. 1–14.

Akan H, Gurol Y, Izbirak G, et al. (2010). Knowledge and attitudes of university students toward pandemic influenza: a cross-sectional study from Turkey. *BMC Public Health,* 10:413. doi:10.1186/1471-2458-10-413.

Author. (2013). Self-reported attitudes and beliefs of University and College Students for failing to receive an influenza vaccine. APNM, 38:1082.

Daly P, Gustafson R. (2011). Public health recommendations for athletes attending sporting events. *Clin J Sport Med.,* 21(1):67–70. doi:10.1097/JSM.0b013e31820758dc.

Eichner ER. (1995). Contagious Infections. *In Competitive Sports. Sports Science Exchange*, 8(3).

Godin G, Kok G. (1996). The theory of planned behavior: A review of its applications to health-related behaviors. *Am J Heal Promot.*,11:87–98.

Health Canada. Influenza (Flu) [Health Canada Influenza (flu) website]. April 8, 2013. http://www.hc-sc.gc.ca/hc-ps/dc-ma/influenza-eng.php#flu. Accessed March 31, 2014.

Levy DJ, Ambrose CS, Oleka N, Lewin EB. (2009). A survey of pediatricians' attitudes regarding influenza immunization in children. *BMC Pediatrics,* 9:8. doi:10.1186/1471-2431-9-8]

Mavros MN, Mitsikostas PK, Kontopidis IG, Moris DN, Dimopoulos G, Falagas ME. (2011). H1N1v influenza vaccine in Greek medical students. *Eur J Public Health*, 329–32. doi:10.1093/eurpub/ckq109.

Merriam-Webster's Collegiate Dictionary. 10th ed. Springfield, MA: Merriam-Webster INC; 2012. Retrieved from: http://search.credoreference.com.ezproxy.lib.ucalgary.ca/content/entry/mwcollegiate/knowledge/0?searchId=3299a679-36ad-11e4-9be7-12c1d36507ee&result=0

Merrill R, Kelley T, Cox E. (2010). Factors and barriers influencing influenza vaccination among students at Brigham Young University. *Med J.,* 16(2):29–34. Available at: http://www.ncbi.nlm.nih.gov/pubmed/20110927. Accessed October 21, 2013.

Milunic SL, Quilty JF, Super DM, Norritz GH. (2013). Patterns of influenza vaccination among medical students. *Infect Control Hosp Epidemiol.,* 31:85–88. doi:10.1086/649219.

Naing C, Tan RYP. (2011). Knowledge about the pandemic influenza A (H1N1) and willingness to accept vaccination: a cross-sectional survey. *J Public Health (Bangkok),* 19(6):511–516. doi:10.1007/s10389-011-0434-2.

Nieman DC. (1994). Exercise, upper respiratory tract infection, and the immune system. *Med Sci Sports Exerc.* Available at: http://www.setantacollege.com/wp-content/uploads/Journal_db/Exercise, upper respiratory tract infection.pdf. Accessed November 18, 2013.

Nieman DC. (1997). Immune response to heavy exertion. *J Appl Physiol.,* 82(5):1385–94. Available at: http://www.ncbi.nlm.nih.gov/pubmed/9134882.

Plans-Rubió P. (2012). The vaccination coverage required to establish herd immunity against influenza viruses. *Prev Med (Baltim),* 55(1):72–77. doi:10.1016/j.ypmed.2012.02.015.

Ramsey M, Marczinski C. (2011). College students' perceptions of H1N1 flu risk and attitudes toward vaccination. *Vaccine,* 29(44):7599–601. doi:10.1016/j.vaccine.2011.07.130.

Rickert D, Santoli J, Shefer A, Myrick A. (2006). Influenza vaccination of high-risk children: what the providers say. *Am J Prev Med.*, 30(2):111-118].

Rodas JR, Lau CH, Zhang ZZ, Griffiths SM, Luk WC, Kim JH. (2012). Exploring predictors influencing intended and actual acceptability of the A/H1N1 pandemic vaccine: a cohort study of university students in Hong Kong. *Public Health,* 126:1007–12. doi:10.1016/j.puhe.2012.09.011.

Valenciano M, Kissling E, Cohen J-M, Oroszi B, Barret A-S, Rizzo C, et al. (2011). Estimates of pandemic influenza vaccine effectiveness in Europe, 2009-2010: results of Influenza Monitoring Vaccine Effectiveness in Europe (I-MOVE) multicentre case-control study. *PLoS Med.,* 8(1):e1000388. doi:10.1371/journal.pmed.1000388.

WHO. (2011). Manual for the laboratory diagnosis and virological surveillance of influenza. World Health Organization.

Young M, Fricker P, Maughan R, MacAuley D. (1998). The travelling athlete: issues relating to the Commonwealth Games, Malaysia, 1998. *Br J Sports Med.,* 32(1). 77–81.

21

Effects of Short-Term Jump Squat Training With and Without Chains on Strength and Power in Recreational Lifters

David C. Archer
Center for Sport Performance and Human Performance Lab, Department of Kinesiology, California State University, Fullerton, CA, USA
E-mail: dvdarcher@csu.fullerton.edu

Lee E. Brown (Corresponding author)
Center for Sport Performance and Human Performance Lab, Department of Kinesiology, California State University, Fullerton, 800 N. State College Blvd., Fullerton, CA 92834-6870, USA
E-mail: leebrown@fullerton.edu

Jared W. Coburn
Center for Sport Performance and Human Performance Lab, Department of Kinesiology, California State University, Fullerton, CA, USA
E-mail: jcoburn@fullerton.edu

Andrew J. Galpin
Center for Sport Performance and Human Performance Lab, Department of Kinesiology, California State University, Fullerton, CA, USA
E-mail: agalpin@fullerton.edu

Phillip C. Drouet
Center for Sport Performance and Human Performance Lab, Department of Kinesiology , California State University, Fullerton, CA, USA
E-mail: phillip.drouet@yahoo.com

Whitney D. Leyva
Center for Sport Performance and Human Performance Lab, Department of Kinesiology , California State University, Fullerton, CA, USA
E-mail: whitleyva@gmail.com

Cameron N. Munger
Center for Sport Performance and Human Performance Lab, Department of Kinesiology, California State University, Fullerton, CA, USA
E-mail: cammunger@gmail.com

Megan A. Wong
Center for Sport Performance and Human Performance Lab, Department of Kinesiology , California State University, Fullerton, CA, USA
E-mail: mwong52493@csu.fullerton.edu

Abstract

Background: The use of chains in resistance training is a way to accommodate the muscular strength curve. Short-term training and jump squats have been shown to increase back squat strength, but not in conjunction with each other or with chains. Jump squats have also been used to increase jump height and power. **Objectives:** The purpose of this study was to investigate the effects of short-term jump squat training with and without chains on strength and power. **Methods:** Thirty-one resistance-trained men volunteered to participate (age = 23.87 ± 2.2 years, height=174.87 ± 6.94 cm, mass = 82.74 ± 14.95 kg) and were randomly assigned to one of three groups [control (C) = 10, no chains (NC) =10, or chains (CH) = 11]. Participants had their jump height (VJ) and back squat strength (BS) tested before and after a week of training. The NC and CH groups performed three training sessions consisting of five sets of three reps of jump squats at 30% 1RM with 30s rest between sets. The CH group had 20% of their load added by chains when standing erect. The C group did not train. **Results:** A 3 (group: CH, NC, C) x 2 (time: pre, post) mixed factor ANOVA revealed a significant ($p = 0.006$) interaction for back squat 1RM. Both the CH (pre 142.56 ± 20.40 kg; post 145.66 ± 19.59 kg) and NC (pre 150.00 ± 15.23 kg; post 154.77 ± 15.09 kg) groups significantly increased while the C (pre 157.27 ± 25.35 kg; post 156.36 ± 24.85 kg) group showed no difference. There were no significant interactions (p =0.32) or main effects for VJ (C = pre 50.59 ± 9.39cm; post 51.29 ± 9.68cm; NC = pre 55.29 ± 5.23cm; post 57.39 ± 5.22cm; CH = pre 46.19 ± 5.02; post 47.45 ± 4.62.) **Conclusions:** The CH group was able to increase strength while lifting less overall weight. Coaches may use short-term training with chains to yield a similar increase in back squat strength as without chains.

Keywords: variable resistance, back squats, novel, vertical jump

1. Introduction

Strength and power are vital for performance in sport. Jumping high utilizes strength to increase power and the vertical jump test is an easy and reliable way to measure power (McLellan, Lovell, & Gass, 2011). Traditional resistance training has been implemented in many programs to increase strength, power, and vertical jump height. One of the standard exercises used is the back squat as it increases lower body strength and power (Neelly, Terry, & Morris, 2010). Jump squats are another exercise that results in an increase in performance (Dalen, Welde, Van Den Tillaar, & Aune , 2013; MacKenzie, S.J., Lavers, R.J., Wallace, 2014). Plyometric exercises utilize the stretch shortening cycle (Adibpour, Bakht, & Behpour, 2012; Alemdaroglu, Dundar, Koklu, & Findikoglu, 2013; Arabatzi, Kellius, & Saez-Saez De Villarreal, 2010). Jump squats use loads from 0-80% of one repetition maximum (1RM) (Bevan, Bunce, Owen, Bennett, Cook, Cunningham, Newton, & Kilduff, 2010; Cormie, McGuigan, & Newton, 2010; Hoffman, Ratamess, Cooper, Kang, Chilakos, & Faigenbaum, 2005; Sleivert, & Taingahue, 2004; Smilios, Pilianidis, Sotiropoulos, Antonakis, & Tokmakidis, 2005; Turner, Unholz, Potts, & Coleman, 2012). However, many training studies have used 30%1RM (Cormie, McGuigan, & Newton, 2010; Thomas, Kraemer, Spiering, Volek, Anderson, & Maresh, 2007).

A popular program, variable resistance training, has also been shown to increase strength and power. Variable resistance training uses elastic bands or chains to add resistance during different parts of the lift depending on where they are applied. Specifically, in a back squat, resistance is added during the concentric phase due to more chain coming off the floor (McMaster, Cronin, & McGuigan, 2009; McMaster, Cronin, & McGuigan, 2010; Neelly, Terry, & Morris, 2010). Elastic bands and chain length and width alter resistance (McMaster, Cronin, & McGuigan, 2009; McMaster, Cronin, & McGuigan, 2010; Wallace, Winchester, & McGuigan, 2006). However, bands have a curvilinear length/tension relationship while chains have a linear length/tension relationship (McMaster, Cronin, & McGuigan, 2009; McMaster, Cronin, & McGuigan, 2010).

Long term training can increase strength and power but short-term training has also has shown to increase strength and speed (Brown & Whitehurst, 2003; Coburn, Housh, Malek, Weir, Cramer, Beck, & Johnson, 2006). Brown demonstrated that two visits increased velocity of isokinetic knee extensions; while Coburn found that three visits increased isokinetic knee strength. However, limited research has combined power training in the short-term.

Powerlifters have implemented variable resistance in their training to increase strength (Swinton, Stewart, Lloyd, Aqouris, & Keogh, 2012). Additionally, it has been shown to increase force, strength, and power of the upper (Ghigiarelli, Nagle, Gross, Robertson, Irrgang, & Myslinski, 2009) and lower body (Israetel, McBride, Nuzzo, Skinner, & Dayne, 2010; Rhea, Kenn, & Dermody, 2009; Wallace, Winchester, & McGuigan, 2006). However, limited research has examined short-term variable resistance training to specifically increase jump height. Therefore, the purpose of this study was to investigate the effects of short-term jump squat training with and without chains on strength and power.

2. Methods

2.1 Participants

Thirty-one healthy males (age=23.87± 2.2 years, mass= 82.74 ± 14.95kg, height =174.87±6.94 cm) volunteered to participate and were randomly assigned to either a chain (CH=11), no chain (NC=10), or control group (C=10). The requirements for participation were that each subject had been resistance training for at least one year, at least three times a week, and could squat at least 1.5 times their body weight with a minimum of 200 lbs. On testing and training days they were asked to not perform any lower body exercises or strenuous activities and not supplement with creatine. All subjects were kinesiology students recruited from classes. All testing was performed in a laboratory setting. On the first day they read and signed a university Institutional Review Board approved informed consent document.

2.2 Procedures

Prior to testing, participants' mass (ES Series Bench Scale, Ohaus Corporation, Pine Brook, NJ) and height (ProDoc Series DHRWM Digital Height Rod, Cardinal Scale MFG, Webb City, MO) were measured. Participants then performed a dynamic warm up consisting of walking knee hugs, lunges, and Frankenstein's for 20 m each. These exercises were used to warm up the lower body (Brown, Weir, 2001).

2.3 Vertical Jump Testing

After the warm up, participants performed two practice countermovement jumps before three maximal jumps using a vertical jump test apparatus (Jones, Brown, Coburn, Noffal, 2015) (Epic Combine Jump Station). If they touched any vanes on the third attempt, they continued jumping until they could not jump any higher. The best trial was used for data analysis. Reliability of the vertical jump test was ICC = 0.98.

2.4 1RM Back Squat Testing

For the back squat, a safety squat device (Safety Squat; Bigger Faster Strong, Salt Lake City, UT) was used to ensure that each participant squatted to parallel at the top of the quadriceps. They warmed up by squatting 10 repetitions at 50% of their predicted 1RM, five repetitions at 70%, three repetitions at 80%, and one repetition at 90%. They then had a max of five attempts to reach their 1RM. There were 3 min of rest between warm up and max attempts (Brown, Weir, 2001).

2.5 Training

There were three training sessions total and the NC and CH groups performed jump squats for five sets of three repetitions with 30 s rest (Moreno, Brown, Coburn, Judelson, 2014). They were instructed to perform a quarter squat and jump as high as possible. Each session was separated by 48 hrs. The C group was instructed to not do any lower body training for the entire week.

2.6 Load

The load for the CH and NC group was matched at approximately 30%1RM (Nijem, Coburn, Brown, Lynn, Ciccone, 2016). The weight for the CH group was quantified by having subjects stand upright with an unloaded barbell. Large chains were suspended from smaller chains in a double loop method (Figure 1). Chains were then added to each side until the desired load of 20% was reached. The remaining weight was then added to the bar via weight plates to equal the prescribed 30% 1RM load. The weight for the NC group came entirely from weight plates on the bar.

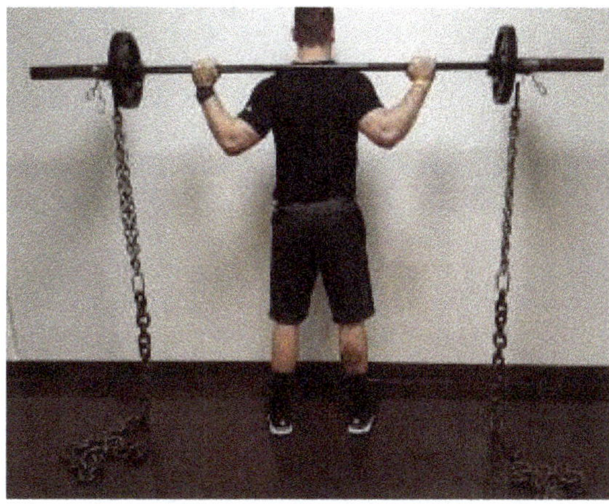

Figure 1. Barbell with double loop chain load

2.7 Statistical Analyses

A 3 (group = C, NC, CH) x 2 (time = pre, post) mixed factor ANOVA was used. Alpha level was set at 0.05. Follow up tests were paired samples t-tests. SPSS version 22 was used for all analyses.

3. Results

3.1 Back Squat 1RM

There was a significant (p = 0.006) interaction of group x time. Both the CH and NC groups showed a significant increase from pre to post while the C group showed no change (Table 1). There were no significant differences between the CH and NC group.

Table 1. Mean (SD) of one repetition maximum (1RM) back squat (BS) with p-value and 95% confidence interval (95% CI) between control (C), no chain (NC), and chain (CH) groups.

	C			NC			CH		
	Pre	Post	p-value, (95% CI)	Pre	Post	p-value, (95% CI)	Pre	Post	p-value, (95% CI)
1RM BS (kg)	157.27 (25.35)	156.36 (24.85)	0.46 (-3.89 - 7.89)	150.00 (15.23)	154.77* (15.09)	0.001 (15.4 - -5.6)	142.56 (20.40)	145.66* (19.59)	0.031 (12.88 - -.76)

*Significantly greater than pre.

3.2 Vertical Jump

There were no significant (p = 0.32) interactions or main effects for time (p = 0.63) or condition (p = 0.11) (table 2).

Table 2. Mean (SD) of EPIC vertical jump (VJ) with p-value and 95% confidence interval (95% CI) between control (C), no chain (NC), and chain (CH) groups.

	C			NC			CH		
	Pre	Post	p-value, (95% CI)	Pre	Post	p-value, (95% CI)	Pre	Post	p-value, (95% CI)
VJ (cm)	50.59 (9.39)	51.29 (9.68)	0.6, (-2.01 - 3.28)	55.29 (5.23)	57.39 (5.22)	0.047, (-2.78 - -.02)	46.19 (5.02)	47.45 (4.62)	0.99, (-1.89 - -1.89)

4. Discussion

The purpose of this study was to determine the effects of short-term jump squat training with and without chains on strength and power. The major finding was that 1RM back squat strength increased for both the CH and NC groups with no change in the control group. These results may be due to neurological adaptations such as increased motor unit recruitment or firing rate (Aagaard, Simonsen, Andersen, Magnusson, Dyhre-Poulsen, 2002; Cormie, McGuigan, & Newton, 2010; Cormie, McGuigan, & Newton, 2011; Gabriel, Kamen, & Frost, 2006).

Short-term resistance training can result in neural adaptations in the absence of hypertrophic changes, such as increased motor unit firing rate (Gabriel, Kamen, & Frost, 2006). Increasing firing rate has been shown to increase muscular force (Cormie, McGuigan, & Newton, 2010; Gabriel, Kamen, & Frost, 2006). High firing rates are also important for increasing rate of force development (Aagaard, Simonsen, Andersen, Magnusson, Dyhre-Poulsen, 2002; Ratamess). Another adaptation is motor unit recruitment. Motor units move from smaller slow-twitch to larger fast-twitch depending on the load or speed of the movement (Gabriel, Kamen, & Frost, 2006, Ratamess). Movements that are slow and light use primarily small motor units while heavy, fast, and explosive require large motor units (Ratamess). Previous research has shown that these adaptations can occur in only one week. Brown (Brown & Whitehurst, 2003) and Coburn (Coburn, Housh, Malek, Weir, Cramer, Beck, & Johnson, 2006) studied the effects of short-term training with two or three visits respectively. Brown found that two visits showed an increase in velocity, but not force, while Coburn found that three visits showed an increase in force. Tillin et al. (Tillin & Folland 2014) examined the short-term effects of maximal vs. explosive strength training in an isometric knee extension. They found that maximal training resulted in greater improvement in voluntary contractions, but explosive training had a greater increase in early phase force. Both of these adaptations occurred at the onset of training and promoted strength gains. The current study supports this as short-term explosive training increased strength gains and early phase force.

Variable resistance has been used in different types of training. The use of bands or chains are designed to alter the strength curve of an exercise. This causes the load to increase as the lifter rises during the concentric action and can be more explosive (McMaster, T., Cronin, J., McGuigan, 2009). Rhea (Rhea, Kenn, & Dermody, 2009) found that the use of bands with fast movements increased peak power greater than slow heavy movements yet both similarly increased maximal strength. The current study also demonstrated that variable resistance increased strength. However, power was unaffected in their study, which may have been due to the relatively heavy loads used. Galpin (Galpin et al., 2015) also examined the effects of different loads using variable resistance. Their study used banded deadlifts at 60% and 85% 1RM using different resistances (B1=15% resistance, B2 = 35% resistance.) Results showed that force decreased as tension increased. However, velocity was greater for the two banded deadlift conditions at 60% than the free weight deadlift, but B2 was greatest at 85% 1RM. Peak power was also higher for the banded conditions than with free weights. This current study used a lighter intensity and found an increases in strength for the CH and NC groups, but no changes in power for any group.

McCurdy (McCurdy, Langford, Ernest, Jenkerson, & Doscher, 2009) also found that training with and without chains increased strength. They compared the bench press with chains supplying all of the weight to plate loaded alone. Both increased strength with no significant differences between conditions. In the current study, the CH group trained with less overall weight, but still showed a significant increase in strength. We hypothesized that the chain group would have a greater increase in vertical jump height due to lifting less weight with greater speed and acceleration. However, this was not the case as no group demonstrated a change in vertical jump height. The weight that the chains provided was a relatively light load, so there may have only been a small increase in acceleration during the concentric phase.

There have been few studies examining the load that chains supply to a lift. A study by Nijem (Nijem, Coburn, Brown, Lynn, & Ciccone, 2016) had subjects perform deadlifts using a load of 20% of the weight supplied by chains at the top of the lift. The current study used the same loading scheme, but used the double loop method to suspend the chains from a standing position which supplied more variable resistance than having the larger chains hanging directly to the floor (Neelly, Terry, & Morris, 2010). The load supplied by the chains for the CH group was matched to the NC at 30%1RM. One possible reason why there were no significant differences was that the CH group lifted less total weight. Matching the total weight at the bottom of the jump squat may have resulted in greater power or strength gains.

Training intensity plays a key role in the adaptation of power. Many studies have examined 30%1RM for peak power in jump squats (Cormie, McGuigan, & Newton, 2010, Thomas, Kraemer, Spiering, Volek, Anderson, & Maresh, 2007). McBride (McBride, Triplett-McBride, Davie, & Newton, 2002) examined the effects of eight weeks of jump squat training using light loads (30%1RM) or heavy loads (80%1RM). Both groups had an increase in strength, but the lighter load group also increased velocity. However, other studies have identified different intensities for optimal peak power.

Turner (Turner, Unholz, Potts, & Coleman, 2012) found that jump squat peak power for rugby players was at 20-30%1RM while Slievart (41) found it was between 50-70%. Finally, Bevan (Bevan, Bunce, Owen, Bennett, Cook, Cunningham, Newton, & Kilduff, 2010) and Jimenez-Reyes (Jimenez-Reyes, Pareja-Blanco, Balsalobre-Fernandez, Cuadrado-Penafiel, Ortega-Becerra, & Gonzalez-Badillo, 2015) found peak power at 0%1RM. The current study used 30%1RM but did not see a significant increase in vertical jump height. This could be due to not enough volume.

Adequate volume and frequency are required to increase power. Cormie (Cormie, McGuigan, & Newton, 2010) examined the effects of 10 weeks of power training and found that seven sets of six repetitions at 0%1RM twice a week with five sets of five repetitions at 30%1RM once a week caused an increase in power for both strong and weak individuals. The current study used five sets of three repetitions for only three visits resulting in an increase in strength for both groups, but not explosiveness. Perhaps a longer study may have positively influenced power.

Variability is needed in a training program to decrease staleness. One way to add variety to a program is by using novel training as it provides a new type of stressor (Haff, Hobbs, Haff, Sands, Pierce, & Stone, 2008). Resistance training is novel to untrained individuals, and they will normally experience some type of improvement (Gamble, 2008). Another type of novel stressor is kettlebell training. Otto (Otto, Coburn, Brown, & Spiering, 2012) compared the effects of kettlebell swings to Olympic weightlifting during a 6-week training program. They found that both forms of training increased strength in the back squat, but the increase with weightlifting was greater. The current study was not as long as Otto, but also showed that novel training can increase strength.

Specificity of training is also needed for a training program. Transferability is how well the specific training transfers to a movement or skill (Gamble, 2008). Studies have shown that specific training has greater transferability (Barak, Ayalon, & Dvir, 2004, Cale-Benzoor, Dickstein, Arnon, & Ayalon, 2014). The current study demonstrated that jump squats had greater transferability to the back squat than to the vertical jump. The squatting portion of the jump squat directly resembles the back squat. Although the jump squat utilizes triple extension of the knee, hip, and ankle, the training did not transfer to an increase in jump height. This could be due to the load of the jump squats being more than body weight, so acceleration, force, and power were altered.

5. Conclusion

The findings of the current study demonstrate that short-term jump squat training with or without chains increased 1RM back squat strength. The chain group, while lifting less overall weight, was still able to increase their 1RM strength. However, the training intensity, volume, or duration was not sufficient to increase power. Further research should focus on a longer duration of training and also examine matching chain loads at different positions of the lift. Coaches and athletes may use short-term training with chains to yield a similar increase in back squat strength as traditional loaded jump squats. Coaches and athletes can also use this type of training as a taper to reduce volume without risking a decrease in back squat strength. This jump squat training scheme may be beneficial if time is limited as the training was only approximately three to five minutes.

References

Aagaard, P., Simonsen, E.B., Andersen, J.L., Magnusson, P., & Dyhre-Poulsen, P. (2002). Increased rate of force development and neural drive of human skeletal muscle following resistance training. *Journal of Applied Physiology, 93, 1318-1326.*

Adibpour, N., Bakht, H.N., & Behpour, N. (2012). Comparison of the effect of plyometric and weight training programs on vertical jumps in female basketball players. *World Journal of Sport Sciences, 7(2), 99-104.*

Alemdaroglu, U., Dundar, U., Koklu, Y., Findikoglu, G. (2013). The effect of exercise order incorporating plyometric and resistance training on isokinetic leg strength and vertical jump performance: A comparative study. *Isokinetics and Exercise Science, 21, 211-21.*

Arabatzi, F., Kellius, E., Saez-Saez De Villarreal, E. (2010). Vertical jump biomechanics after plyometric, weight lifting, and combined weight lifting + plyometric training. *Journal of Strength and Conditioning Research, 24(9), 240-2448.*

Barak, Y., Ayalon, M., & Dvir, Z. (2004). Transferability of strength gains from limited to full range of motion. *Medicine and Science in Sports Medicine, 36(8), 1413-1420.*

Bevan, H.R., Bunce, P.J., Owen, N.J., Bennett, M.A., Cook, C.J., Cunningham, D.J., Newton, R.U., & Kilduff, L.P. (2010). Optimal loading for the development of peak power output in professional rugby players. *Journal of Strength and Conditioning Research, 24(1), 43-47.*

Brown, L.E., & Weir, J.P. (2001). ASEP procedures recommendation I: Accurate assessment of muscular strength and power. *Journal of Exercise Physiology Online, 4(3), 1-21.*

Brown, L.E., & Whitehurst, M. (2003). The effect of short-term isokinetic training on force and rate of velocity development. *Journal of Strength and Conditioning Research, 17(1), 88-94.*

Cale-Benzoor, M.C., Dickstein, R., Arnon, M., & Ayalon, M. (2014). Strength enhancement with limited range closed kinetic chain isokinetic exercise of the upper extremity. *Isokinetics and Exercise Science, 22, 37-46.*

Coburn, J.W. Housh, T.J., Malek, M.H., Weir, J.P., Cramer, J.T., Beck, T.W., & Johnson, G.O. (2006). Neuromuscular responses to three days of velocity-specific isokinetic training. *Journal of Strength and Conditioning Research, 20(4), 892-898.*

Cormie, P., McGuigan, M.R., & Newton, R.U. (2010). Adaptations in athletic performance after ballistic power versus strength training. *Medicine & Science in Sport & Exercise, 42(8), 1582-1598.*

Dalen, T., Welde, B., Van Den Tillaar, R., & Aune, T.K. (2013). Effect of single vs. multi joint ballistic resistance training upon vertical jump performance. *Acta Kinesiologiae Tartuensis, 19, 86-97.*

Gabriel, D.A., Kamen, G., & Frost, G. (2006). Neural adaptations to resistive exercise: Mechanisms and recommendations for training practices. *Sports Medicine, 36(2), 133-149.*

Galpin, A.J., Malyszek, K.K., Davis, K.A., Record, S.M., Brown, L.E., Coburn, J.W., Harmon, R.A., Steele, J.M., & Manolovitz, A.D. (2015.) Acute effects of elastic bands on kinetic characteristics during the deadlift at moderate and heavy loads. *Journal of Strength and Conditioning Research,29(12), 3271-3278.*

Gamble, P. (2008). Implications and applications of training specificity for coaches and athletes. *Strength and Conditioning Journal, 28(3), 54-58.*

Ghigiarelli, J.J., Nagle E.F., Gross, F.L., Robertson, R.J., Irrgang, J.J., & Myslinski, T. (2009). The effects of a 7-week heavy elastic band and weight chain program on upper-body strength and upper-body power in a sample of division 1-AA football players. *Journal of Strength and Conditioning Research, 23(3), 756-764.*

Haff, G.G., Hobbs, R.T., Haff, E.E., Sands, W.A., Pierce, K.C., & Stone, M.H. (2008). Cluster training: A novel method for introducing training program variation. *Strength Conditioning Journal, 30, 67-76,*

Hoffman J.R., Ratamess, N.A., Cooper, J.J., Kang, J, Chilakos, A., & Faigenbaum, A.D. (2005). Comparison of loaded and unloaded jump squat training on strength/power performance in college football players. *Journal of Strength and Conditioning Research, 19(4), 810-815.*

Israetel, M. A., McBride, J.M., Nuzzo, J.L., Skinner J.W., & Dayne, A.M. (2010). Kinetic and kinematic differences between squats performed with and without elastic bands. *Journal of Strength and Conditioning Research, 24(1), 190-194.*

Jimenez-Reyes, P., Pareja-Blanco, F., Balsalobre-Fernandez, C., Cuadrado-Penafiel, V., Ortega-Becerra, M.A., & Gonzalez-Badillo, J.J. (2015). Jump-squat performance and its relationship with relative training intensity in high-level athletes. *International Journal of Sports Physiology and Performance, 10, 1036-1040.*

Jones, A., Brown, L.E., Coburn, J.W., & Noffal, G.J. (2015). Effects of foam rolling on vertical jump performance. *International Journal of Kinesiology & Sport Science, 3(3), 38-42.*

MacKenzie, S.J., Lavers, R.J., & Wallace, B.B. (2014). A biomechanical comparison of the vertical jump, power clean, and jump squat. *Journal of Sports Sciences, 1-10.*

McBride, J, Triplett-McBride T, Davie, A, & Newton, R. (2002). The effect of heavy- vs. Light-load jump squats on the development of strength, power, and speed. *Journal of Strength and Conditioning Research, 16, 75-82.*

McCurdy, K., Langford, G., Ernest, J., Jenkerson, D., & Doscher, M. (2009). Comparison of chain- and plate-loaded bench press training on strength, joint pain, and muscle soreness in division II baseball players. *Journal of Strength and Conditioning Research, 23(1), 187-195.*

McLellan, C.P., Lovell, D.I., & Gass, G.C. (2011). The role of rate of force development on vertical jump performance. *Journal of Strength and Conditioning Research, 25(2), 379-385.*

McMaster, T., Cronin, J., & McGuigan, M. (2009). Forms of variable resistance training. *Strength and Conditioning Journal, 31(1), 50-64.*

McMaster, T., Cronin, J., & McGuigan, M. (2010). Quantification of rubber and chain-based resistance modes. *Journal of Strength and Conditioning Research,24(8), 2056-2064.*

Moreno, S.D., Brown, L.E., Coburn, J.W., & Judelson, D.A. (2014.) Effect of cluster sets on plyometric jump power. *Journal of Strength and Conditioning Research, 28(9), 2424-2428.*

Neelly, K.R., Terry, J. G., & Morris, M.J. (2010). A mechanical comparison of linear and double-looped hung supplemental heavy chain resistance to the back squat: A case study. *Journal of Strength and Conditioning Research, 24(1), 278-281.*

Nijem, R.M., Coburn, J.W., Brown, L.E., Lynn, S.K., & Ciccone, A.B. (2016). An electromyographic and force plate analysis of the deadlift performed with and without chains. *Journal of Strength and Conditioning Research, 30(5), 1177-1182.*

Otto, W.H., Coburn, J.W., Brown, L.E., & Spiering, B.A. (2012). Effects of weightlifting vs. kettlebell training on vertical jump, strength, and body composition. *Journal of Strength and Conditioning Research, 26(5), 1199-1202.*

Ratamess, N.A. adaptations to anaerobic training programs. In Baechle, T.R., & Earle, R.W. (Eds.), *Essentials of Strength Training and Conditioning* (pp. 90-113). Human Kinetics.

Rhea, M.R., Kenn, J.G., & Dermody, B.M. (2009). Alterations in speed of squat movement and the use of accommodated resistance among college athletes training for power. *Journal of Strength and Conditioning Research, 23(9), 2645-2650.*

Sleivert,G., & Taingahue, M. (2004). The relationship between maximal jump-squat power and sprint acceleration in athletes. *European Journal of Applied Physiology, 91, 46-52.*

Smilios, I., Pilianidis, T., Sotiropoulos, K., Antonakis, M., & Tokmakidis, S.P. (2005). Short-term effects of selected exercise and load in contrast training on vertical jump performance. *Journal of Strength and Conditioning Research, 19(1), 135-139.*

Swinton, P.A., Stewart, A.D., Lloyd, R., Aqouris, I., & Keogh, J.W. (2012). Effect of load positioning on the kinematics and kinetics of weighted vertical jumps. *Journal of Strength and Conditioning Research, 26(4), 906-913.*

Thomas, G.A., Kraemer, W.J., Spiering, B.A., Volek, J.S., Anderson, J.M., & Maresh, C.M. (2007). Maximal power at different percentages of one repetition maximum: influence of resistance and gender. *Journal of Strength and Conditioning Research, 21(2), 336-342.*

Tillin, N.A., & Folland, J.P. (2014). Maximal and explosive strength training elicit distinct neuromuscular adaptations, specific to the training stimulus. *European Journal of Applied Physiology, 114, 365-374.*

Turner, A.P., Unholz, C.N., Potts, N., & Coleman, S.G.S. (2012). Peak power, force, and velocity during jump squats in professional rugby players. *Journal of Strength and Conditioning Research, 26(6), 1594-1600.*

Wallace, B.J., Winchester, J.B, & McGuigan, M.R. (2006). Effects of elastic bands on force and power characteristics during the back squat exercise. *Journal of Strength and Conditioning Research, 20(2), 268-272.*

The Influence of Physical Training on Blood Levels of Human Growth Hormone, Testosterone and Procollagen in Young Rowers

Kaloupsis Socratis
Department of Aquatic Sports, University of Athens, PO box 17237, Dafni, Athens, Greece
E-mail: skaloups@phed.uoa.gr

Ditsios Kostas
A` Orthopaedics Department, Aristotle University of Thessaloniki, PO box 54124, Thessaloniki, Greece
E-mail: ditsiosk@otenet.gr

Dessypris Athanasios
Department of Biochemistry and Molecular Biology, University of Athens, PO Box 17237, Dafni, Athens, Greece

Dimakopoulou Eleni (Corresponding author)
Department of Aquatic Sports, University of Athens, PO box 17237, Dafni, Greece
E-mail: edimakop@phed.uoa.gr

Kapoutsis Dimitrios
A` Orthopaedics Department, Aristotle University of Thessaloniki, PO box 54124, Thessaloniki, Greece

Abstract

Objective: The purpose of this study was to investigate muscle strength and skeletal age in trained and untrained pubertal boys and its relationship to the levels of Testosterone (T), Growth Hormone (GH) and Procollagen (PICP). **Methods:** Both the exercise and control groups consisted of 24 (mean 12.91, sd = 0.63) and 17 (mean 12.91, sd = 0.48) year old boys, respectively. The exercise group (EG), in addition to school activities, participated in a rowing training program for six months (rowing technique, strength & aerobic exercises, 60 min/day, three days/week). The control group (CG) only participated in the school physical education program, two to three times/week. Hormonal concentrations were measured by radioimmunoassay techniques. Venus blood samples were taken at rest from both groups. **Results:** Testosterone was increased in both groups ($p<0.001$). Significant differences were found within groups in T before training ($p<0.01$) There was an increase of PICP in EG after training ($p<0.01$). Differences on GH were observed before the training period in both groups ($p<0.01$). Both groups significantly differed in upper and lower limbs strengths. Significant correlation was found between PICP and skeletal age in both ($p<0.05$ and $p<0.02$, respectively) **Conclusions:** The gains in muscle strength in both groups may partly be explained by the increase in the concentrations of hormone levels and the changes in body size.

Key words: skeletal age, muscle strength, anabolic hormones, rowing

1. Introduction

Participation in sport attracts many young people for a variety of reasons. Rowing is a demanding physical and mental workout. Along with rowing skills, young people can develop teamwork, unselfishness and initiative. It is well known in the world of sport sciences that the potential of physical training is related to hormones (Mero et al., 1990, Eliakim and Nemet, 2013, Nemet et al., 2012, Ramson et al., 2012). In addition, hormonal changes are also related to behavioral changes (Mansoubi et al., 2013). Hormones are biochemical indexes which help us diagnose an unsafe situation for the athlete, for instance overtraining and prevent it (Kuipers & Keizer, 1988, Lehmann et al., 1993). Hormones are also related to the changes of body constitution, distribution of fat tissue and muscular strength (Rogol, 1994). There have been long term studies of the physiology of the athletes' endocrine system (Galbo, 1983, Hakkinen et al., 1989). Growth Hormone and T are both anabolic hormones, with T contributing to growth and function of reproductive tissues and to the increase of muscle and bone mass, and GH, being essential for the growth and the development of bones, liver and other organs. PICP is the most abundant type of collagen in most soft tissues and accounts for >90% of the organic matrix of bone. In rowing, there have been studies investigating hormone concentrations referring to hormonal levels before and after a training program and a competitive effort, or throughout the different phases of a training season

(Purge et al., 2006, Maestu et al., 2005). Vervoorn et al., (1991) found that prolonged heavy endurance training causes an increase and a decrease in the fasting levels of Cortisol and T, respectively. In another study improvement of performance was associated with increased GH and Cortisol (Snegovskaya & Viru, 1993). Few studies have investigated the effect of PICP and its relation to skeletal age.

Therefore, the purpose of the present study was a) to investigate the concentration levels of T, GH and PICP in young adolescent athletes participating in a six months rowing training program b) to examine the relation of these hormones to both strength and skeletal age.

2. Methods

2. 1 Participants

Forty-one healthy male high school students, attending a school with special emphasis on physical education and sports (athletic high-school) volunteered to participate in this study. They were randomly assigned into 2 groups: an EG and a CG. A lottery system was used to randomly assign participants into these groups. All students and their parents received full information about the procedure of the study and gave their written consent. The study was approved by the Department of Physical Education of the University of Athens.

2.1.1 Exercise Group (EG)

This group consisted of 24 students (age: 12.8 ± 0.63yrs, height: 166.67 ± 8.22cm, body mass: 58.42± 9.37kg) who followed a six-month rowing training program, appropriately designed for this age group. They trained at least 3 times a week, enabling them to learn the basic rowing technique. The exercise program was designed for both upper and lower extremities. Duration of the training session was approximately 60 minutes. Each session was supervised by a coach. The training regimen of rowers was similar for each week of the study and consisted of 25% strength training, 60% endurance training and 15% technique training in single sculls, pair and in Concept II rowing ergometer (Morrisvile, USA).

2.1.2 Control Group (CG)

The CG consisted of 17 adolescent males (age: 12.91± 0.47yrs, height:156.77± 6.9cm, body mass: 47.89± 8.38kg), who participated regularly in physical exercise classes at school and other leisure-time sports activities, without following a special training program.

2.2 Procedure

2.2.1 Anthropometry

Students' bare-foot standing height was measured with a special height measuring apparatus (Sega se v 91) to the nearest 0.1 cm and weight was determined using a scale (Sega 770) with a precision of 0.1 kg. All anthropometric data were gathered by a single experienced investigator. Body Mass Index (BMI) was determined as the second power of body weight in kilograms divided by height in meters. Each student underwent a left hand and wrist X-ray in order to evaluate the skeletal age, according to the well known method of Greulich and Pyle (1959). The evaluation was conducted by an experienced doctor.

2.2.2 Muscle Strength Measuring

Students were tested after breakfast between 8 and 9 o'clock. On testing day, after a period of warm up, subjects were verbally encouraged to produce a maximal force at an angle of 90^0 degree. Subjects were asked to sit on a Concept II rowing ergometer (Morrisvile, USA). A belt was adjusted around their back and a chain was connected with a strain gauge sensor (Dynamometer, ADW 15, Mantraweigh, UK 2000). All data was recorded in a portable pc. The knee joint was positioned at 90^0 degree of flexion. Subjects then performed one maximum voluntary isometric contraction. The same procedure was followed for upper limb strength (biceps) as subjects lay prone in a gymnastic bench. The elbow joint was positioned at 90^0 flexion. Subjects performed one maximum voluntary isometric contraction.

2.2.3 Blood Tests

After one day of rest from muscle strength measurement and 12 hours of fasting, T, GH and PICP levels were determined by Ria (Orion Diagnostica, Espoo, Finland). All hormones were analyzed on radioimmunoassay in the biochemical lab of the university.. Approximately 10mL of blood was drawn from the antecubital vein using a gauge needle Vacutainer setup. Blood samples were centrifuged two times, each time for ten minutes (speed: 1500/ minute) in order to separate the red blood cells and serum. Serum was distributed into three different vacutainers which were frozen to -20 ^{0}C. In order to minimize the influence of diurnal fluctuation all samples were obtained between 8.30 and 11.00 am.

2.3 Data Analyses

Mean Values and Standard deviations were calculated for all variables. Differences between groups were determined using Repeated Measures Anova followed by Bonferroni post hoc comparisons. Paired Sample t- test was used to detect the differences before and after the study period. For every correlation analysis, Pearson's coefficient was calculated. The data in the tables are presented as mean ± SD. Statistical significance was set at $p<0.05$. Data was analyzed using the IBM SPSS 19.0 (SPSS, Chicago, LII, USA).

3. Results

General characteristics of both EG and CG are shown in Table 1. Significant differences were observed in both groups during the study period regarding skeletal age (p=0.001), height (p=0.001) and body weight (p=0.001). BMI changed significantly in the EG (p=0.01), but not in the CG (p=0.088). Both groups exhibited significant differences before the six-month training period in: skeletal age (p=0.021), in height (p=0.001) and in body weight (p=0.001). After the study period, significant differences were also observed (skeletal age (p=0.002), height (p=0.001), body weight (p=0.001) and BMI (p=0.039)). Chronological age and skeletal age differed before (p=0.001) and after (p=0.000) the study period in EG. In addition, in the CG the chronological age and skeletal age were not different before (p=0.964) but were after (p= 0.009).

Table 1. General characteristics of EG and CG (Mean±*SD*)

Variables	*EG (n=24)*		CG (*n*=17)	
	Pre	**Post**	**Pre**	**Post**
Chron. age(yrs)	12.8 ± 0.63	13.4±0.63	12.9±0.5	13.5±0.5
Skeletal Age	13.5±0.91	14.2±1.06	12.9±0.7	13.3±0.7
Height (cm)	166.6±8.22	170.3±7.94	156.7±6.9	160.9±6.5
Weight (Kg)	58.4±9.37	62.1±8.39	47.8±8.4	51.5±7.8
BMI (Kg/ m^2)	20.6±2.36	21.3±2.02	19.4±2.7	19.8±2.6

T mean concentrations and significant difference, of the EG and CG, before and after the training period, are shown in figure 1.

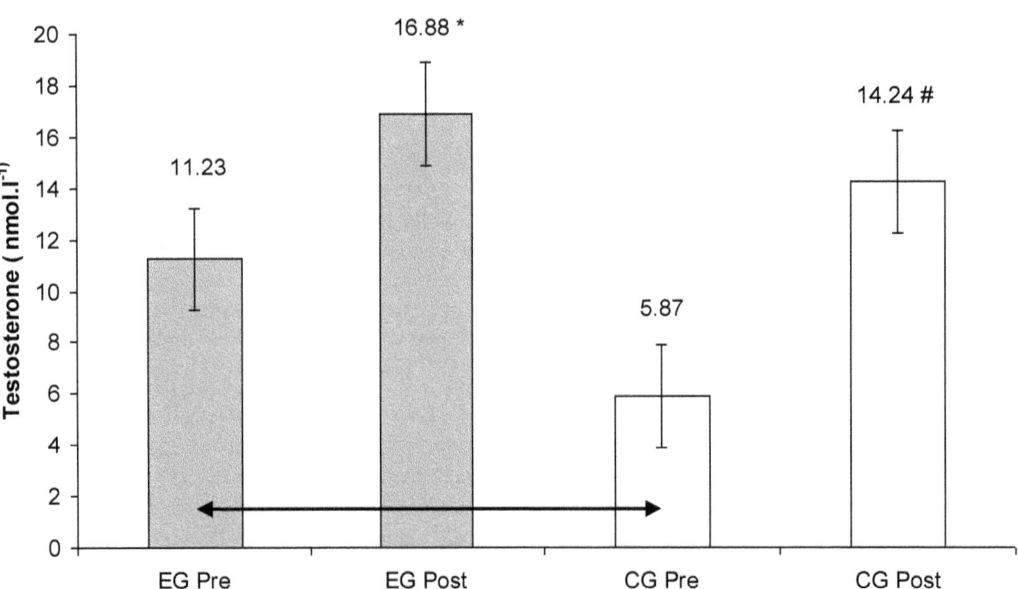

Figure1. Concentrations and differences of T in EG and CG before and after the training period (Mean± Sd). significant difference p< 0.05, * EG pre-post, # CG pre-post,

Figure 2 presents GH mean concentrations and significant difference, of the EG and CG, before and after the study period.

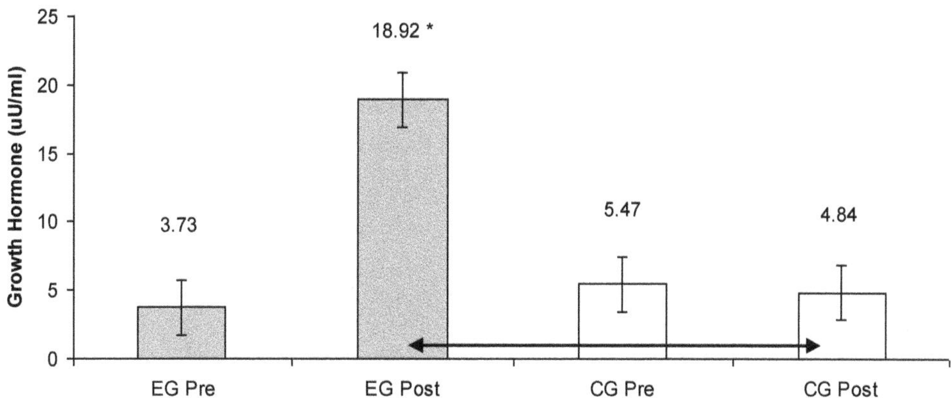

Figure 2. Concentrations and differences of GH in EG and CG before and after the training period (Mean± Sd).significant difference p<0.05, * EG pre-post

In figure 3 PICP mean concentration before and after the training period for both groups is shown (and significant differences). EG and CG had significant differences in T concentrations (p=0.013) in the beginning of the study. After the training period, they had significant differences in GH (p=0.001). Table 2 summarizes the upper and lower limbs strength of the EG and the CG in the start and in the end of the six-month training period. The two groups had significant differences in upper limbs strength (p=0.001) and in lower limbs strength (p=0.001) in the start of the study and at the end of the training period also differed in upper (p=0.001) and lower (p=0.001) limb strength.

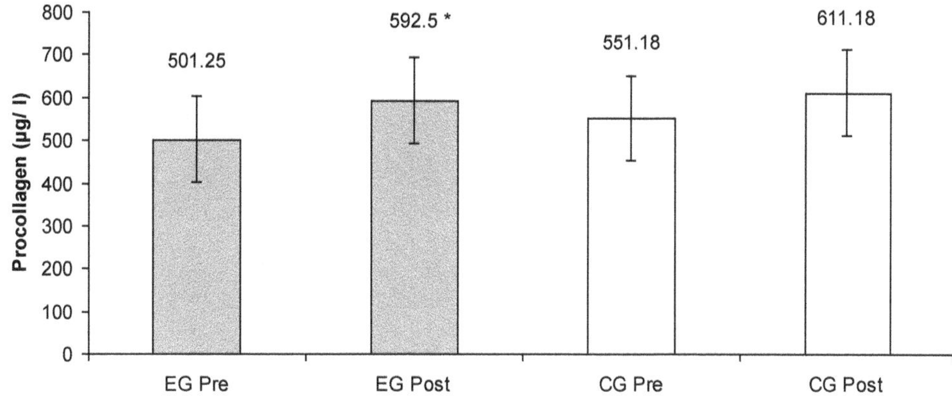

Figure 3. Concentration of PICP and differences in each group before and after the training program (Mean± Sd). significant difference p< 0.05, EG pre-post

Table 2. Differences of Upper and Lower limbs' strength of EG and CG before and after a six-month training period (Mean± *SD*).

Variables/Groups	*Pre training*	*Post training*	*t*	p
Upper Limb Strength / EG	41.83±10.34*	50.39±10.61#	9.71	0.001
Lower Limb Strength / EG	87.08±16.29	106.87±18.69	7.48	0.001
Upper Limb Strength / CG	29.38±5.17	31.94±6.55	4.86	0.001
Lower Limb Strength / CG	60.73±10.48	64.85±11.74	9.67	0.001

* p<0.05 EG-CG (upper, lower limb strength pre), # p<0.05 EG-CG (upper, lower limb strength post)

Significant correlation was observed between T and upper limbs strength (before 0.009, r=0.5, after p< 0.010, r= 0.7) and T and lower limbs strength (before p< 0.039, after p<0.004, r=0.7) in the EG. This correlation was significant before and after the study period. In the CG, significant correlations were found between GH and upper limbs strength

($p<0.043$, r=0.5) before training and after ($p<0.009$, r=0.6). Significant correlation between GH and lower limb strength was found only after the training program ($p<0.008$, r=0.6) in CG. No significant correlation was found between PICP and strength in both groups. In the EG significant correlation was found between PICP and skeletal age, after training ($p<0.004$, r=0.5). Significant correlation was observed before and after training between PICP and skeletal age in CG. The correlations were 0.05 and 0.016, respectively. No significant correlations were found between chronological age and hormones concentrations neither in EG nor in CG.

4. Discussion

Primary findings demonstrated that both groups had a significant increase in skeletal age, height and body weight. BMI significantly increased only in EG. The EG anthropometric characteristics compared to a reference group of untrained Greek children by means of percentiles (P) (Kaloupsis et al., 2008) presented high percentile values for height (P83), weight (P70) and BMI (P52). Significant differences between the two groups was noticed as far as skeletal age, height, body weight and BMI were concerned. The EG had advanced skeletal age. Bouchard and Malina (1977) found that athletes of various sports had advanced skeletal compared to chronological age. Similar results are reported by Hale (1956) and Szabo et al. (1972). Malina et al. (1982) found that children participating in basketball, football, rowing and swimming had advanced skeletal age compared to sedentary children of the same chronological age. Advanced skeletal age is also reported for Polish and Czech boys regularly involved in sports (Parizkova, 1974). The increase in height for both groups was expected as a result of somatic growth and maturation (Kobayashi et al.,1978, Prader, 1983, Rogol et al., 2000). Similarly, body weight was significantly different. Study group was heavier. According to Malina and Bouchard (1991) children with advanced biological maturity tend to present increased body weight.

A significant increase in T levels was observed in both groups. Before training, T levels differed significantly ($p=0.013$) between the two groups. After training period, there were no significant differences ($p=0.324$). The results of Mero et al. (1990) suggested that T concentration increased in boy athletes during a 1- year training period. Cacciari et al. (1990) who studied football players found the same results as Mero et al. (1990). Ramos et al. (1998) found increased T levels in older boys and a specific gain in muscle strength. Frasier et al. (1969) studied boys during childhood and adolescence and found T levels rising significantly after the age of 11. Similar findings are reported in Wieland et al. (1971). Another study, demonstrated that 2 months of strength training resulted in significant increase in the level of T (Tsolakis et al., 2007). In the present study, the GH concentrations increased after the study period in EG. Steinacker et al. (2000) found a 10% increase in human GH during a high load training phase. The two groups differed significantly only after the training period in GH. No correlation was found between GH and chronological age (Greenwood et al., 1964). According to Hartley (1975) and Bunt et al. (1986), GH levels increase during training period. Tsolakis et al. (2003) found significant differences in T and GH among athletes group (handball, rowing, running, basketball, fencing etc.). The mean T of the control group (sedentary boys) did not differ from those of the corresponding exercise group. The study by Tsolakis et al. (2003) demonstrated the importance of the specificity of the training stimulus in the hormonal adaptations of pre-pubertal sedentary subjects.

In another study (Kaloupsis, 1996), 61 subjects were studied. They were arranged randomly in 4 groups (2 exercise and 2 control groups). The study groups consisted of subjects of different chronological ages (13-14yrs) and rowing experience (novice and more experienced). For each exercise group there was a corresponding group of the same age who did not exercise systematically. The subjects of the study group underwent a 6-month rowing training program. The results of this study showed a post exercise increase in T concentration in all groups which is in line with the findings of our results. PICP was increased only in EG and was found to be correlated with skeletal age in both groups. This result was expected, as PICP is the most abundant type of collagen in most soft tissues and accounts for > 90% of the organic matrix of bones. Assessment of the turnover rhythm of this collagen is particularly relevant to bone metabolism. The assay of the carboxyterminal propeptide of type I procollagen provides a method of estimating the rate of type I collagen synthesis in the body (Melkko et al., 1990). Another study by Fujimura et al. (1997) in males (23-31yrs) reports slight increase of PICP in the training group (4 months, weight training) after the first month of resistance training. The PICP returned to baseline thereafter. In the sedentary group the PICP significantly decreased. These results are in line with our study.

A significant increase of muscle strength of upper (biceps) and lower limbs was observed in both groups. In EG (quadriceps, biceps femoris, gastrocnemious), T was positively correlated to muscle strength of upper and lower extremities. Testosterone has been shown to stimulate anabolic processes in skeletal muscles and appears to be the principal hormone responsible for the development of strength (Hakkinen and Parakin, 1993). Our results are in agreement with another study (Ramos et al., 1998) which found a positive correlation between T levels and absolute muscle strength in boys (11-12yrs). Increase in strength can be due to several factors including changes in body size and composition. Gregory et al. (1992) found that height, weight, and muscle mass increase with age and are correlated with gains in muscle strength. Age and weight is suggested to be the most important factors (Falker, 1978). The increase in muscle strength can be explained also by the context of the specific training (rowing technique), endurance and resistance training. The rowers (EG) probably recruited both fast and slow twitch muscle fibres in their training, which induced effects in both cell types. Synchronous strength training and increased T levels may affect muscle growth (Richter, 1986).

In this study, training can be a stimulus for increased hormone levels. The increase is observed in puberty (13yrs) and in the EG hormone levels increased more. Our results are in agreement with the study of Zakas et al. (1994) who suggested that training elevates serum T and GH concentrations in puberty (13yrs), when there is a stimulus such as a high intensity and duration in exercise. In summary, significant increases in muscle strength occurred in both groups. The gains in muscle strength may partly be explained by the increase in the concentrations of hormonal levels and the changes in body size.

5. Conclusion

Puberty is a dynamic period of development in body size, shape and composition. Our study concludes that either mild or high training can change the levels of T, GH and PICP in puberty. The significant increase in hormonal levels of T, GH and PICP concentrations during the six-month training program are of great importance as this information might be useful to coaches for designing training programs for these age groups.

References

Bouchard C. and Malina R.M. (1977). Skeletal maturity in a Pan American Canadian Team. *Canadian Journal of Applied Sport Science,* 2, 109-114.

Bunt J.C., Boileau R.A., Bahr J.M., Nelson R.A. (1986). Sex and training differences in human growth hormone levels during prolonged exercise. *Journal of Applied Physiology*, 61(5), 1796-801.

Cacciari E., Mazzanti L., Tassinari D., Bergamaschi R., Magnani C., Zappula F., Nanni G., Codianchi C., Ghini T., Pini R., Tani G. (1990). Effects of sport (football) on growth : auxological, anthropometric and hormonal aspects. *European Journal of Applied Physiology and Occupational Physiol*ogy, 61(1-2), 149-158.

Eliakim A., Nemet D. (2013). The endocrine response to exercise and training in young athletes. *Pediatric Exercise Science*, 25, 605-615.

Falker J. (1978). Plantar flexor strength testing using the Cybex isokinetic dynamometer. *Physical Therapy*, 58, 847-50.

Frasier S.D., Gafford F., Horton R. (1969). Plasma androgens in childhood and adolescence. *Journal of Clinical Endocrinology and Metabolism*, 29, 1404-8.

Fuzimura R., Ashizawa N., Watanabe M., Mukai N., Amagai H., Fukubayashi T., Hayashi K., Tokuyama K., Suzuki M. (1997). Effect of resistance exercise training on bone formation and resorption in young male subjects assessed by biomarkers of bone metabolish. *Journal of Bone and Mineral Research*, 12(4), 656-662.

Galbo H. (1983). Hormonal and metabolic adaptations to exercise. Stuttgart: Thieme, p. 2-27.

Greenwood F.C., Hunter W.M., Marrian V.J. (1964). Growth hormone levels in children and adolescents. *British Medical Journal*, 1, 25-6.

Gregory J.W., Greene S.A., Thompson J., Scrimgeour C.M., Rennie M.J. (1992). Effects of oral testosterone undecanoate on growth, body composition, strength and energy expenditure of adolescents boys. *Clinical Endocrinology*, 37, 207-13.

Greulich W.W., Pyle S.I. (1959). Radiographic atlas of skeletal development of the hand and wrist. Stanford University Press.

Hakkinen K., Keskinen K.L., Alen M., Komi P.V., Kauhanen H. (1989). Serum hormone concentrations during prolonged training in elite endurance trained and strength trained athletes. *European Journal of Applied Physiology and Occupational Physiology*, 59, 233-238.

Hakkinen K., Pakarinen A. (1993). Muscle strength and serum testosterone, cortisol and SHBG concentrations in middle-aged and elderly men and women. *Acta Physiologica Scandinavica*, 148, 199-207.

Hale J. (1956). Physiological maturity of Little League Baseball players. *Research Quarterly*, 27, 276-284.

Hartley L. (1975). Growth hormone and catecholamine response to exercise in relation to physical training. *Medicine and Science in Sports*, 7(1), 34-36.

Kaloupsis S. (1996). The effect of rowing training of male rowers of adolescence age on the levels of selective anthropometrics ergometric and hormonal parameters with the rate of biological maturation. Phd Thesis.

Kaloupsis S., Bogdanis G.C., Dimakopoulou E., Maridaki M. (2008). Anthropometric characteristics and somatotype of young Greek rowers. *Biology of Sport*, 25(1), 57-68.

Kobayashi K., Kitamura K., Miura M., Sodeyama H., Murasa Y., Miyashita M., Matsui H. (1978). Aerobic power as related to body growth and training in Japanese boys. A longitudinal study. *Journal of Applied Physiology*, 44, 666-672.

Kuipers H., Keizer A. (1988). Overtraining in elite athletes. *Sports Medicine*, 6, 79-92.

Lehmann M., Forster C., Keul J. (1993). Overtraining in endurance athletes: a brief review. *Medicine and Science in Sports and Exercise*, 25, 854-61.

Maestu J., Jurimae J., Jurimae T. (2005). Hormonal response to maximal rowing before and after heavy increase in training volume in highly trained male rowers. *Journal of Sports Medicine & Physical Fitness*, 45(1), 121-6.

Malina R., Meeleski B., Shoup R. (1982). Anthropometric, body composition and Maturity characteristics of selected school age athletes. *Pediatric Clinics of North America*, 29 (6), 1305-23.

Malina R.M., Bouchard C. (1991). Physical activity as a factor in growth, maturation and performance. Growth, maturation, and physical activity. Human Kinetics, Champaign I 11, p. 371-390.

Mansoubi M., Hojjat S., Shojaei M. (2013). Effect of national preparation training on salivary testosterone, cortisol, and some psychological factors on Iranian female rowers. *European Journal of Experimental Biology*, 3(2), 13-17.

Melkko J., Niemi S., Risteli L., Risteli J. (1990). Rarioimmunoassay of the Carboxyterminal propeptide of Human Type I Procollagen. *Clinical Chemistry*, 36(6):1328-1332.

Mero A., Jaakkola L., Komi P.V. (1990). Serum hormones and physical performance capacity in young boy athletes during a 1-year training period. *European Journal of Applied Physiology*, 60: 32-37.

Nemet D., Portal S., Zadik Z., Pliz-Burstein R., Adler-Portal D., Meckel Y., Eliakim A. (2012). Training increases anabolic response and reduces inflammatory response to a single practice in elite male adolescent volleyball players. *Journal of Pediatric Endocrinology and Metabolism*, 25 (9-10), 875-880.

Parizkova J. (1974). Particularities of lean body mass and fat development in growing boys as related to their motor activity. *Acta Pediatrica belgica*, 28(Suppl): 233-243.

Prader A. (1983). Biomedical and endocrinological aspect of normal growth and development. *Biomedical Aspects of Normal Growth*, 1-21.

Purge P., Jurimae J., Jurimae T. (2006). Hormonal and psychological adaptation in elite male rowers during prolonged training. *Journal of Sports Science*, 24(10), 1075-1082.

Ramos E., Frontera W.R., Liopart A., Feliciano D. (1998). Muscle strength and Hormonal Levels in Adolescents: Gender Related Differences. *International Journal of Sports Medicine*, 19: 526-531.

Ramson R., Jurimae J., Jurimae T., Maestu J. (2012). The effect of 4-week training period on plasma neyropeptide Y, leptin and ghrelin response in male rowers. European Journal of applied Physiology, 112(5), 1873-1880.

Richter E.A. (1986). Hormones, exercise and skeletal muscle. *Scandinavian Journal of Sports Science,* 8, 35-41.

Rogol A.D. (1994). Growth at puberty: interaction of androgens and growth hormone. *Medicine and Science in Sports and Exercise*, 26, 767-70.

Rogol A.D., Clark P.A., Roemmich J.N. (2000). Growth and pubertal development in children and adolescents: effects of diet and physical activity. *American Journal of Clinical Nutrition*, 72 (suppl), 521S-8S.

Snegovskaya V., Viru A. (1993). Elevation of cortisol and growth hormone levels in the course of further improvement of performance capacity in trained rowers. *International Journal of Sports Medicine*, 14, 202-207.

Steinacker J.M., Lormes W., Kellmann M., et al. (2000). Training of junior rowers before world championships: effects on performance, mood state and selected hormonal and matabolic responses. *Journal of Sports Medicine and Physical Fitness*, 40, 327-35.

Szabo S., Doka J., Apor P., Somogyvar K. (1972). Die Beziehugh zwischen Knochenlebensalter funktionel anthropometrischen Daten und der aeroben kapazitat. *Schweizerische Zeitschhrift Sportmedizin*, 20, 109-115.

Tsolakis C., Bogdanis G.C. (2007). Influence of resistance training on anabolic hormones in prepubertal and pubertal males. *Journal of Exercise Science and Physiology*, 3(1), 1-11.

Tsolakis C., Messinis D., Stergioulas A., Dessypris A. (2000). Hormonal responses after training and detraining in prepubertal and pubertal boys. *Journal of Strength and Conditional Research*, 14(4), 399-404.

Tsolakis C., Xekouki P., Kaloupsis S., Karas D., Messinis D., Vagenas G., Dessypris A. (2003). The influence of exercise on growth hormone and testosterone in prepubertal and early-pubertal boys. *Hormones*, 2(2), 103-112.

Vernoorn C., Quist A.M., Vermulst L.J., et al. (1991). The bahavior of the plasma free testosterone/cortisol ratio during a season of elite rowing training. *International Journal of Sports Medicine*, 12(3), 257-63.

Wieland R.G., Chen J.C., Zorn E.M., Hallberg M.C. (1971). Correlation of growth pubertal staging, growth hormone, gonadotropins, and testosterone levels during pubertal growth spurt in males. *Journal of Pediatrics*. 79, 999-1002.

Zakas A., Mandroukas K., Karamouzis M., Panagiotopoulou G. (1994). Physical training, growth hormone and testosterone levels and blood pressure in prepubertal, pubertal and adolescent boys. *Scandinavian Journal of Medicine and Science in Sports*, 4, 113-118.

Permissions

All chapters in this book were first published in IJKSS, by Australian International Academic Centre PTY. LTD.; hereby published with permission under the Creative Commons Attribution License or equivalent. Every chapter published in this book has been scrutinized by our experts. Their significance has been extensively debated. The topics covered herein carry significant findings which will fuel the growth of the discipline. They may even be implemented as practical applications or may be referred to as a beginning point for another development.

The contributors of this book come from diverse backgrounds, making this book a truly international effort. This book will bring forth new frontiers with its revolutionizing research information and detailed analysis of the nascent developments around the world.

We would like to thank all the contributing authors for lending their expertise to make the book truly unique. They have played a crucial role in the development of this book. Without their invaluable contributions this book wouldn't have been possible. They have made vital efforts to compile up to date information on the varied aspects of this subject to make this book a valuable addition to the collection of many professionals and students.

This book was conceptualized with the vision of imparting up-to-date information and advanced data in this field. To ensure the same, a matchless editorial board was set up. Every individual on the board went through rigorous rounds of assessment to prove their worth. After which they invested a large part of their time researching and compiling the most relevant data for our readers.

The editorial board has been involved in producing this book since its inception. They have spent rigorous hours researching and exploring the diverse topics which have resulted in the successful publishing of this book. They have passed on their knowledge of decades through this book. To expedite this challenging task, the publisher supported the team at every step. A small team of assistant editors was also appointed to further simplify the editing procedure and attain best results for the readers.

Apart from the editorial board, the designing team has also invested a significant amount of their time in understanding the subject and creating the most relevant covers. They scrutinized every image to scout for the most suitable representation of the subject and create an appropriate cover for the book.

The publishing team has been an ardent support to the editorial, designing and production team. Their endless efforts to recruit the best for this project, has resulted in the accomplishment of this book. They are a veteran in the field of academics and their pool of knowledge is as vast as their experience in printing. Their expertise and guidance has proved useful at every step. Their uncompromising quality standards have made this book an exceptional effort. Their encouragement from time to time has been an inspiration for everyone.

The publisher and the editorial board hope that this book will prove to be a valuable piece of knowledge for researchers, students, practitioners and scholars across the globe.

List of Contributors

Yumeng Li
Department of Kinesiology, University of Georgia, Athens, Georgia, USA
330 River Rd, Athens, GA30605, USA

Marion J. L. Alexander
Faculty of Kinesiology and Recreation Management, University of Manitoba, Winnipeg, Canada
306 Max Bell Center, Winnipeg, R3T 2N2, Canada

Cheryl M. Glazebrook
Faculty of Kinesiology and Recreation Management, University of Manitoba, Winnipeg, Canada
319 Max Bell Center, Winnipeg, R3T 2N2, Canada

Jeff Leiter
Pan Am Clinic, Winnipeg, Canada
75 Poseidon Bay, Winnipeg, R3M 3E4, Canada

Nathan J Washington and Kylie A Steel
School of Science and Health, Western Sydney University, Sydney New South Wales, Australia

Sera Dogramaci
New South Wales Institute of Sport, Figtree Drive, Olympic Park, Sydney, NSW, Australia

Eathan Ellem
School of Science and Health, Western Sydney University Sydney New South Wales, Australia

Robert Rietjens, Tori M. Stone, Jeffrey Montes, John C. Young, Richard D. Tandy and James W. Navalta
Department of Kinesiology and Nutrition Sciences, University of Nevada, Las Vegas 4505 S. Maryland Parkway, Las Vegas, NV, USA

Jenifer C. Utz
School of Life Sciences, University of Nevada, Las Vegas 4505 S. Maryland Parkway, Las Vegas, NV, USA

Tajul Arifin Muhamad and Mohd Radzani Abd Razak
Departemant Sport Management, Faculty of Education, Universiti Kebangsaan Malaysia, Kajang 43600, Malaysia

Fatemeh Golestani
Departemant Sport Management, Faculty of Education, Universiti Kebangsaan Malaysia, Kajang 43600, Malaysia
Enghelab Tennis Club, Enghelab Sport Complex, Tehran, Iran

Joel Jackson, Alex Game, Pierre Gervais and Gordon Bell
Faculty of Physical Education and Recreation, University of Alberta, Edmonton T6G 2H9, Canada

Gary Snydmiller
Augustana Faculty, University of Alberta, Camrose T4V 2R3, Canada

Andrew L. Shim
Department of Kinesiology & Human Performance, Briar Cliff University 3303 Rebecca Street, Sioux City, IA. USA

Kristin Steffen
Department of Physical Therapy, University of South Dakota 414 Cherry Street, Vermillion, SD. USA

Patrick Hauer and Patrick Cross
Department of Physical Therapy, Briar Cliff University 3303 Rebecca Street, Sioux City, IA. USA

Guido Van Ryssegem
Department of Recreational Sports, Oregon State University 211 Dixon Recreation Center, Corvallis, OR. USA

Fatemeh Pasand, Heydar Fooladiyanzadeh and Gholamhossien Nazemzadegan
Department of physical Education, Shiraz University, Iran

Amr Ali Shady
Sport Training Department, Faculty of Sport Education, Mansoura University, Mansoura, Egypt

Dean M. Cordingley
Pan Am Clinic Foundation, 75 Poseidon Bay, Winnipeg R3M 3E4, Canada

Gordon J. Bell and Daniel G. Syrotuik
Faculty of Physical Education & Recreation, University of Alberta, Edmonton T6G 2H9, Canada

Thomas W. Nesser and Neil Fleming
Kinesiology, Recreation, and Sport, Indiana State University 401 N. 4th Street, Terre Haute, IN 47809 USA

Matthew J. Gage
Department of Health Professions, Liberty University 1971 University Blvd, Lynchburg, VA 24515 USA

Nico Nitzsche
Chemnitz University of Technology, Department of Human Movement Science and Health Thüringer Weg 11, 09130 Chemnitz, Germany

Norman Stutzig and Tobias Siebert
University of Stuttgart, Department of Sport and Motion Science Allmandring 28, 70569 Stuttgart, Germany

Achim Walther
University Hospital Carl Gustav Carus Dresden, Department of Sports medicine Fetcherstraße 74, 01307 Dresden, Germany

Charles Allen
Exercise Science Program, Florida Southern College, 111 Lake Hollingsworth Drive, Lakeland, FL 33801, USA

Yang-Chieh Fu
Department of Health, Exercise Science and Recreation Management, University of Mississippi, University, Mississippi 38677, USA

John C. Garner
Department of Kinesiology and Health Promotion, Troy University, 600 University Avenue, Troy, Alabama 36082, USA

Mike R. Hellyer
TESTify Performance, Winnipeg, Canada
91 Lowson Crescent, Winnipeg, R3P 0T3, Canada

Vanessa L. Cazás-Moreno, Jacob R. Gdovin, Charles C. Williams, Charles R. Allen, Yang-Chieh Fu and John C. Garner III
School of Applied Sciences, University of Mississippi, 215 Turner Center, University, MS 38677-1848

Lee E. Brown
College of Health and Human Development, California State University, Fullerton, 800 North State College Blvd., Fullerton, CA 92834

Adam Michael Szlezak
Division of Sports Science, School of Allied Health Sciences, Griffith University, Parklands Dr, Southport QLD 4215, Australia

Lotti Tajouri, James Keane and Siri Lauluten Szlezak
Faculty of Health Science & Medicine, Bond University, Gold Coast QLD 4229, Australia

Clare Minahan
Division of Sports Science, School of Allied Health Sciences, Griffith University, Parklands Dr, Southport QLD 4215, Australia

Dan Newmire
Exercise Physiology and Biochemistry Laboratory Department of Kinesiology Texas Woman's University, Denton, Texas, USA 304 Administration Drive, Denton, TX 76204

Darryn S. Willoughby
Exercise and Biochemical Nutrition Laboratory Department of Health, Human Performance, and Recreation Baylor University, Waco, Texas, USA 1312 South 5th Street, Waco, TX, USA

Jeff R. Leiter
Pan Am Clinic Foundation, 75 Poseidon Bay, Winnipeg R3M 3E4, Canada

Adam J. Zeglen and Glenn D. Carnegie
Focus Fitness, 3969 Portage Ave, Winnipeg R3K 1W4, Canada

Peter B. MacDonald
Pan Am Clinic, 75 Poseidon Bay, Winnipeg R3M 3E4, Canada

Elham Shakoor, Mohsen Salesi, Maryam Koushki, Enayatollah Asadmanesh and Ahmad Qassemian
Department of Sport Physiology, School of Physical Education and Sport Sciences, Shiraz University, Shiraz, Iran

Darryn S. Willoughby
Department of Health, Human Performance, and Recreation, Exercise and Biochemical Nutrition Laboratory, Baylor University, Waco, TX, USA

Iván González-García, Luis Casáis Martínez and Jorge Viaño Santasmarinas
Faculty of Education and Sport Sciences, University of Vigo A Xunqueira Campus, Pontevedra, Spain

Miguel A. Gómez Ruano
Faculty of Physical Activity and Sport Sciences, University of Madrid Central building, 7th floor, Madrid, Spain

Janell Lautermilch, Andrew Stewart and Patricia K. Doyle-Baker
Faculty of Medicine, University of Calgary 2500 University Drive, Calgary, T2N 1N4, Canada

Tak Fung
Research Consulting Services, Information Technologies, University of Calgary 2500 University Drive, Calgary, T2N 1N4, Canada

David C. Archer, Jared W. Coburn, Andrew J. Galpin and Cameron N. Munger
Center for Sport Performance and Human Performance Lab, Department of Kinesiology, California State University, Fullerton, CA, USA

Lee E. Brown
Center for Sport Performance and Human Performance Lab, Department of Kinesiology, California State University, Fullerton, 800 N. State College Blvd., Fullerton, CA 92834-6870, USA

Phillip C. Drouet, Whitney D. Leyva and Megan A. Wong
Center for Sport Performance and Human Performance Lab, Department of Kinesiology, California State University, Fullerton, CA, USA

Kaloupsis Socratis
Department of Aquatic Sports, University of Athens, Dafni, Athens, Greece

Ditsios Kostas and Kapoutsis Dimitrios
A` Orthopaedics Department, Aristotle University of Thessaloniki, Thessaloniki, Greece

Dessypris Athanasios
Department of Biochemistry and Molecular Biology, University of Athens, Dafni, Athens, Greece

Dimakopoulou Eleni
Department of Aquatic Sports, University of Athens, Dafni, Greece

Index

R

S

T

V

W

www.ingramcontent.com/pod-product-compliance
Lightning Source LLC
Chambersburg PA
CBHW050450200326
41458CB00014B/5124
9781641163378